全国高等中医药院校中药学类专业双语规划教材

Bilingual Planned Textbooks for Chinese Materia Medica Majors in TCM Colleges and Universities

物理化学

Physical Chemistry

（供中药学类、药学类及相关专业使用）

(For Chinese Materia Medica, Pharmacy and other related majors)

主　编　邵江娟

副主编　冯　玉　李晓飞　张明波　申　蕊

编　者　（以姓氏笔画为序）

申　蕊（天津中医药大学）　　　　冯　玉（山东中医药大学）

刘　强（浙江中医药大学）　　　　刘靖丽（陕西中医药大学）

李晓飞（河南中医药大学）　　　　何玉珍（湖北中医药大学）

邵江娟（南京中医药大学）　　　　张明波（辽宁中医药大学）

张洪江（南京中医药大学翰林学院）　张彩云（安徽中医药大学）

林　舒（福建中医药大学）　　　　赵晓娟（甘肃中医药大学）

姚薇薇（南京中医药大学）　　　　钱　坤（江西中医药大学）

黄宏妙（广西中医药大学）　　　　曹姣仙（上海中医药大学）

韩　宁（北京中医药大学）

中国健康传媒集团

中国医药科技出版社

内 容 提 要

　　本教材是"全国高等中医药院校中药学类专业双语规划教材"之一，根据物理化学教学大纲的基本要求和课程特点编写而成，内容上涵盖化学热力学、化学动力学、相平衡、电化学、表面现象、溶胶、大分子溶液等内容。本教材具有逻辑严谨、简明清晰、具有"药味"以及中英双语结合等特点。本教材为书网融合教材，即纸质教材有机融合电子教材、教学配套资源（PPT、微课、视频、图片等）、题库系统、数字化教学服务（在线教学、在线作业、在线考试），使教学资源更加多样化、立体化。

　　本教材供从事双语教学的中药学、药学类及相关专业师生使用。

图书在版编目（CIP）数据

物理化学：汉英对照 / 邵江娟主编 . —北京：中国医药科技出版社，2021.8

全国高等中医药院校中药学类专业双语规划教材

ISBN 978-7-5214-1886-6

Ⅰ.①物… Ⅱ.①邵… Ⅲ.①物理化学 – 双语教学 – 中医学院 – 教材 – 汉、英 Ⅳ.①O64

中国版本图书馆 CIP 数据核字（2020）第 100518 号

美术编辑	陈君杞
版式设计	辰轩文化
出版	中国健康传媒集团 | 中国医药科技出版社
地址	北京市海淀区文慧园北路甲 22 号
邮编	100082
电话	发行：010-62227427　邮购：010-62236938
网址	www.cmstp.com
规格	889 × 1194 mm $\frac{1}{16}$
印张	18 $\frac{1}{4}$
字数	467 千字
版次	2021 年 8 月第 1 版
印次	2021 年 8 月第 1 次印刷
印刷	三河市万龙印装有限公司
经销	全国各地新华书店
书号	ISBN 978-7-5214-1886-6
定价	49.00 元

获取新书信息、投稿、为图书纠错，请扫码联系我们。

近些年随着世界范围的中医药热潮的涌动，来中国学习中医药学的留学生逐年增多，走出国门的中医药学人才也在增加。为了适应中医药国际交流与合作的需要，加快中医药国际化进程，提高来中国留学生和国际班学生的教学质量，满足双语教学的需要和中医药对外交流需求，培养优秀的国际化中医药人才，进一步推动中医药国际化进程，根据教育部、国家中医药管理局、国家药品监督管理局等部门的有关精神，在本套教材建设指导委员会主任委员成都中医药大学彭成教授等专家的指导和顶层设计下，中国医药科技出版社组织全国 50 余所高等中医药院校及附属医疗机构约 420 名专家、教师精心编撰了全国高等中医药院校中药学类专业双语规划教材，该套教材即将付梓出版。

本套教材共计 23 门，主要供全国高等中医药院校中药学类专业教学使用。本套教材定位清晰、特色鲜明，主要体现在以下方面。

一、立足双语教学实际，培养复合应用型人才

本套教材以高校双语教学课程建设要求为依据，以满足国内医药院校开展留学生教学和双语教学的需求为目标，突出中医药文化特色鲜明、中医药专业术语规范的特点，注重培养中医药技能、反映中医药传承和现代研究成果，旨在优化教育质量，培养优秀的国际化中医药人才，推进中医药对外交流。

本套教材建设围绕目前中医药院校本科教育教学改革方向对教材体系进行科学规划、合理设计，坚持以培养创新型和复合型人才为宗旨，以社会需求为导向，以培养适应中药开发、利用、管理、服务等各个领域需求的高素质应用型人才为目标的教材建设思路与原则。

二、遵循教材编写规律，整体优化，紧跟学科发展步伐

本套教材的编写遵循"三基、五性、三特定"的教材编写规律；以"必需、够用"为度；坚持与时俱进，注意吸收新技术和新方法，适当拓展知识面，为学生后续发展奠定必要的基础。实验教材密切结合主干教材内容，体现理实一体，注重培养学生实践技能训练的同时，按照教育部相关精神，增加设计性实验部分，以现实问题作为驱动力来培养学生自主获取和应用新知识的能力，从而培养学生独立思考能力、实验设计能力、实践操作能力和可持续发展能力，满足培养应用型和复合型人才的要求。强调全套教材内容的整体优化，并注重不同教材内容的联系与衔接，避免遗漏和不必要的交叉重复。

三、对接职业资格考试，"教考""理实"密切融合

本套教材的内容和结构设计紧密对接国家执业中药师职业资格考试大纲要求，实现教学与考试、理论与实践的密切融合，并且在教材编写过程中，吸收具有丰富实践经验的企业人员参与教材的编写，确保教材的内容密切结合应用，更加体现高等教育的实践性和开放性，为学生参加考试和实践工作打下坚实基础。

四、创新教材呈现形式，书网融合，使教与学更便捷更轻松

全套教材为书网融合教材，即纸质教材与数字教材、配套教学资源、题库系统、数字化教学服务有机融合。通过"一书一码"的强关联，为读者提供全免费增值服务。按教材封底的提示激活教材后，读者可通过 PC、手机阅读电子教材和配套课程资源（PPT、微课、视频等），并可在线进行同步练习，实时收到答案反馈和解析。同时，读者也可以直接扫描书中二维码，阅读与教材内容关联的课程资源，从而丰富学习体验，使学习更便捷。教师可通过 PC 在线创建课程，与学生互动，开展在线课程内容定制、布置和批改作业、在线组织考试、讨论与答疑等教学活动，学生通过 PC、手机均可实现在线作业、在线考试，提升学习效率，使教与学更轻松。此外，平台尚有数据分析、教学诊断等功能，可为教学研究与管理提供技术和数据支撑。需要特殊说明的是，有些专业基础课程，例如《药理学》等 9 种教材，起源于西方医学，因篇幅所限，在本次双语教材建设中纸质教材以英语为主，仅将专业词汇对照了中文翻译，同时在中国医药科技出版社数字平台"医药大学堂"上配套了中文电子教材供学生学习参考。

编写出版本套高质量教材，得到了全国知名专家的精心指导和各有关院校领导与编者的大力支持，在此一并表示衷心感谢。希望广大师生在教学中积极使用本套教材和提出宝贵意见，以便修订完善，共同打造精品教材，为促进我国高等中医药院校中药学类专业教育教学改革和人才培养做出积极贡献。

全国高等中医药院校中药学类专业双语规划教材
建设指导委员会

数字化教材编委会

主　编　邵江娟

副主编　张彩云　冯　玉　李晓飞　张明波　申　蕊

编　者（以姓氏笔画为序）

申　蕊（天津中医药大学）　　　　　冯　玉（山东中医药大学）

刘　强（浙江中医药大学）　　　　　刘靖丽（陕西中医药大学）

李晓飞（河南中医药大学）　　　　　何玉珍（湖北中医药大学）

邵江娟（南京中医药大学）　　　　　张明波（辽宁中医药大学）

张洪江（南京中医药大学翰林学院）　张彩云（安徽中医药大学）

林　舒（福建中医药大学）　　　　　赵晓娟（甘肃中医药大学）

姚薇薇（南京中医药大学）　　　　　钱　坤（江西中医药大学）

黄宏妙（广西中医药大学）　　　　　曹姣仙（上海中医药大学）

韩　宁（北京中医药大学）

物理化学是高等院校药学类、医学类各专业的基础课，是继无机化学、有机化学、分析化学课程后开设的重要理论化学课程，是培养药学类、医学类各专业人才知识结构与能力素质的重要组成部分。通过本课程的教学，使学生能比较系统地掌握物理化学的基本原理、基本概念、基本定律，熟悉或了解其在药学、医学等专业方面的应用，为后续相关专业课程的学习打好基础，并使学生得到一般科学方法的训练以及逻辑思维能力、知识应用能力和实验技能的提高，能够运用物理化学的原理、方法指导医药研究、生产。目前国内物理化学双语教材很少，主要适用于化工专业，内容与医药学类院校适用的教学大纲不太相符。因此，基于高等院校双语教学的趋势，以及中外合作办学专业的发展，迫切需要出版一本适合医药学类专业的双语教材。

本教材根据药学类、医学类专业本科生的培养目标及特点，本着系统和重点相结合的原则，以教材大纲为基本框架，对大纲所要求的基本理论作简明清晰的阐述，各章节联系逻辑紧密，与医药的应用有机结合，是一本带有"药味"的教材。本教材的编写以英文为主，在必要的专业词汇处标注中文。教材各章编写模块包括：学习目标、正文、重点小结、目标检测、参考答案。本教材英文专业术语的表达，主要参考了《中华人民共和国药典》2015年版英文版，同时也参考了其他英文版教材及论文要求。双语形式有助于学生掌握英语专业词汇和提升英语阅读能力，为以后论文撰写奠定基础，另一方面也有利于提升参与对外交流与合作的能力。

本教材主要分为8章，内容包括热力学第一定律与热化学、热力学第二定律与化学平衡、相平衡、电化学、化学动力学、表面现象、溶胶、大分子溶液。本教材力求简单明了，全面准确地阐述了物理化学的基本概念、基本原理、重要定律及其应用，以满足药学、医学类各专业学生对物理化学课程教学的要求。本教材可供中药学类、药学类及相关专业学生使用。

本教材的编写工作分工：绪论及第一章，邵江娟、姚薇薇、林舒；第二章，李晓飞、钱坤；第三章，冯玉、曹姣仙；第四章，赵晓娟、刘强；第五章，申蕊、黄宏妙；第六章，张明波、韩宁；第七章，张彩云、何玉珍；第八章，张洪江、刘靖丽；附录，邵江娟。

在编写修订过程中得到参编院校领导和各位同行的大力支持，在此表示衷心的感谢！由于编者知识水平所限，不足之处在所难免，敬请各校师生在使用过程中，予以指正。

编　者

2021.5

目录 | **Contents**

Contents | 目录 ■■

Introduction

Section 1　Research Objects, Methods and Contents of Physical Chemistry

Physical chemistry is the study of the underlying physical principles that govern the properties and behavior of chemical system. It is a branch or a component part of chemistry.

Physical chemistry can be studied into three levels: the macroscopic level, the transition level from microscope to macroscopic, and the microscope level. The microscopic level viewpoint is based on the conception of molecules. The macroscopic level viewpoint study large-scale properties of matter without considering molecules.

We can dive physical chemistry into four areas: thermodynamics, quantum chemistry, statistical chemistry, and kinetics.

For the macroscopic level, thermodynamic is a macroscopic science that studies the interrelationship of the various equilibrium characteristics of a system. It also studies the changes in equilibrium characteristics in process.

For the microscopic level, quantum chemistry studies the atomic structure, molecular bonding, and spectroscopy based on the quantum mechanics which differs from classic mechanics.

For the transition level from microscopic to macroscopic, statistical chemistry plays the role of a bridge from the microscopic approach of quantum chemistry to the macroscopic approach of thermodynamic.

Kinetics studies the rate processes such as chemical reactions, diffusion, or the flow of charge in an electrochemical cell. Kinetics uses relevant portions of thermodynamics, quantum chemistry, and statistical chemistry.

In its early years, physical chemistry research was done mainly at the macroscopic level. With the discovery of the laws of quantum mechanics in 1925-1926, emphasis began to shift to the molecular level. Nowadays, the power of physical chemistry has been greatly increased by experimental techniques that study properties chemistry and processes at the molecular level and by fast computers that ① process and analyze data of spectroscopy and x-ray crystallography experiments, ② accurately calculate properties of molecules that are not too large, and ③ perform simulations of collections of hundreds of molecules.

As a basic course in a medical college, we can only combine the characteristics of various specialties to select the appropriate contents for teaching. For the curriculum of the specialty of traditional Chinese medicine, we choose the following parts in the whole book.

Thermodynamics (热力学): As a component part of physics, thermodynamics is a branch of science with the task to study various macroscopic changes of state and the corresponding energy transformation concerning the thermal phenomena in nature.

Phase equilibrium (相平衡): It is a branch of thermodynamics, which studies the rule of phase changes via phase diagrams.

Chemical kinetics (化学动力学): It studies the effects of various factors on reactions rates. Briefly, there are three kinds of factors. The first concerns concentrations of reactants, products, catalysts, and other substances. The second is the temperature and pressure of the system. The third is the external fields such as light, electric field and magnetic field.

Surface phenomenon (界面现象): All the physical and chemical phenomena concerning surfaces are called the surface phenomenon. Macroscopically, they can be distinguished as two categories, equilibria and rates. Microscopically, the structure of the surface if the main concern.

Colloid chemistry (胶体化学): It studies the stabilization mechanism, the preparation and destruction, various properties and applications of colloidal system.

By employing the theories and experimental methods of the basic sciences of physics and mathematics, the task of the physical chemistry lies in studying the principles of equilibria and rates in chemical reactions including phase and p、V、T changes, and the relations between those principles and the microscopic structures of substances. It severs as the theoretical basis of the whole chemistry science.

Section 2　Learning Methods of Physical Chemistry

As mentioned above, physical chemistry is a basic theoretical course for studying the material changes and the laws of material changes. Therefore, the physical chemistry course has been put in a very important position for students of many majors. In order to learn this course to get well, every beginner should explore a set of learning methods suitable for their own characteristics according to their own majors, and the next suggestions can be used for students to learn.

1. Strive to understand abstract concepts of physical chemistry. The concepts in physical chemistry are so numerous and profound that beginners often find it hard to understand and remember them. In fact, these concepts and theories are summarized from objective reality, and if they can be linked to the objective phenomenon of life, you will not feel difficult to understand them, and even more you will feel them vivid.

2. Master mathematics. Physical chemistry is a very logical subject, so that mathematics is very important for studying of Thermodynamics and kinetics. You will develop a scientific approach of seeking truth and a scientific method of logical thinking. You will be trained to calculate in the correct and tidy way.

3. Pay attention to the special conditions of the formulas. This book applies a large number of mathematical deductions and draws some conclusions used under different conditions. Mathematical derivation process is to let us understand the origin of the formula. It is only the necessary means to obtain results, but is not the purpose, so students do not spend much time on the complicated derivation

PPT

process, but pay attention to the special conditions and physical significance of the conclusions which you use. In addition to some important theories, the formula and its derivation process only require understanding and generally do not require strong memory except some more important principles.

4. Do plenty of exercises. To help you prepare for the exam, it is recommended that doing some basic exercises is necessary. If you have spare time and are interested in physical chemistry, you can increase training and do some remedial exercises. The concepts within the lectures are strengthened with the aid of exercises. Beginners need to go through enough repeated learning, in order to gradually deepen understanding.

5. Pay attention to the lab. Experiments are key important part of physical chemistry, they will help us to understand the theories. Physical chemistry is a subject of both theories and experiments, and the development of theories cannot be separated from the enlightenment and test of experiments. Physical chemistry experiment methods are often physical methods and more devices are used. So it requires students to fully preview before the experiment, understand what the purpose of the experiment is and know which formula it examines. Don't forget to do the pre-experiment seriously. This lab should help you connect theory with the real world. You will be concentrating on the correct use of various kinds of laboratory equipment and procedures, but the lab will reinforce chemical principles covered in your lecture.

Be aware that your ability to learn and understand is limited, and it's best to acknowledge the fact that there are some things that you may not fully understand. No one can fully understand everything, even experts in this field. But at the end of the course, students will have gained a general understanding of Thermodynamics and kinetics, and their ability of analyzing, problem solving and self-learning in physical chemistry will have been greatly improved.

Section 3　Applications of Physical Chemistry to Medicine

PPT

The theory of physical chemistry is generalized from production practice, and it will serve production and scientific research in turn. With the development of medical technology and the deepening of medical research, there are more and more interpenetration and mutual connection between disciplines, and the combination of pharmacy and Physical chemistry is more and more close.

The extraction and separation of effective components in natural drugs is an important aspect of inheriting and carrying forward the heritage of traditional Chinese medicine. In this work, distillation, extraction, emulsification, adsorption and other operations are often needed, which requires knowledge of thermodynamics, phase equilibrium, surface phenomena, colloidal chemistry and other aspects.

In the pharmaceutical production, it is necessary to master the theoretical knowledge of chemical thermodynamics and chemical kinetics to select the appropriate process route, process conditions, explore the mechanism of pharmaceutical reaction, study the stability of drugs, and the conditions and duration of drug preservation. For example, can chemical reactions be carried out? If it can be carried out, what is the reaction rate? Various factors, such as temperature, reactant concentration, catalyst and so on how to affect the chemical reaction rate, and so on.

In the study of drug synthesis, we should understand the relationship between the structure and properties of drugs, in order to find the most effective drugs, which requires the knowledge of material structure. In the process of synthesis, knowledge of chemical kinetics is also needed.

In the aspect of pharmaceutical preparation, when studying the reform of dosage form, we should understand the content of surface phenomenon and the influence of dispersion degree on drug performance. For the same drug, the smaller the main drug particles, the better the efficacy. For example, the development of nanotechnology will play a very important role in the reform of pharmaceutical formulations.

From the perspective of the development trend, it is very necessary for pharmaceutical workers to master the principles and methods of physical chemistry.

Chapter 1　The First Law of Thermodynamics and Thermochemistry

📖 学习目标

知识要求

1.掌握

（1）热和功、热力学能、热力学第一定律的数学表达式。

（2）焓、定容热、定压热、定容热容、定压热容。

（3）热力学第一定律对理想气体的应用（理想气体的定温过程、C_p和C_v的关系）。

（4）化学反应热的计算（定容反应热与定压反应热的关系、盖斯定律、生成热、燃烧热）。

2.熟悉

（1）热力学基本概念（体系和环境、广度性质和强度性质、状态和状态函数、过程和途径、热和功）。

（2）可逆过程的概念和特点。

3.了解

（1）理想气体的绝热过程。

（2）基尔霍夫定律。

能力要求

1. 能够运用热力学第一定律分析某些实际问题。

2. 会选择合适的方法计算化学反应热。

Thermodynamics (热力学) (from the Greek words for "heat" and "power") is the study of **heat (热)**, **work (功)**, energy and the changes they produce in the states of systems. In a broad sense, thermodynamics studies the relationships between the macroscopic properties of a system.

This chapter introduces some of the basic concepts of thermodynamics. It concentrates on the conservation of energy——the experimental observation that energy can neither created nor destroyed and shows how the principle of the conservation of energy can be used to assess the energy changes that accompany physical and chemical processes.

Section 1　The Basic Concepts

1.1　System and surroundings

For the purposes of physical chemistry, the universe is divided into two parts: system and its surroundings.

System (系统): The system adopted here is an abbreviation of a macroscopic system. It contains all the objects studied including the matter and the space.

Surroundings (环境): The matter and the space outside and related to the system are called the surroundings.

In distinguishing the system from the surroundings, it is demanded that there is no interaction between them or the interaction is negligible. The system is separated from its surroundings by a real or an imagined dividing interface, through which the matter comes in or out, and the energy gains or losses between the system and the surroundings. The system can be divided into three types.

Open system (敞开系统): If matter and energy can both be transferred through the boundary between the system and its surroundings, the system is classified as open system.

Closed system (封闭系统): Only energy can pass through the boundary, the matter cannot pass through the boundary between the system and its surroundings, the system is classified as closed system.

Isolated system (孤立系统): Neither the energy nor the matter is transported between the system and its surroundings, the system is classified as isolated system.

1.2　Extensive and intensive properties

What properties does thermodynamics use to characterize a system? The composition must be specified. This can be done by stating the mass of each chemical species that is present in each phase. The volume V is a property of the system, the pressure p is another thermodynamic variable. If external electric or magnetic fields act on the system, the field strengths are thermodynamic variables.

Extensive property (广度性质): An extensive property is one whose value is equal to the sum of its values for the parts of the system. For example, the mass of the system is the sum of the masses the parts. Mass is an extensive property. It exhibits the "quantity" of the system.

Intensive property (强度性质): An intensive property is one whose value does not depend on the size of the system. If dividing the system into several parts, for each part, the property still keeps the value of the original system. It exhibits the "quality" of the system. Density and pressure are examples of intensive properties.

1.3　Equilibrium

If any change will not happen for quite a long time in each part of the system, and without any macroscopic exchange of energy and materials with the surroundings, the system is at an equilibrium state. Equilibrium thermodynamics deals with systems in equilibrium. An isolated system is in equilibrium when its macroscopic properties remain constant with time. A non-isolated system is in equilibrium when the following two conditions hold: ① the system's macroscopic properties remain constant with time; ② removal of the system from contact with its surroundings causes no change in the properties of the system.

These equilibria can be divided into the following four kinds of equilibrium.

Mechanical equilibrium (机械平衡): No unbalanced forced act on or within the system; hence the system undergoes no acceleration, and there is no turbulence within the system. The pressure is identical when the system is in the equilibrium.

Thermal equilibrium (热平衡): There must be no change in the properties of the system or its surroundings when they are separated by a thermally conducting wall. The temperature is identical when the system is in the equilibrium.

Phase equilibrium (相平衡): Every phase of the system coexists for a long time and compositions and amounts of each phase do not change with time. The chemical potential is identical when the system is in the equilibrium.

Chemical equilibrium (化学平衡): When there is chemical reaction between the substances, the composition of the system will not change with time after reaching the equilibrium.

For thermodynamic equilibrium, all four kinds of equilibrium must be present.

1.4　State and state function

State (状态): The sum of all the properties of the system is called the state. The state of a system is determined when all the properties of the system are fixed, and the state changes when anyone of the properties changes.

State function (状态函数): The properties solely determined by the equilibrium state are called the state functions. The value of a state function is fixed if the state is fixed. If the state changes, the change in the value of a state function depends only on the initial and the final state of the system independent of the concrete path travelled.

The characteristics of the state function are as follows:

(1) For a homogeneous system with a given constant composition, an arbitrary macroscopic property of the system is function of two other self-governed macroscopic properties, that is, $z=f(x,y)$. For instance, the perfect gas: $V=nRT/p$, that is, the volume of the perfect gas can be determined by T and p with n is constant.

(2) If the state is constant, state function is constant. State function changes with state, however, the changing value is independent of the way the state was prepared. That is, Δ(state function) = the final value-the initial value. For instance: $\Delta T=T_2-T_1$.

(3) In mathematical treatment, we can use the complete differential for the state function, the infinitesimal change in a state function X is the complete differential dX. From an initial state to a final state for a system, the variation of the state function ΔX is expressed by

$$\Delta X=\int_{X_1}^{X_2}dX=X_2-X_1$$

If the state recovers by a cyclic process, $\oint dX=0$, the state function does not change.

(4) The set of the state functions (sum, difference, product, and quotient) are also state functions.

1.5　Process and path

Process (过程): When a thermodynamic system changes from one state to another, the operation is called a process. Process of the system consists of: simple p, V and T change process, phase transformation process, and chemical change process.

Several important pVT change processes are as follows:

(1) Isothermal process: T is constant throughout the process, that is $T_1=T_2=T_{su}=$constant, $dT=0$, $\Delta T=0$.

(2) Isobaric process: p is constant throughout the process, that is $p_1=p_2=p_{su}=$constant, $dp=0$, $\Delta p=0$.

(3) Isochoric process: V is constant throughout the process, that is $V_1=V_2=$constant, $dV=0$, $\Delta V=0$.

(4) Adiabatic process: This can be achieved by surrounding the system with adiabatic walls. $Q=0$.

(5) Cyclic process: The final state of the system is the same as the initial state, so the change in all state functions is zero, that is Δ (state function) = 0, such as $\Delta p=0$, and $\Delta H=0$.

(6) Expansion against constant external pressure: $p_{su}=$constant.

(7) Free expansion process or expansion into a vacuum process: $p_{su}=0$.

Path (途径): The change of the system from the initial state to the final state can be completed by one or more different steps. The specific steps (or processes) to complete a process are called pathways.

1.6　Heat and work

There are two different forms for the energy transport: transferring heat and doing work.

Heat: The energy exchange caused by the temperature difference between the system and surroundings is called heat.

Symbol: Q; unit: J.

An exothermic process is a process that releases energy as heat ($Q<0$). All combustion reactions are exothermic process.

An endothermic process is a process that absorbs energy as heat ($Q>0$). An example of an endothermic process is the vaporization of water.

Work: In thermodynamics, all forms of energy transfer between the system and surroundings other than heat are called work.

Symbol: W; unit: J.

When the system works on the surroundings, W is taken as negative value; when the system obtains work from the surroundings, W is taken as positive value.

Various kinds of work: Work is well defined in classical mechanics. The most fundamental one is the mechanical work defined by multiplying the force f and the displacement dl. Work of other forms can be defined by multiplying the generalized force and the generalized displacement. We list various kinds of work in Table 1–1.

Table 1–1　Various kinds of work

Various kinds of work	Extensive property	the change of intensive property
Mechanical work ($F\mathrm{d}l$)	F(force)	$\mathrm{d}l$ (displacement)
Lumetric work ($-p_{su}\mathrm{d}V$)	p_{su} (pressure)	$\mathrm{d}V$ (the volume change)
Interfacial work ($\sigma\mathrm{d}A$)	σ(interfacial tension)	$\mathrm{d}A$ (the change in interfacial area)
Electrical work ($E\mathrm{d}q$)	E (the electric potential)	$\mathrm{d}q$ (the change in electric charge)

Section 2　Work and Process

The expansion work arises from a change in volume. This type of work includes the work done by a gas as it expands and drives back the atmosphere. The term "expansion work" also includes work associated with negative changes of volume, that is, compression (Fig. 1–1).

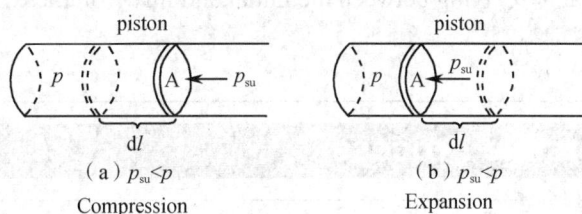

(a) $p_{su}<p$　　　　　(b) $p_{su}<p$
Compression　　　　　　Expansion

Fig. 1–1　Compression (a) and expansion (b) process

2.1　The general expression for work

The calculation of expansion work starts from the definition used in the physics, which states that the work required to move an object a distance $\mathrm{d}l$ against an opposing force of magnitude F is

$$\mathrm{d}W=-F\mathrm{d}l$$

The negative sign tells us that, when the system moves an object against an opposing force, the internal energy of the system doing the work will decrease. If external pressure is p_{su}, the magnitude of the force acting on the outer face of the piston is $F=p_{su}A$. When the system expands through a distance $\mathrm{d}l$ against an external pressure, it follows that the work done is $\mathrm{d}W=-p_{su}A\mathrm{d}l$. But $A\mathrm{d}l$ is the change in volume, $\mathrm{d}V$, in the course of the expansion. Therefore, the work done when the system expands by $\mathrm{d}V$ against a pressure is

$$\mathrm{d}W=-p_{su}\mathrm{d}V$$

To obtain the total work done when the volume changes from V_1 to V_2, we integrate this expression between the initial and final volumes:

$$W=-\int_{V_1}^{V_2}p_{su}\mathrm{d}V \tag{1-1}$$

If the system is compressed instead, the above equation can be still used, but now $V_2<V_1$. It is

important to note that it is still the external pressure that determines the magnitude of the work.

2.2 Free expansion

By free expansion, we mean expansion against zero opposing force. It occurs when $p_{su}=0$, so $W=0$. That is, no work is done when a system expands freely. Expansion of this kind occurs when a system expands into vacuum.

2.3 Expansion against constant pressure

Suppose that the external pressure is constant throughout the expansion. For example, the piston may be pressed on by the atmosphere, which exerts the same pressure throughout the expansion. We can take the constant p_{su} outside the integral.

$$W=-\int_{V_1}^{V_2}p_{su}dV=-p_{su}\int_{V_1}^{V_2}dV=-p_{su}(V_2-V_1) \qquad (1-2)$$

This result is illustrated graphically in the Fig. 1–2, which make use of the fact that an integral can be interpreted as an area. The magnitude of W is equal to the area beneath the horizontal line at $p=p_{su}$ lying between the initial and final volumes.

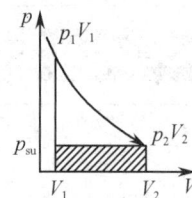

Fig. 1–2 The work done against constant pressure

Section 3　Reversible Process

3.1 Reversible expansion

A **reversible process (可逆过程)** in thermodynamics is a change that can be reversed by an infinitesimal modification of a variable. The system is always infinitesimally close to equilibrium, and an infinitesimal change in conditions can reverse the process to restore both system and surroundings to their initial states. A reversible process is obviously an idealization.

Suppose a gas is confined by a piston and that the external pressure, p_{su}, is set equal to the pressure, p, of the confined gas. Such a system is in mechanical equilibrium with its surroundings because an infinitesimal change in the external pressure in either direction causes changes in volume in opposite directions. If the external pressure is reduced infinitesimally, then the gas expands slightly. If the external pressure is increased infinitesimally, then the gas contracts slightly. In either case the change is reversible in the thermodynamic sense. If on the other hand, the external pressure differs measurably from the internal pressure, then changing p_{su} infinitesimally will not decrease it below the pressure of the gas and so will not change the direction of the process. Such a system is not in mechanical equilibrium with its surroundings and expansion is thermodynamically irreversible.

To achieve reversible expansion we set p_{su} equal to p at each stage of the expansion. In practice, this equalization could be achieved by gradually removing weights from the piston so that the downward force due to the weights always match the changing upward force due to the pressure of the gas. When set

$p_{su}=p$,

$$dW=-p_{su}dV=-pdV$$

Although the pressure inside the system appears in this expression for the work, it does so only because p_{su} has been set equal to p to ensure reversibility. The total work of reversible expansion is

$$W=-\int_{V_1}^{V_2}pdV \tag{1-3}$$

3.2   Isothermal reversible expansion

Consider the isothermal, reversible expansion of a perfect gas. The expansion is made isothermal by keeping the system in thermal contact with its surroundings. Because the equation of state is $p=nRT/V$, with the volume at that stage of the expansion. The temperature T is constant in an isothermal expansion, so it may be taken outside the integral. It follows that the work of reversible isothermal expansion of a perfect gas from V_1 to V_2 at a temperature T is

$$W=-nRT\int_{V_1}^{V_2}\frac{dV}{V}=-nRT\ln\frac{V_2}{V_1} \tag{1-4}$$

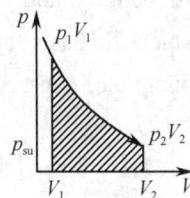

Fig. 1–3   The work done by perfect gas when it expands reversibly and isothermally

We can express the work done is equal to the area under the isotherm $p=nRT/V$ (Fig. 1–3).

3.3   Features of reversible processes

(1) The process is carried out with infinitesimal changes, and the system is always infinitely close to the equilibrium state. That is to say, the whole process is composed of a series of states which are infinitely close to equilibrium. To realize a finite process reversibly, it takes an infinite time.

(2) The system and environment can be restored completely by following the opposite direction of the original process.

(3) The system does the maximum work (absolute value) in the reversible process and the environment does the minimum work (absolute value) in the reversible process. The reverse process has the highest efficiency.

Reversible process is an ideal process and a scientific abstraction. In fact, there is no real reversible process in nature, and the actual process can only approach it infinitely. But the concept of reversible process is very important. The reversible process occurs when the system is close to equilibrium, so it is closely related to the equilibrium state. In the future, we can see some important changes of thermodynamic functions, which can only be obtained through reversible process.

In addition to the expansion and compression of gas, there are many processes close to the reversible process. For example, the phase transformation process (evaporation of liquid at its boiling point, melting process of solid at its melting point), chemical reaction under equilibrium conditions, charging and discharging of reversible battery in infinite hours of electromotive force difference, etc. can be approximately regarded as reversible process.

Section 4   The First Law of Thermodynamics and Thermodynamic Energy

All matter in nature has energy, which has many forms. It has been proved that energy can be transformed from one form to another, but in the process of transformation, energy can neither be created out of nothing nor destroyed by itself, that is, the sum of energy before and after transformation is unchanged. This is the principle of energy conservation, which is summed up by people through numerous experiments and practices. Joule et al. made a series of experiments on heat and work conversion in the 19th century, and put forward the famous heat work equivalent, i.e. 1cal = 4.184J (joule), which provides a scientific basis for the principle of energy conservation. The first law of thermodynamics is to apply the principle of conservation of energy to the macroscopic thermodynamic system.

4.1   Empirical expression of the first law of thermodynamics

There are many ways to express **the first law of thermodynamics(热力学第一定律)**. From one way to another, we can deduce another way, but all of them explain a problem, that is, the conservation of energy. Common expressions are as follows:

(1) The first law of thermodynamics is the law of conservation of energy.

(2) All substances in nature have energy, which can be transformed from one form to another in various forms, and the total amount of energy remains unchanged during the transformation.

The first type of perpetual motion machine is a kind of heat engine which does not need to obtain energy from the outside, does not consume its own energy, and can circulate and do more than work. The first type of perpetual motion machine has never been created.

Numerous facts have proved the correctness of the first law of thermodynamics. Up to now, there has been no contradiction between the first law of thermodynamics and nature.

4.2   Thermodynamic energy

Thermodynamic energy(热力学能), is also known as internal energy. It is the sum of all the energy in the system, but it does not include the kinetic energy and potential energy of the system as a whole. Thermodynamic energy refers to the sum of energy in the system, including translational energy, rotational energy, vibrational energy, electronic energy, nuclear energy and potential energy of molecular motion. Thermodynamic energy is denoted by the symbol U. The energy of each particle in the system is the microscopic property of the particle, and the thermodynamic energy is the overall expression of this microscopic property.

Thermodynamic energy has the following basic characteristics:

(1) The absolute value of the thermodynamic energy can not be determined, only the change value between two states can be obtained.

(2) The thermodynamic energy is the extensive property of the system, which is proportional to the

number of substances in the system.

The thermodynamic energy U of the system divided by the quantity n of the substance, i.e. $U/n=U_m$, is called the molar thermodynamic energy. The unit of U_m is $J \cdot mol^{-1}$.

(3) The thermodynamic energy is a state function whose value depends on the state of the system.

The thermodynamic energy is a single value function of the state of the system. The change value of thermodynamic energy is only related to the state but not to the path, which completely conforms to the characteristics of the state function.

Since the thermodynamic energy is the state function, dU is the total differential. For the homogeneous closed system of pure matter (the following are all closed systems), U can be regarded as a function of T, p or T, V. If there is a small state change in the system, the small change in the thermodynamic energy can be expressed by the full differential dU, and the following equation can be obtained.

$$U=f(T, V)$$

The total differential can be written as

$$dU = \left(\frac{\partial U}{\partial T}\right)_V dT + \left(\frac{\partial U}{\partial V}\right)_T dV \tag{1-5}$$

Or

$$dU = \left(\frac{\partial U}{\partial T}\right)_p dT + \left(\frac{\partial U}{\partial p}\right)_T dp \tag{1-6}$$

The motion mode and interaction of particles in the system are extremely complex, which has not been fully understood by people. Therefore, the absolute value of the thermodynamic energy of the system in a certain state cannot be determined, but this does not hinder the practical application of the concept of thermodynamic energy. Because in the calculation of thermodynamics, we only need to know the change of thermodynamic energy, ΔU, when the system is in a certain process.

4.3　Mathematical equation of the first law of thermodynamics

In a closed system, from state 1 to state 2, if the system absorbs the heat of Q from the surroundings and obtains the work of W from the surroundings, the increment of thermodynamic energy of the system must be equal to the heat Q absorbed from the surroundings plus the work W obtained from the surroundings. According to the first law of thermodynamics, the change of thermodynamic energy of the system is as follows.

$$\Delta U=U_2-U_1=Q+W \tag{1-7}$$

U_1 and U_2 are the internal energy of the initial and final states of the system. If the system changes slightly, then

$$dU=\delta Q+\delta W \tag{1-8}$$

Equation (1-7) is the mathematical expression of the first law of thermodynamics for a closed system. It shows the quantitative relation of the conversion of thermodynamic energy, heat and work. In fact, it also tells us that when the initial and final states are specified, although heat and work are related to the process, their sum is not related to the path.

In the first law, work should include volume work and non volume work.

[Example 1–1] Suppose that the state of a certain system changes from the initial state to the final state via route A, and the system absorbs 100J of heat. When the system follows another path B from the final state to the original initial state, the system does 600J of work to the environment, while the system absorbs 400J of heat. Find the work done by the system in path A.

Solution: After the system passes through path A, $\Delta U_A = Q_A + W_A$

After the system passes through path B, $\Delta U_B = Q_B + W_B$

Since the system returns to its original initial state, $\Delta U = \Delta U_A + \Delta U_B = 0$

$\Delta U_A = -\Delta U_B$

$Q_A + W_A = -(Q_B + W_B)$

$100 + W_A = -[(-600) + 400]$

$W_A = 100J$

That is, in path A, the environment works 100J on the system.

Section 5   Enthalpy

5.1   Special significance of heat in constant volume and constant pressure process

The heat transfer between the system and the surroundings is not a state function, but the heat of some specific processes can have the characteristics of a state function. The thermal effects of constant volume process and constant pressure process are discussed below.

5.1.1   Constant volume heat(定容热)

For a closed system, when the non volume work is zero, if it is a constant volume process, the volume work of the process is zero, $\delta W = 0$.

The first law of thermodynamics, $dV = \delta Q + \delta W$, can be written as follows.

$$dU = \delta Q_V \qquad (1-9)$$

Or
$$\Delta U = Q_V \qquad (1-10)$$

In the above equation, Q_V is the thermal effect of constant volume process. Since the thermodynamic energy is a state function, its increment only depends on the initial and final states of the system, so the constant volume heat Q_V also depends on the initial and final states of the system, independent of the specific path of the process. Equation (1–10) shows that when the non volume work is zero, the heat absorbed by the closed system is used to increase the internal energy of the system. Therefore, the ΔU value of the system can be calculated from the Q_V measured experimentally.

5.1.2   constant pressure heat (定压热)

In the process of constant pressure for a closed system which only does volume work, from state 1 to state 2, the first law of thermodynamics can be written as follows.

$$\Delta U = U_2 - U_1 = Q_p - p(V_2 - V_1)$$
$$U_2 - U_1 = Q_p - p_2 V_2 + p_1 V_1$$

Or
$$Q_p=(U_2+p_2V_2)-(U_1+p_1V_1)$$

5.2   Definition and properties of enthalpy

Because U, p and V are all state functions, so $(U+pV)$ is also a state function, its change only depends on the initial and final states of the system. In thermodynamics, $(U+pV)$ is defined as **enthalpy(焓)**, expressed as H.

$$H=U+pV \tag{1-11}$$

So
$$Q_p=H_2-H_1$$

$$\Delta H=Q_p \tag{1-12}$$

For small changes, then

$$dH=\delta Q_p \tag{1-13}$$

In the above equation, Q_p is the thermal effect of constant pressure process. Because enthalpy is a state function, which only depends on the initial and final states of the system, the constant pressure heat Q_p must also only depend on the initial and final states of the system, regardless of the specific path of the process. Equation (1–12) shows that under the condition that the non volume work is zero, the heat absorbed by the closed system through a certain pressure process is used to increase the enthalpy of the system. Therefore, the value ΔH of the system can be calculated by Q_p. There is no definite physical meaning of enthalpy.

Because the absolute value of thermodynamic energy cannot be determined, the absolute value of enthalpy cannot be determined. Enthalpy is also extensive properties, and has the dimension of energy.

Although the absolute values of the thermodynamic energy and enthalpy of the system are not known yet, under certain conditions, we can obtain the change values of the thermodynamic energy and enthalpy of the system from the heat exchanged and transferred between the system and the surroundings, i.e. $\Delta U=Q_V$, $\Delta H=Q_p$. Because most of the chemical reactions are carried out under the condition of zero non volume work and constant pressure, the introduction of enthalpy as a state function will bring great convenience to the calculation of thermal effect, and enthalpy has more practical significance.

Section 6   Heat Capacity

The **heat capacity(热容)** is a kind of basic heat data measured by experiments, which is used to calculate the constant volume heat, constant pressure heat, ΔU and ΔH of the system in such changes when the system has a simple state change.

6.1   Definition of heat capacity

Under the condition of zero non volume work, for a homogeneous closed system without chemical

PPT

and phase changes, if the system absorbs heat Q from the environment and the temperature rises from T_1 to T_2, the average heat capacity of the system is defined as.

$$\overline{C} = \frac{Q}{T_2 - T_1} = \frac{Q}{\Delta T}$$

$\overline{C}$ is called average heat capacity, that is, the heat that the system needs to absorb when the average temperature rises 1K in the ΔT range. It is known that the heat capacity changes with the temperature. If the temperature changes infinitely small, you can write:

$$C = \frac{\delta Q}{dT} \tag{1-14}$$

The unit of heat capacity is $J \cdot K^{-1}$.

Because the heat capacity is related to the amount of material in the system, the specific heat capacity and molar heat capacity are commonly used.

The heat capacity of 1kg substance is called specific heat capacity (or specific heat), expressed in C, and the unit is $J \cdot K^{-1} \cdot kg^{-1}$.

The heat capacity of 1 mole of material is called molar heat capacity, which is expressed in C_m, and the unit is $J \cdot K^{-1} \cdot mol^{-1}$.

$$C_m = C/n \quad (n \text{ is the amount of substance}) \tag{1-15}$$

6.2 Constant volume heat capacity and constant pressure heat capacity

Because heat is not a state function, the value of Q is related to the process, so the heat capacity of the system is also related to the process.

6.2.1 Constant volume heat capacity （定容热容）

Constant volume heat capacity C_V is the heat required for a closed system at constant volume only due to temperature rise of 1K.

$$C_V = \frac{\delta Q_V}{dT} \tag{1-16}$$

The results of C_V measurement of various substances show that it varies not only with species and their aggregation state, but also with temperature.

The constant volume heat capacity of 1mol substance is called the constant volume molar heat capacity, expressed in $C_{V,m}$.

$$C_{V,m} = \frac{C_V}{n} \tag{1-17}$$

For a constant volume process in which the non volume work of a closed system is zero,

$$dU = \delta Q_V$$

So

$$C_V = \frac{\delta Q_V}{dT} = \left(\frac{\partial U}{\partial T}\right)_V$$

It can be seen that C_V is equal to the rate of change of internal energy with temperature in the constant volume process with zero non volume work.

Hence
$$dU = C_V dT \tag{1-18}$$

Integral on both sides of the equation,
$$\Delta U = Q_V = \int_{T_1}^{T_2} C_V dT \tag{1-19}$$

Since $C_V = nC_{V,m}$, the above equation can also be written as
$$\Delta U = Q_V = n\int_{T_1}^{T_2} C_{V,m} dT \tag{1-20}$$

Equation (1-20) provides an effective method to calculate the change value of internal energy in a closed system without chemical change or phase change and only volume work. If it can be regarded as a constant in the integral temperature range, equation (1-20) can be written as
$$\Delta U = Q_V = nC_{V,m}(T_2 - T_1) \tag{1-21}$$

6.2.2　Constant pressure heat capacity（定压热容）

The constant pressure heat capacity C_p is the heat required by the system under constant pressure only due to the temperature rise of 1K. The properties of C_p changing with species, phase and temperature are similar to those of C_p. The mathematical expression of C_p definition is
$$C_p = \frac{\delta Q_p}{dT} \tag{1-22}$$

The constant pressure heat capacity of 1mol substance is called the constant pressure molar heat capacity, expressed in $C_{p,m}$.
$$C_{p,m} = \frac{C_p}{n} \tag{1-23}$$

For a constant pressure process in which the non volume work of a closed system is zero,
$$dH = \delta Q_p$$

So
$$C_p = \frac{\delta Q_p}{dT} = \left(\frac{\partial H}{\partial T}\right)_p$$

It can be seen that C_p is equal to the rate of change of enthalpy with temperature in the constant pressure process with zero non volume work.

Hence
$$dH = C_p dT \tag{1-24}$$

Integral on both sides of the equation,
$$\Delta H = Q_p = \int_{T_1}^{T_2} C_p dT \tag{1-25}$$

Since $C_p = nC_{p,m}$, the above formula can also be written as
$$\Delta H = Q_p = n\int_{T_1}^{T_2} C_{p,m} dT \tag{1-26}$$

Equation (1-26) provides an effective method to calculate the change value of enthalpy in a closed system without chemical change or phase change and only volume work. If it can be regarded as a constant in the integral temperature range, equation (1-26) can be written as
$$\Delta H = Q_p = nC_{p,m}(T_2 - T_1) \tag{1-27}$$

[Example 1-2] At a constant pressure of 1.00×10^5Pa, 2mol of water at 30℃ becomes water vapor at 140℃, and the heat absorbed in this process is calculated. It is known that the average molar constant pressure heat capacities of water and steam are 75.31 and 33.47J · K⁻¹ · mol⁻¹ respectively. At 100℃ and 1.00×10^5Pa, the heat of vaporization from liquid water to steam is 40.70kJ · mol⁻¹.

Solution: From 30℃ water to 100℃ water, then

$$Q_{p,1} = nC_{p,\text{m(l)}}(T_2 - T_1) = 2 \times 75.31 \times (373 - 303) = 10543\text{J} = 10.54\text{kJ}$$

The transformation heat from 100℃ liquid water to 100℃ water vapor is as follows:

$$Q_{p,2} = n \cdot \Delta H_{\text{vaporization}} = 2 \times 40.70 = 81.40\text{kJ}$$

The transformation heat from 100℃ water vapor to 140℃ water vapor is as follows:

$$Q_{p,3} = nC_{p,\text{m(g)}}(T_2 - T_1) = 2 \times 33.47 \times (413 - 373) = 2678\text{J} = 2.68\text{kJ}$$

The heat absorbed in the whole process is:

$$Q_p = Q_{p,1} + Q_{p,2} + Q_{p,3} = 10.54 + 81.40 + 2.68 = 94.62\text{kJ}$$

6.3 Empirical equation of heat capacity

The change of heat capacity with temperature is measured by experiment. As there is a certain relationship between $C_{V,\text{m}}$ and $C_{p,\text{m}}$, as long as one of them is measured, the other can be deduced. The most commonly used empirical equation are as follows.

$$C_{p,\text{m}} = a + bT + cT^2 + \cdots \tag{1-28}$$

$$C_{p,\text{m}} = a + bT + \frac{c'}{T^2} + \cdots \tag{1-29}$$

In the equation, T is absolute temperature; a, b, c are empirical constants, which vary with different substances and temperature ranges. If $C_{p,m}$ changes with temperature, and $C_{p,m} = a + bT + cT^2$, Q_p or ΔH can be calculated from the following equation.

$$\Delta H = Q_p = n\int_{T_1}^{T_2} C_{p,\text{m}}\,\mathrm{d}T = n\int_{T_1}^{T_2}(a + bT + cT^2)\,\mathrm{d}T \tag{1-30}$$

Section 7　Application of the First law of Thermodynamics to Ideal Gas

When we study the laws of thermodynamics, we find it most convenient to describe a special system, i.e. ideal gas, because gas is the simplest in the state of matter aggregation, and it is the easiest to study with molecular model.

7.1 Ideal gas

There are four basic states of matter: gas, solid, liquid and plasma. Gas can be a single atom (such as inert gas), a single substance composed of one element, or a compound composed of many elements. The significant difference between gas, liquid and solid is that there is a large gap between gas particles. Gas is a fluid, which can flow, deform and diffuse when its volume is not limited. Volume, temperature and pressure are three factors commonly used in the description of gas.

7.1.1   Ideal gas state equation（理想气体状态方程）

For a long time, people have summed up a number of empirical laws for the results of gas observation in the early stage. For example:

Boyle's Law: at a constant temperature, the volume of a certain amount of gas is inversely proportional to the pressure;

Gay-lussac's Law: under constant pressure, the volume of a certain amount of gas is directly proportional to the absolute temperature;

Avogadro's Law: when the temperature of any two gases is the same, they have the same average kinetic energy. At the same time, it can be inferred that under the same temperature and pressure, all gases of the same volume contain the same number of molecules.

These laws describe the relationship between the quantity n of gas substance and their properties of pressure, volume and temperature under different specific conditions. Their mathematical equation are as follows.

Boyle's Law: pV=constant (Under the condition of constant n and T)
Gay-lussac's Law: V/T=constant (Under the condition of constant n and p)
Avogadro's Law: V/n=constant (Under the condition of constant p and T)

These empirical laws are summed up under the condition that the temperature is not too low and the pressure is not too high. Although the measurement accuracy is not high, they all objectively reflect the simple relationship between p, V and T that the low pressure gas obeys. The ideal gas state equation can be obtained by combining the three laws.

$$pV=nRT \tag{1-31}$$

The lower the pressure is and the higher the temperature is, the more the gas conforms to this relationship. We call the gas with zero molecular volume and no interaction force between molecules under any pressure and temperature as **ideal gas** (理想气体).

In fact, ideal gas is a scientific abstract concept. There is no ideal gas objectively. It can only be regarded as a kind of limit case of actual gas at a very low pressure. But it is useful to introduce the concept of ideal gas. On the one hand, it reflects the commonness of any gas under low pressure; on the other hand, different gases have their own particularity, and the relationship between p, V and T of ideal gas is relatively simple. Some relations derived from the ideal gas equation can be applied to any gas as long as they are properly modified.

In the definition of ideal gas, in addition to four physical quantities p, V, T and n, there is also a constant R, which is a general applicable proportional constant in the equation of state of ideal gas. It is called molar gas constant, which is short for gas constant, and its unit is J·mol^{-1}·K^{-1}.

7.1.2   Molar gas constant R（摩尔气体常数 R）

It is very important to accurately determine the gas constant R of ideal gas. In principle, the values of p, V and T can be measured directly for a certain amount of gas, and then substituted into one form to calculate R. However, since the gases used for measurement are all actual gases, when the pressure is very small and the volume is very large, the experimental data are not easy to measure accurately. So it is necessary to use extrapolation method to extrapolate the $(pV)_{p\to 0}$ value of the actual gas under different pressure p, and then the pV value of the actual gas strictly follows the ideal gas state equation, that is

$$\lim_{p \to 0} pV_m = RT \qquad (1-32)$$

Fig. 1–4 shows the extrapolation of several gases under different pressures at 273.15K.

$$(pV_m)_{p \to 0} = 22.414 \text{L·atm} = 2271.10 \text{J}$$

Using the extrapolation value, the accurate value of gas constant can be obtained

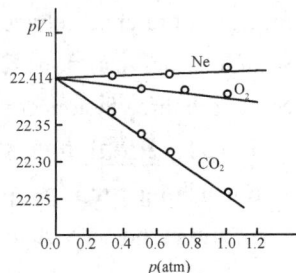

Fig. 1–4 pV_m–p isotherms of N_e, O_2 and CO_2

$$R = \frac{(pV_m)_{p \to 0}}{nT} = \frac{22.414 \times 10^{-3} \times 101325}{1 \times 273.15} = 8.314 \text{J·mol}^{-1}\text{·K}^{-1}$$

R is a very important constant, not only in the calculation of the values of n, p, V, T of gases, but also in the calculation of many problems in physical chemistry.

7.1.3 Law of mixed ideal gas（混合理想气体定律）

The gases encountered in production and scientific research are often a mixture of many components, such as air. Therefore, the question is often asked: what is the contribution of each component in the gas mixture to some properties of the system (such as pressure)? By studying the mixed gas, J. Dalton proposed the concept of partial pressure and Dalton's law.

In 1810, Dalton found that the total pressure of a gas mixture is equal to the sum of the pressures produced by placing each gas in a container separately (this law is accurate only under the limit of zero pressure). If we have A gas of n_A mole, B gas of n_B mole, etc, and we put them in the container separately, the pressure produced by any kind of gas B conforms to the ideal gas state equation n_iRT/V (here we assume that the pressure is low enough to make the gas basically ideal). If all gases are put into one container, Dalton's law holds that the total pressure p of the mixed gas is as follows.

$$p = \frac{nRT}{V} = (n_A + n_B + \cdots + n_J)\frac{RT}{V}$$
$$= \frac{n_A RT}{V} + \frac{n_B RT}{V} + \cdots + \frac{n_J RT}{V}$$
$$= p_A + p_B + \cdots + p_J$$

This is **Dalton's law of partial pressure**(道尔顿分压定律), that is, the total pressure of a gas mixture is equal to the sum of the **partial pressures**(分压力) of each gas. The so-called partial pressure is the pressure with which individual gases exist alone and occupy the same volume as the mixed gas at the same temperature.

Dalton's law of partial pressure can be explained by the molecular model of gas. There is no interaction between ideal gas molecules, so the existence of B, C and other gases has no effect on gas A, and its contribution to the total pressure is the same as when A exists alone. The mixture of gases satisfying Dalton's law of partial pressure is called ideal gas mixture.

In view of the need of thermodynamic calculation, a definition of partial pressure which is suitable for both ideal gas mixture and non ideal gas mixture is also proposed, that is, in the mixed gas with total pressure p, the partial pressure p_B of any component B is the product of its mole fraction y_B in the gas and the total pressure p of the mixed gas.

$$p_B = y_B p \tag{1-33}$$

If the pressure of each component in the mixed gas is summed, because of $\sum y_1 = 1$, we get the following equation.

$$\sum p_B = p \tag{1-34}$$

That is, in any mixed gas, the total pressure is equal to the sum of the pressure of each component.

7.2　The relationship between C_p and C_V of ideal gas

At the same temperature, C_p and C_V of the same substance are usually different, especially for gaseous substances. For any closed system with no phase change or chemical change and only volume work, the relationship between them can be deduced as follows.

$$C_p - C_V = \left(\frac{\partial H}{\partial T}\right)_p - \left(\frac{\partial U}{\partial T}\right)_V$$

$$= \left(\frac{\partial (U + pV)}{\partial T}\right)_p - \left(\frac{\partial U}{\partial T}\right)_V$$

$$= \left(\frac{\partial U}{\partial T}\right)_p + p\left(\frac{\partial V}{\partial T}\right)_p - \left(\frac{\partial U}{\partial T}\right)_V$$

Let $U = f(T, V)$, then the total differential of U is

$$\mathrm{d}U = \left(\frac{\partial U}{\partial T}\right)_V \mathrm{d}T + \left(\frac{\partial U}{\partial V}\right)_T \mathrm{d}V$$

Under constant pressure, divide both sides by $\mathrm{d}T$,

$$\left(\frac{\partial U}{\partial T}\right)_p = \left(\frac{\partial U}{\partial T}\right)_V + \left(\frac{\partial U}{\partial V}\right)_T \left(\frac{\partial V}{\partial T}\right)_p$$

So
$$C_p - C_V = \left(\frac{\partial U}{\partial V}\right)_T \left(\frac{\partial V}{\partial T}\right)_p + p\left(\frac{\partial V}{\partial T}\right)_p = \left[\left(\frac{\partial U}{\partial V}\right)_T + p\right]\left(\frac{\partial V}{\partial T}\right)_p \tag{1-35}$$

There is no condition introduced in the derivation of equation (1-35), so it can be applied to any homogeneous pure component system.

For liquid or solid systems, their volume changes very little with temperature, so $\left(\frac{\partial V}{\partial T}\right)_p$ is approximated to 0 and $C_p \approx C_V$.

For ideal gases, because $\left(\frac{\partial U}{\partial V}\right)_T = 0$, $\left(\frac{\partial V}{\partial T}\right)_p = \frac{nR}{p}$

So
$$C_p - C_V = nR \tag{1-36}$$

Divided both sides by n to get

$$C_{p,m} - C_{V,m} = R \tag{1-37}$$

The above equation shows that there is a constant difference between the constant pressure molar heat capacity and the constant volume molar heat capacity of any ideal gas, that is, the molar gas constant R, R = 8.314J · mol^{-1} · K^{-1}. It can be proved that the physical meaning of R is the work done at constant pressure when the ideal gas of 1mol is heated up to 1K.

According to statistical thermodynamics, it can be proved that under normal temperature, For monatomic molecules, $C_{V,m}=\frac{3}{2}R$, $C_{p,m}=\frac{5}{2}R$; For diatomic molecules, $C_{V,m}=\frac{5}{2}R$, $C_{p,m}=\frac{7}{2}R$; For polyatomic molecules (non linear), $C_{V,m}=3R$, $C_{p,m}=4R$.

7.3 Joule experiment（焦耳实验）

In 1843, Joule carried out the following experiments with the device shown in Fig. 1–5. Two containers with equal capacity connected by cocks in the middle were placed in a water bath with an insulating wall. Fill the container A with air (Pressure not higher than 100kPa), and the container B is vacuumized. After the heat balance is reached, open the middle cock to make the gas expand freely to the vacuum, from vessel A to vessel B, until the gas in the two vessels reaches the balance.

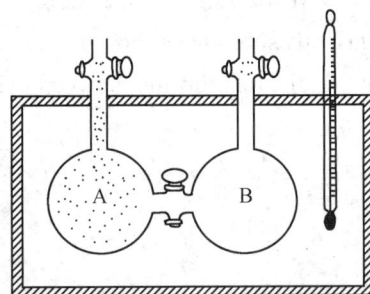

Fig. 1–5   Schematic diagram of Joule experimental device

The experimental results show that there is no change in the temperature of water. Taking gas as the system and water bath as the environment, no change of water temperature was observed, $dT = 0$,

that is, there was no heat exchange between the system and the environment, $\delta Q = 0$. Because this process was expansion to vacuum, $p_{su} = 0$, $\delta W = 0$, according to the first law of thermodynamics, $dU = \delta Q + \delta W = 0$. It can be seen that when the gas expands to vacuum, the internal energy will remain unchanged if the temperature remains unchanged.

For homogeneous systems of pure components, $U = f(T,V)$, the total differential is:

$$dU = \left(\frac{\partial U}{\partial T}\right)_V dT + \left(\frac{\partial U}{\partial V}\right)_T dV$$

Because $dT = 0$ and $dU = 0$, $\left(\frac{\partial U}{\partial V}\right)_T dV = 0$.

The volume of the gas has changed, $dT \neq 0$, so it can only be

$$\left(\frac{\partial U}{\partial V}\right)_T = 0 \qquad (1–38)$$

The above equation shows that the internal energy of gas does not change with volume at constant temperature. It can also be proved that

$$\left(\frac{\partial U}{\partial p}\right)_T = 0 \qquad (1–39)$$

That is to say, the internal energy of the above experimental gas does not change with the pressure at a constant temperature. It is shown from equations (1–38 and 1–39) that the internal energy of the above gases is only a function of temperature, independent of volume and pressure.

$$U = f(T) \qquad (1–40)$$

In fact, these experiments are not accurate enough. Further accurate experiments show that the temperature will change slightly when the real gas expands to vacuum. This is because when the actual gas pressure is large, the intermolecular gravity increases, and when the gas expands freely, it resists the internal pressure and works, so the internal energy changes. The temperature change of real gas decreases with the decrease of gas initial pressure. Therefore, it can be inferred that the above conclusion of Joule experiment is completely correct only when the initial pressure of gas tends to zero, that is, the gas tends to ideal gas. Therefore, only the internal energy of an ideal gas is a function of temperature, independent of volume or pressure.

Because there is no gravity between ideal gas molecules, when increasing the volume to increase the distance between molecules at a certain temperature, it is not necessary to overcome the gravity between molecules and consume the kinetic energy of molecules. Therefore, the temperature of ideal gas is unchanged, and the gas expansion does not need to absorb energy, so the internal energy of ideal gas remains unchanged, that is, the internal energy of ideal gas is only a function of temperature, independent of pressure and volume.

For the enthalpy of an ideal gas:

$$H = U + pV = U + nRT = f(T) \tag{1-41}$$

That is to say, the enthalpy of ideal gas is only a function of temperature, independent of volume or pressure.

$$\left(\frac{\partial H}{\partial V}\right)_T = 0 \tag{1-42}$$

$$\left(\frac{\partial H}{\partial p}\right)_T = 0 \tag{1-43}$$

Because
$$C_p = \left(\frac{\partial H}{\partial T}\right)_p, \quad C_V = \left(\frac{\partial U}{\partial T}\right)_V$$

So, C_p and C_V of ideal gas is only a function of temperature.

7.4　Isothermal process of ideal gas

The process in which the temperature of the system keeps constant with the ambient temperature from the initial state to the final state is called the **isothermal process** (等温过程). Because the internal energy and enthalpy of the ideal gas are only functions of temperature, that is,

$$\Delta U = 0, \quad \Delta H = 0$$

Since
$$\Delta U = Q + W$$

So
$$Q = -W$$

Because heat and work are related to processes, the values of Q and W are different for different processes.

7.4.1　Heat and work in constant temperature reversible process

For the constant temperature reversible process of ideal gas, the heat Q absorbed by the system from the environment is all used to work on the environment. At this time, the maximum work done by the gas is: $Q_R = -W_R = -nRT \ln\dfrac{V_2}{V_1} = -nRT \ln\dfrac{p_1}{p_2}$

7.4.2 Heat and work in irreversible process of constant temperature

At constant temperature, the finite expansion (or compression) of gas in any finite time is an irreversible process at constant temperature.

(1) Free expansion　If the ideal gas is allowed to expand (free expansion) against zero external pressure, it is an irreversible process. According to the Joule experiment, $dT = 0$, because $p_{su} = 0$, $Q_{IR} = -W_{IR} = 0$.

(2) Constant external pressure expansion　Under constant external pressure p_{su}, the ideal gas will expand at constant temperature.

$$Q_R = -W_R = p_{su}(V_2 - V_1)$$

(3) Constant temperature expansion　The absolute values of W_{IR} and Q_{IR} of the ideal gas in the constant temperature irreversible compression process are greater than W_{IR} and Q_{IR} in the constant temperature reversible compression process.

When the ideal gas passes through a reversible cycle at constant temperature, both the system and the environment are completely restored to the original state, then ΔU and ΔH in the state function is equal to zero, and the heat and work of the reversible cycle process is equal to zero.

$$Q_R = -W_R = 0$$

As long as one step of the system is irreversible, the cycle process is irreversible. During the constant temperature irreversible cycle,

$$Q_{IR} = -W_{IR} \neq 0$$

That is to say, the environment makes the net work of the system, and the system transfers the net heat to the environment.

[Example 1–3] At 298K, the ideal gas of 1mol single atom expands from 15.00dm^3 to 40.00dm^3 in the following three ways: (1) free expansion; (2) Constant temperature reversible expansion; (3) Constant temperature expansion at 100kPa. Solve Q, W, ΔU and ΔH of the above three processes.

Solution: (1) Free expansion process, $W = -p_{su}(V_2 - V_1) = 0 \times (V_2 - V_1) = 0$

Because the thermodynamic energy and enthalpy of ideal gas are only functions of temperature, while the temperature of free expansion process of ideal gas is constant,

$$\Delta U = \Delta H = f(T) = 0, \quad Q = \Delta U - W = 0$$

(2) Because of the ideal gas isothermal process: $\Delta U = \Delta H = 0$

$$W = -nRT\ln\frac{V_2}{V_1} = -2 \times 8.314 \times 298 \times \ln\frac{40.00}{15.00} = -4860J$$

$$Q = -W = 4860J$$

(3) Similarly, $\Delta U = \Delta H = 0$

$$W = -p_{su}(V_2 - V_1) = -100000 \times (40.00 - 15.00) \times 10^{-3} = -2500J$$

$$Q = -W = 2500J$$

7.5　Adiabatic process of ideal gas

7.5.1　Adiabatic reversible process equations（绝热可逆过程方程式）

For the adiabatic process, $\delta Q = 0$, according to the first law of thermodynamics,

$$dU = \delta W$$

For the adiabatic reversible process of ideal gas, if only volume work is done, $W' = 0$,

Then
$$\delta W = -p_{su}\,dV = -p\,dV = -\frac{nRT}{V}\,dV$$

Because of the ideal gas
$$dU = C_V\,dT$$

So
$$-\frac{nR\,dV}{V} = C_V\,\frac{dT}{T}$$

The integral on both sides is
$$\int_{V_1}^{V_2}\frac{nR\,dV}{V} = -\int_{T_1}^{T_2}C_V\,\frac{dT}{T}$$

$$nR\ln\frac{V_2}{V_1} = -C_V\ln\frac{T_2}{T_1}$$

For ideal gas, $C_p - C_V = nR$, substituting the above equation, we can get

$$\left(C_p - C_V\right)\ln\frac{V_2}{V_1} = C_V\ln\frac{T_1}{T_2}$$

Divided both sides of the equation by C_V, and let $C_p / C_V = C_{p,\mathrm{m}} / C_{V,\mathrm{m}} = \gamma$ (adiabatic index), so the above equation can be written as

$$(\gamma-1)\ln\frac{V_2}{V_1} = \ln\frac{T_1}{T_2}$$

So
$$T_1 V_1^{\gamma-1} = T_2 V_2^{\gamma-1}$$

Or
$$TV^{\gamma-1} = \text{constant} \tag{1-44}$$

If $T = \dfrac{pV}{nR}$ is substituted into equation (1-44), we can get

$$pV^{\gamma} = \text{constant} \tag{1-45}$$

If $V = \dfrac{nRT}{P}$ is substituted into equation (1-45), the following results can be obtained

$$T^{\gamma}p^{1-\gamma} = \text{constant} \tag{1-46}$$

Equation (1-44), (1-45) and (1-46) are all process equations of adiabatic reversible process of ideal gas under the condition of zero non volume work. They show the relationship between p, V and T in the adiabatic reversible process of ideal gas.

7.5.2　Calculation of work in adiabatic process

In the adiabatic process, $\delta Q = 0$, then
$$\delta W = dU$$

For ideal gas,
$$dU = C_V\,dT$$

Therefore, the work done in the adiabatic process is

$$W = \int_{T_1}^{T_2} C_V\,dT$$

If C_V is constant, the integral is

$$W = C_V\,(T_2 - T_1) \tag{1-47}$$

Since
$$C_p - C_V = nR, \quad C_p / C_V = \gamma$$

Then
$$\gamma - 1 = \frac{nR}{C_V}$$

So equation (1-47) can be written as

$$W = \frac{nR(T_2 - T_1)}{\gamma - 1} \tag{1-48}$$

$$= \frac{p_2 V_2 - p_1 V_1}{\gamma - 1} \tag{1-49}$$

Equation (1–48) and (1–49) can be used to calculate the adiabatic work of ideal gas, including reversible and irreversible processes.

[**Example 1–4**] In the adiabatic cylinder with frictionless piston, there is 5mol ideal gas with two atoms, the pressure is 1000kPa and the temperature is 298.2K.

(1) If the gas is adiabatically and reversibly expanded to 100kPa, calculate the work done by the system.

(2) If the external pressure suddenly decreases from 1000kPa to 100kPa, what is the work done by the system?

Solution: (1) $C_{V,m} = \frac{5}{2}R, C_{p,m} = \frac{7}{2}R, \gamma = C_{p,m}/C_{V,m} = 1.4$

$$T_2 = T_1^{\gamma} p_1^{1-\gamma} / p_2^{1-\gamma}$$

$$T_2 = (298^{1.4} \times 10^{-0.4} \times 1^{0.4})^{1/1.4} = 154.4K$$

$$Q_1 = 0, \ W_1 = \Delta U_1 = nC_{V,m}(T_2 - T_1)$$

$$W_1 = 5 \times \frac{5}{2} \times 8.314 \times (154.4 - 298.2) = -14.94kJ$$

(2) $Q_2 = 0, \ W_2 = \Delta U_2$

$$W_2 = -p_{su}(V_2 - V_1) = -p_{su}\left(\frac{nRT_2}{p_2} - \frac{nRT_1}{p_1}\right) = -5 \times 8.314 \times \left(T_2 - \frac{298.2}{10}\right)$$

$$\Delta U_2 = nC_{V,m}(T_2 - T_1) = 5 \times \frac{5}{2} \times 8.314 \times (T_2 - 298.2)$$

$$T_2 = 221.5K$$

$$W_2 = -5 \times 8.314 \times \left(221.5 - \frac{298.2}{10}\right) = -7.97kJ$$

By comparing the results of (1) and (2), it can be seen that from the same initial state, the same final state can not be achieved through the adiabatic reversible and adiabatic irreversible processes. When the volume of the final state of the two processes is the same, because the work of the reversible process is greater, the thermodynamic energy is reduced more, resulting in the lower temperature of the final state.

Section 8　Thermal Effects of Chemical Reaction

It is noticed that energy in the form of heat (thermal energy) is generally evolved or absorbed as a result of a chemical change. The study of the energy transferred as heat during the course of chemical reactions is called **thermochemistry(热化学)**. Thermochemistry is the branch of physical chemistry.

Heat of reaction(反应热) may be defined as the amount of heat absorbed or evolved in a reaction when the number of moles of reactants as represented by the balanced chemical equation change completely into the products at constant temperature in a closed system only with work done due to a volume change.

The heat of a reaction is simply the amount of heat absorbed or evolved in the reaction. Although the values of Q for a change from state 1 to state 2 depend on the process used, under some particular conditions, the value of Q, which is constant. Let's talk about Q for constant- volume and constant-pressure processes respectively. These are discussed below.

8.1　Relationship between reaction heat at constant volume and reaction heat at constant pressure

Reaction heat at constant volume(定容反应热) may be defined as the amount of heat absorbed or evolved in a reaction when the number of moles of reactants as represented by the balanced chemical equation change completely into the products. It is denoted by Q_V .The value of Q_V, which equals ΔU, is constant.

$$Q_V = \Delta_r U = (\sum U)_{products} - (\sum U)_{reactants}$$

Q_V can be determined by experiment. The most common device for measuring Q_V is an adiabatic bomb calorimeter. It follow that, by measuring the energy supplied to a constant - volume system as heat ($Q_V > 0$) or released from it as heat ($Q_V < 0$) when it undergoes a reaction, we are in fact measuring the change in its internal energy.

Reaction heat at constant pressure(定压反应热) may be defined as the amount of heat absorbed or evolved in a reaction when the number of moles of reactants as represented by the balanced chemical equation change completely into the products. It is denoted by Q_p.

We also know that the amount of heat absorbed or evolved at constant temperature and pressure is called enthalpy. Therefore the amount of heat change during a reaction at constant temperature and pressure may also be called enthalpy change. Although Q is generally path-dependent, it is path-independent for constant-pressure processes, for which $Q_p = \Delta_r H$.

$$Q_p = \Delta_r H = (\sum H)_{products} - (\sum U)_{reactants}$$

Although ΔH is the same for any process with the same initial and final states as the overall process, Q is dependent on the path of a particular process. If the pressure is not constant during the entire process, Q is not necessarily equal to ΔH.

Q_p can be determined by experiment. The most common device for measuring Q_p is an isobaric calorimeter. By measuring the energy supplied to a constant pressure system as heat ($Q_p > 0$) or released from it as heat ($Q_p < 0$) when it undergoes a reaction, we are in fact measuring the change in its enthalpy.

Another route to $\Delta_r H$ is to measure the internal energy change by using bomb calorimeter, and then to convert $\Delta_r U$ to $\Delta_r H$. So it is important to know the relationship of $\Delta_r U$ and $\Delta_r H$.

Let us consider a general reaction which occurs at constant temperature and pressure or at constant temperature and volume respectively (Fig. 1–6).

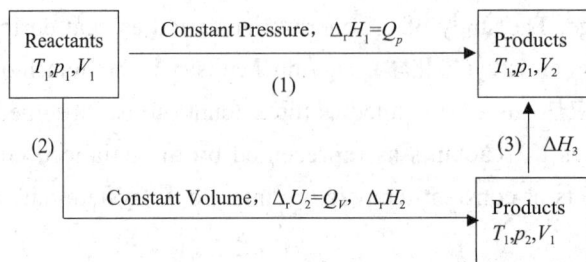

Fig. 1-6 Relationship between reaction heat at constant pressure and reaction heat at constant volume

Since enthalpy is state function:

$$\Delta_r H_1 = \Delta_r H_2 + H_3$$

From the definition of the enthalpy we can write an expression for ΔH for a chemical reaction

$$\Delta_r H_1 = \Delta_r H_2 + \Delta_r H_3 = \Delta_r H_2 + \Delta(pV)_2 + \Delta H_3$$

where $\Delta(pV)_2$ is equal to pV of final state minus pV of initial state on the process 2

$$\Delta(pV)_2 = (pV)_{2,\text{ final}} - (pV)_{2,\text{ initial}}$$

Because

$$pV = p(V(s) + V(l) + V(g))$$

where $V(s)$ is the volume of all of the solid phases, $V(l)$ is the volume of all of the liquid phases, and $V(g)$ is the volume of the gas phase.

If a process involves only solids or liquids, because solids or liquids have small molar volumes, $\Delta(pV)$ is so small that the change of enthalpy and the change of internal energy are identical ($\Delta_r H_2 = \Delta_r U_2 + \Delta(pV)_2 \approx \Delta_r U_2$). And $\Delta_r H_3$ is much smaller than $\Delta_r H_2$, so that a less accurate calculation of $\Delta_r H_2$ might suffice. That is, $Q_p = Q_V$.

Under ordinary conditions the molar volume of a gas is several hundred to a thousand times larger than the molar volume of a solid or liquid. If there is at least one gaseous product or reactant we can ignore the volume of the solid and liquid phases to an adequate approximation,

$$pV \approx pV(g)$$

So

$$\Delta(pV) \approx \Delta[pV(g)]$$

If the products and reactants are at the same temperature and if we use the ideal gas equation as an approximation,

$$\Delta(pV)_2 = p_2 V_1 - p_1 V_1 = \Delta n(g)RT_1$$

where $\Delta n(g)$ is the change in the number of moles of gaseous substances in the reaction equation.

$$\Delta_r H = \Delta_r U + \Delta n(g)RT \tag{1-50}$$

Or

$$Q_p = Q_V + \Delta n(g)RT \tag{1-51}$$

If 1 mol of reaction occurs, then

$$\Delta_r H_m = \Delta_r U_m + \Delta \nu(g)RT \tag{1-52}$$

Which defines the quantity $\Delta \nu(g)$, equal to the number of moles of gas in the product side of the balanced chemical equation minus the numbers of moles of gas in the reactant side of the balanced equation.

[Example 1-5] The heat of combustion of *n*-heptane at constant volume and at 298.2K is $-4.807 \times 10^6 \text{J} \cdot \text{mol}^{-1}$, Calculate its heat of combustion at constant pressure ($R = 8.314\text{J} \cdot \text{mol}^{-1} \cdot \text{K}^{-1}$).

Solution:

$$C_7H_{16}(l) + 11O_2(g) = 7CO_2(g) + 8H_2O(l)$$

$$\Delta n = 7 - 11 = -4$$
$$Q_p = Q_V + (\Delta n)RT$$
$$= -4.807 \times 10^6 - 4 \times 8.314 \times 298.2$$
$$= -4.817 \times 10^6 \, J \cdot mol^{-1}$$

8.2　Thermochemical equation

An equation which indicates the amount of heat change (evolved or absorbed) in the reaction or process is called a **thermochemical equation(热化学方程式)**.

There are a number of factors which affect the quantity of heat evolved or absorbed during a physical or chemical transformation. One of these factors has already been discussed viz., whether the change occurs at constant pressure or constant volume. The other factors are: (a) Amount of the reactants and products; (b) Physical state of the reactants and products; (c) Temperature; (d) Pressure.

So that a Thermochemical equation must essentially: (a) Be balanced; (b) Give the value of ΔU or ΔH corresponding to the quantities of substances given by the equation; (c) Mention the physical states of the reactants and products. The physical states are represented by the symbols (s), (l), (g) and (aq) for solid, liquid, gas and gaseous states respectively.

It is very important to note that heat of reaction varies with the change in temperature or in pressure. Therefore, we must mention the temperature and the pressure at which the reaction is taking place. According to the conventions prevalent in thermodynamics, the standard state of a substance at a specified temperature is its pure form under a pressure of one atmosphere. The heat change accompanying a reaction taking place at a specified temperature and one atmospheric pressure is called the standard heat change or standard enthalpy change. It is denoted by $\Delta_r H_m^\ominus (T)$.

It is also convenient for comparison to fix up some temperature as standard or reference. The convenient temperature for reporting thermodynamics data is 298K (corresponding to 25℃). Unless otherwise mentioned, all thermodynamics data in this text will refer to this convenient temperature. The heat change accompanying a reaction taking place at 298K and one atmospheric pressure is denoted by $\Delta_r H_m^\ominus (298K)$.

Examples of thermochemical equation are as follows:

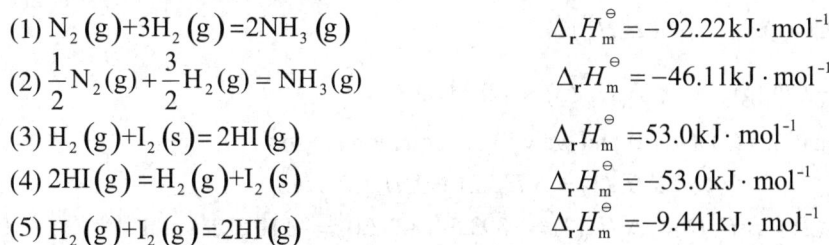

(1) $N_2(g) + 3H_2(g) = 2NH_3(g)$　　　　　　$\Delta_r H_m^\ominus = -92.22 \, kJ \cdot mol^{-1}$

(2) $\dfrac{1}{2}N_2(g) + \dfrac{3}{2}H_2(g) = NH_3(g)$　　　　$\Delta_r H_m^\ominus = -46.11 \, kJ \cdot mol^{-1}$

(3) $H_2(g) + I_2(s) = 2HI(g)$　　　　　　　$\Delta_r H_m^\ominus = 53.0 \, kJ \cdot mol^{-1}$

(4) $2HI(g) = H_2(g) + I_2(s)$　　　　　　　$\Delta_r H_m^\ominus = -53.0 \, kJ \cdot mol^{-1}$

(5) $H_2(g) + I_2(g) = 2HI(g)$　　　　　　　$\Delta_r H_m^\ominus = -9.441 \, kJ \cdot mol^{-1}$

In case $\Delta_r H_m^\ominus$ is negative ($\Delta_r H_m^\ominus < 0$), the sum of enthalpies of the products is less than that of the reactants and the difference in enthalpy is given out in the form of heat. Such reactions which are accompanied by the evolution of heat energy are called exothermic reactions.

When $\Delta_r H_m^\ominus$ is positive ($\Delta_r H_m^\ominus > 0$), the enthalpy or heat content of the reactants and an equivalent of heat is absorbed by the system from the surroundings. Such reactions which are accompanied by absorption of heat are called Endothermic reactions.

Exothermic reaction: $\Delta_r H_m^\ominus < 0$; Endothermic reaction: $\Delta_r H_m^\ominus > 0$.

8.3 Hess's Law

<u>**Hess's Law**(盖斯定律)</u> may be stated as: If a chemical change can be made to take place in two or more different ways whether in one step or two or more steps, the amount of total heat change is same no matter by which method the change is brought about.

The law also follows as a mere consequence of the first law of thermodynamics. We have already seen that heat changes in chemical reactions are equal to the difference in internal energy $\Delta_r U$ or heat content $\Delta_r H$ of the products and reactants, depending upon whether the reaction is studied at constant volume or constant pressure. Since $\Delta_r U$ and $\Delta_r H$ are functions of the state of the system, the heat evolved or absorbed in a given reaction must be independent of the manner in which the reaction is brought about.

Let us suppose that a substance A can be changed to B directly, as well the same change is brought about in several stages (Fig. 1–7):

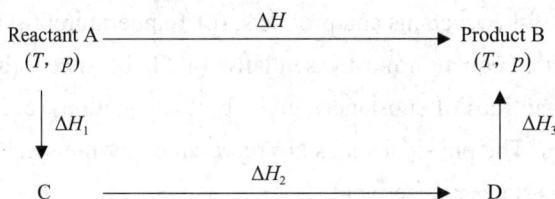

Reactant A $\xrightarrow{\quad\Delta H\quad}$ Product B
$(T, \ p)$ $\qquad\qquad\qquad\qquad\qquad\qquad$ $(T, \ p)$

$\downarrow \Delta H_1$ $\qquad\qquad\qquad\qquad\qquad\qquad$ $\uparrow \Delta H_3$

C $\xrightarrow{\quad\Delta H_2\quad}$ D

Fig. 1–7 Schematic diagram of Hess's law

Since H is state function, ΔH depends only on the initial state and final state of the system and not the manner or the steps in which the change takes place, so that:

$$\Delta H = \Delta H_1 + \Delta H_2 + \Delta H_3 \tag{1-53}$$

Hess's law has been of great service in the indirect determination of heats of formation reactions.

[Example 1–6] Calculate $\Delta_r H_m^\ominus$ of reaction (2):

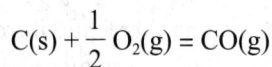

$$C(s) + \frac{1}{2} O_2(g) = CO(g)$$

Given that:

(1) $C(s) + O_2(g) = CO_2(g)$ $\qquad\qquad$ $\Delta_r H_m^\ominus (1) = -393.5 kJ \cdot mol^{-1}$

(2) $C(s) + \frac{1}{2} O_2(g) = CO(g)$ $\qquad\qquad$ $\Delta_r H_m^\ominus (2)$

(3) $CO(g) + \frac{1}{2} O_2(g) = CO_2(g)$ $\qquad\quad$ $\Delta_r H_m^\ominus (3) = -283.0 kJ \cdot mol^{-1}$

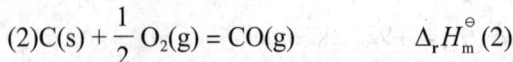

Solution: Adding equations (2) and (3) and we will get equation (1), so

$$\Delta_r H_m(1) = \Delta_r H_m(2) + \Delta_r H_m(3)$$

$$\Delta_r H_m(2) = \Delta_r H_m(1) + \Delta_r H_m(3) = -393.5 - (-283.0) = -110.5 kJ \cdot mol^{-1}$$

It is obvious from the above example that by the addition of a series of chemical equations we can obtain not only the resultant products of this series of reactions but also the net heat effect. It is, therefore, clear that: Thermochemical equations may be multiplied, added or subtracted like ordinary algebraic equations.

The substances like methane, carbon monoxide, benzene, etc., cannot be prepared by uniting their elements. Therefore it is not possible to measure the heats of formation reactions of such compounds directly. These can be determined indirectly by using Hess's law. Hess's law has been of great service in the determination of heat of formation reactions of substances which otherwise cannot be measured experimentally.

Section 9   Several Thermal Effects

In the laboratory most of the chemical reactions are carried out at constant pressure (atmospheric pressure) rather than at constant volume. Enthalpy changes of constant-pressure reactions are sometimes called "heats" of the reactions. So when we talk about heat of a reaction, we will refer to $\Delta_r H$.

As we have known, a change in enthalpy ($\Delta_r H$) accompanying a process can be measured accurately and is given by the expression.

$$\Delta_r H = Q_p = (\sum H)_{products} - (\sum H)_{reactants} \tag{1-54}$$

Just like internal energy, enthalpy is also a function of the state and it is not possible to measure its absolute value. Therefore it is not possible to calculate the $\Delta_r H$ directly and it is not convenient to measure heat of all kinds of reactions experimentally. These can be determined indirectly by using relative value.

For example, if you want to measure the potential energy of something in a gravitational field, you have to define the zero somewhere, because it is arbitrary. You can set it anywhere you want. It's the same with enthalpy.

So there is an arbitrary set point that needs to be defined. Because $\Delta_r H$ is change in enthalpy, just like what you measure when you look at change of potential energy. The relative number that you assign to it is something that's arbitrary. You have to set what the zero is. And so there are two well-understood conventions for what the zero is. These are discussed below.

We choose a convention for the zero of enthalpy, so that we can write entropies of products and reactants always referring to the same standard state. And then we calculate changes, the convention is understood with respect to what is the zero. And so our tabulated statistics values, they'll all work. Adding Hess's law, we'll be able to calculate the heat of most reactions conveniently without any experiment.

The heat or enthalpy changes accompanying chemical reactions are expressed in different ways, depending on the nature of the reaction. These are discussed below.

9.1   Standard Heat of Formation

The **heat of formation(生成热)** of a compound is defined as the change in enthalpy that takes place when one mole of the compound is formed from its elements. It is denoted by $\Delta_r H_m$.

The **standard molar enthalpy of formation(标准摩尔生成焓)** of a compound is defined as: The change in enthalpy that takes place when one mole of a compound is formed from its elements, all substances being in their standard states (298K and 1 atm pressure).

By convention the standard heat of formation of every element which is in its most stable form at 298.15K and 1 atm pressure is assumed to be zero as shown below.

$$\Delta_f H_m^{\ominus}(H_2, g, 298.15K) = 0 \qquad \Delta_f H_m^{\ominus}(O_2, g, 298.15K) = 0$$
$$\Delta_f H_m^{\ominus}(C(graphite), s, 298, 15K) = 0 \qquad \Delta_f H_m^{\ominus}(O_2, g, 298, 15K) = 0$$

$$\Delta_f H_m^{\ominus}(N_2, g, 298, 15K) = 0$$

For example, the standard heat of formation of liquid water at 298.15K may be expressed as:

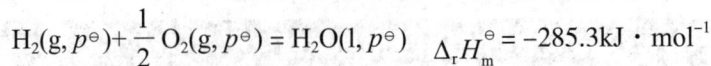

$$H_2(g, p^{\ominus}) + \frac{1}{2} O_2(g, p^{\ominus}) = H_2O(l, p^{\ominus}) \qquad \Delta_f H_m^{\ominus} = -285.3 kJ \cdot mol^{-1}$$

So $\qquad \Delta_r H_m^{\ominus}(298.15K) = \Delta_f H_m^{\ominus}(H_2O, l, 298.15K) = -285.3 kJ \cdot mol^{-1}$

The standard heat of formation of some compounds at 298.15K is given in appendix.

We can calculate the heat of reaction under standard conditions from the values of standard heat of formation of various reactants and products. The standard heat of reaction is equal to the standard heat of formation of products minus the standard heat of formation of reactants.

That is,

$$\Delta_r H_m^{\ominus}(T) = \sum_B (\Delta_f H_m^{\ominus})_{products} - \sum_B (\Delta_f H_m^{\ominus})_{reactants} \qquad (1-55)$$

Let us consider a general reaction at TK and one atmospheric pressure (Fig. 1–8).

$$aA + dD \rightarrow gG + hH$$

Or $\qquad\qquad\qquad\qquad\qquad\qquad 0 = \sum_B v_B B$

For reactants, v_B is negative; for products, v_B is positive.

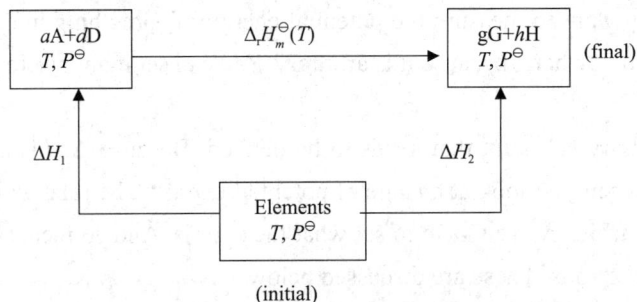

Fig. 1–8　Solution diagram of chemical reaction heat by heat of formation

Because of the Hess's Law $\qquad \Delta H_1 + \Delta_r H_m^{\ominus}(T) = \Delta H_2$

So $\qquad\qquad\qquad\qquad \Delta_r H_m^{\ominus}(T) = \Delta H_2 - \Delta H_1$

Also

$$\Delta H_1 = a \Delta_f H_m^{\ominus}(A) + d \Delta_f H_m^{\ominus}(D) = \sum_B (-v_B \Delta_f H_m^{\ominus})_{reactants}$$

$$\Delta H_2 = g \Delta_f H_m^{\ominus}(G) + h \Delta_f H_m^{\ominus}(H) = \sum_B (v_B \Delta_f H_m^{\ominus})_{products}$$

So $\qquad \Delta_r H_m^{\ominus}(T) = \sum_B (v_B \Delta_f H_m^{\ominus})_{products} - \sum_B (-v_B \Delta_f H_m^{\ominus})_{reactants} = \sum_B v_B \Delta_f H_m^{\ominus} \qquad (1-56)$

The standard heat of reaction is given by

$$\Delta_r H_m^{\ominus}(T) = [g \Delta_f H_m^{\ominus}(G) + h \Delta_f H_m^{\ominus}(H)] - [a \Delta_f H_m^{\ominus}(A) + d \Delta_f H_m^{\ominus}(D)]$$

[Example 1–7] Calculate $\Delta_r H_m^{\ominus}(298.15K)$ for the reaction at 298.15K and 101.325kPa:

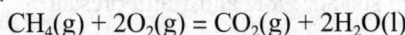

$$CH_4(g) + 2O_2(g) = CO_2(g) + 2H_2O(l)$$

Given that：

$CH_4(g)$	$+$	$2O_2(g)$	$=$	$CO_2(g)$	$+$	$2H_2O(l)$

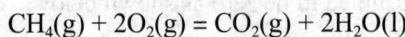

$\Delta_f H_m^{\ominus} / (kJ \cdot mol^{-1})$	-74.8	0	-393.5	-285.3

Solution:

$$\Delta_r H_m^\ominus (298.15K) = \sum_B v_B \Delta_f H_m^\ominus (B) = -393.5 + 2 \times (-285.3) - (-74.8) = -889.3kJ \cdot mol^{-1}$$

9.2　Standard Heat of Combustion

The direct determination of the heats of formation of some organic compounds is often impossible, but the heats of combustion of organic compounds can be determined with considerable ease, these are employed to calculate heats of reactions.

The **heat of combustion(燃烧热)** of a substance is defined as the change in enthalpy of a system when one mole of the substance is completely burnt in excess of air or oxygen. It is denoted by $\Delta_c H_m$.

The **standard molar enthalpy of combustion(标准摩尔燃烧焓)** of a substance is defined as: the change in enthalpy of a system when one mole of the substance is completely burnt in excess of air or oxygen, all substances being in their standard states (298K and 1 atm pressure). It is denoted by $\Delta_c H_m^\ominus$ (298K). As for example, the standard heat of combustion of ethanol at 298.15K is $-1366.8kJ \cdot mol^{-1}$, as shown by the equation

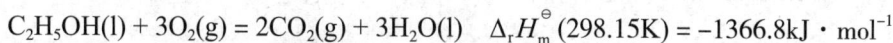

$$C_2H_5OH(l) + 3O_2(g) = 2CO_2(g) + 3H_2O(l) \quad \Delta_r H_m^\ominus (298.15K) = -1366.8kJ \cdot mol^{-1}$$

So

$$\Delta_r H_m^\ominus (298.15K) = \Delta_c H_m^\ominus (C_2H_5OH, l, 298.15K) = -1366.8kJ \cdot mol^{-1}$$

$\Delta_r H_m^\ominus$ is the standard reaction enthalpy for the complete oxidation of an organic compound to CO_2 gas and liquid H_2O if the compound contains C, H, and O, and to N_2 gas and HCl(aq) if N and Cl are also present. It should be noted clearly that oxidation has converted carbon to carbon monoxide and is by no means complete as carbon monoxide can be further oxidised to carbon dioxide.

At 298K and 1atm, the combustion enthalpy of complete oxidation is defined as zero. The standard heat of combustion of some compounds at 298.15K is given in appendix.

We can calculate the heat of reaction under standard conditions from the values of standard heat of combustion of various reactants and products. The standard heat of reaction is equal to the standard heat of combustion of reactants minus the standard heat of combustion of products.

That is,

$$\Delta_r H_m^\ominus (T) = \sum_B (\Delta_c H_m^\ominus)_{reactants} - \sum_B (\Delta_c H_m^\ominus)_{products} \tag{1-57}$$

Let us consider a general reaction at T K and one atmospheric pressure (Fig. 1-9).

$$aA + dD \rightarrow gG + hH$$

Or

$$0 = \sum_B v_B B$$

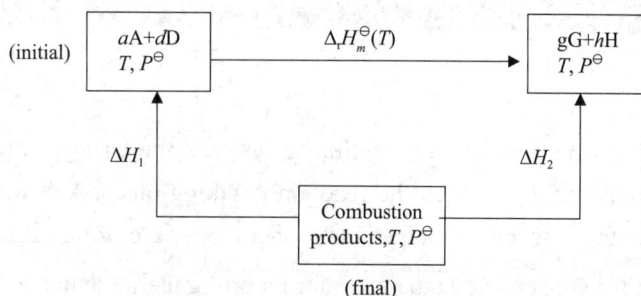

Fig. 1-9　Solution diagram of chemical reaction heat by heat of combustion

Because of the Hess's Law

$$\Delta H_1 = \Delta_r H_m^{\ominus}(T) + \Delta H_2$$

$$\therefore \Delta_r H_m^{\ominus}(T) = \Delta H_1 - \Delta H_2$$

But we have already seen that

$$\Delta H_1 = a\,\Delta_c H_m^{\ominus}(A) + d\Delta_c H_m^{\ominus}(D) = \sum_B (-v_B \Delta_c H_m^{\ominus})_{reactants}$$

$$\Delta H_2 = g\,\Delta_c H_m^{\ominus}(G) + h\Delta_c H_m^{\ominus}(H) = \sum_B (v_B \Delta_c H_m^{\ominus})_{products}$$

So $\qquad \Delta_r H_m^{\ominus}(T) = \sum_B (v_B \Delta_c H_m^{\ominus})_{reactants} - \sum_B (v_B \Delta_c H_m^{\ominus})_{products} = \sum_B - v_B \Delta_f H_m^{\ominus}(B)$ （1–58）

The standard heat of reaction is given by

$$\Delta_r H_m^{\ominus}(T) = [a\Delta_c H_m^{\ominus}(A) + d\Delta_c H_m^{\ominus}(D)] - [g\Delta_c H_m^{\ominus}(G) + h\Delta_c H_m^{\ominus}(H)]$$

[Example 1–8] Given that: at 298.15K and 101.325kPa, $\Delta_c H_m^{\ominus}$ for $H_2(g)$, C(graphite)and

cyclopropane are -285.3, -393.5 and -2091kJ $\cdot$ mol^{-1} respectively; $\Delta_f H_m^{\ominus}$ for propylene is 20.6kJ $\cdot$ mol^{-1}

(1) Calculate $\Delta_f H_m^{\ominus}$(298.15K) for cyclopropane;

(2) Calculate $\Delta_r H_m^{\ominus}$(298.15K) for the reaction C_3H_6(cyclopropane) $\rightarrow CH_3$ — CH = CH_2
Solution:

$$3C(graphite) + 3H_2(g) = C_3H_6(cyclopropane)$$

So

(1) $\qquad \Delta_r H_m^{\ominus}(T) = \Delta_f H_m^{\ominus}(cyclopropane) = -\sum_B v_B \Delta_c H_m^{\ominus}(B)$

$$= 3 \times (-393.5) + 3 \times (-285.3) - 1 \times (-2091) = 54.6\text{kJ} \cdot \text{mol}^{-1}$$

(2) $\qquad C_3H_6$(cyclopropane) $\rightarrow CH_3$ — CH = CH_2

$$\Delta_r H_m^{\ominus}(298.15K) = -\sum_B v_B \Delta_f H_m^{\ominus}(B) = 20.6 - 54.6 = -34.0\text{kJ} \cdot \text{mol}^{-1}$$

Section 10 The Relationship between Heat of Reaction and Temperature—— Kirchhoff's Law

It is very important to note that heat of reaction varies with the change in temperature. Therefore, we must mention the temperature at which the reaction is taking place. According to the conventions prevalent in thermodynamics, a specified temperature under a pressure of one atmosphere has been fixed as the standard state. But the convenient temperature for reporting thermodynamics data is 298K, so $\Delta_r H_m^{\ominus}$

(298K) which we calculate is the heat of reaction taking place at 298K. To calculate Heat of reaction at a specified given temperature when it is known at some other temperature, not at 298K, we ought to know the relationship of heat of reaction with temperature.

The equations representing the variation of heat change of reaction with temperature are known as **Kirchhoff's equations (基尔霍夫定律)**.

Given by the reaction

$$aA + dD \rightarrow gG + hH$$

Or

$$0 = \sum_{B} v_B B$$

Since enthalpy is a state function, at constant pressure the heat of reaction $\Delta_r H$ is

$$\Delta_r H = H_2 - H_1$$

where H_2 is the heat content (enthalpy) of the products and H_1 being that of the reactants. Differentiating this equation with respect to temperature at constant pressure, we get

$$\left(\frac{\partial \Delta_r H}{\partial T} \right)_p = \left(\frac{\partial H_2}{\partial T} \right)_p - \left(\frac{\partial H_1}{\partial T} \right)_p$$

But we have already seen that

$$\left(\frac{\partial H}{\partial T} \right)_p = C_p$$

$$\therefore \left(\frac{\partial \Delta_r H}{\partial T} \right)_p = (C_p)_2 - (C_p)_1 = \Delta C_p$$

where $(C_p)_2$ and $(C_p)_1$ are the heat capacities of products and reactants respectively.

Change in heat of reaction at constant pressure per degree change of temperature is equal to difference in heat capacities of products and reactants at constant pressure.

$$\Delta C_p = (\sum C_p(B))_{products} - (\sum C_p(B))_{reactants} = \sum_B v_B C_{p,m}(B)$$

Or

$$\Delta C_p = [g C_{p,m}^{\ominus}(G) + h C_{p,m}^{\ominus}(H)] - [a C_{p,m}^{\ominus}(A) + d C_{p,m}^{\ominus}(D)]$$

Integrating the equation between temperature T_1 and T_2, we have

$$\int_{\Delta H(T_1)}^{\Delta H(T_2)} d(\Delta_r H) = \Delta_r H(T_2) - \Delta_r H(T_1) = \int_{T_1}^{T_2} \Delta C_p dT$$

where $\Delta_r H(T_1)$ and $\Delta_r H(T_2)$ are the reaction heat at constant pressure of T_1 and T_2 respectively.

Formula (1–54) and (1–55) were first derived by Kirchoff and are called Kirchoff's equations. These equations may be used for calculating heat of reaction at a given temperature when it is known at some other temperature and when the heat capacities of products and reactants are known.

If the heat capacity is independent of temperature:

$$\Delta_r H(T_2) = \Delta_r H(T_1) + \Delta C_p(T_2 - T_1) \quad \text{(if } C_p \text{ is independent of } T) \tag{1-59}$$

If the heat capacity is dependent of temperature:

$$C_{p,m} = a + bT + cT^2$$

So

$$\Delta C_{p,m} = \Delta a + \Delta bT + \Delta cT^2$$

where

$$\Delta a = \sum_B v_B a(B), \Delta b = \sum_B v_B b(B), \Delta c = \sum_B v_B c(B)$$

Integrating the equation between temperature T_1 and T_2, we have

$$\Delta_r H(T_2) = \Delta_r H(T_1) + \Delta a(T_2 - T_1) + \frac{1}{2}\Delta b(T_2^2 - T_1^2) + \frac{1}{3}\Delta c(T_2^3 - T_1^3) \qquad (1-60)$$

[Example 1–9] Given that:

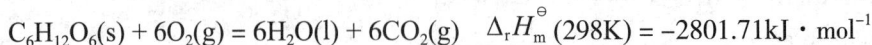

$$C_6H_{12}O_6(s) + 6O_2(g) = 6H_2O(l) + 6CO_2(g) \quad \Delta_r H_m^{\ominus}(298K) = -2801.71 kJ\cdot mol^{-1}$$

At 298K, $C_{p,m}$ of $O_2(g), CO_2(g), H_2O(l)$ and $C_6H_{12}O_6(s)$ are 29.36, 37.13, 75.30, and 218.9 kJ$\cdot$mol^{-1} respectively. If the heat capacity is independent of temperature between 298K to 310K, Calculate $\Delta_r H_m^{\ominus}$ (310K) for the reaction at 310K.

Solution:

$$\Delta C_p = \sum_B \nu_B C_{p,m}(B)$$
$$= 6 \times 75.30 + 6 \times 37.13 - 218.9 - 6 \times 29.36 = 279.52 J\cdot mol^{-1}\cdot K^{-1}$$
$$\Delta_r H_m(310K) = \Delta_r H_m^{\ominus}(298K) + \Delta C_p(T_2 - T_1)$$
$$= -2801.71 + 279.52 \times (310-298) \times 10^{-3} = 2798.3 kJ\cdot mol^{-1}$$

[Example 1–10] Given that: at 298K,

$$N_2(g) + 3H_2(g) = 2NH_3(g)$$

$$\Delta_r H_m^{\ominus}(298K) = -92.22 kJ\cdot mol^{-1}$$

$$C_{p,m}(N_2) = 26.98 + 5.912 \times 10^{-3}T - 3.376 \times 10^{-7}T^2 \qquad (J\cdot K^{-1}\cdot mol^{-1})$$

$$C_{p,m}(H_2) = 29.07 - 0.837 \times 10^{-3}T + 20.12 \times 10^{-7}T^2 \qquad (J\cdot K^{-1}\cdot mol^{-1})$$

$$C_{p,m}(NH_3) = 25.89 + 33.00 \times 10^{-3}T - 30.46 \times 10^{-7}T^2 \qquad (J\cdot K^{-1}\cdot mol^{-1})$$

Calculate the heat of reaction at 398K, $\Delta_r H_m^{\ominus}(398K)$.

Solution:

$$\Delta a = (2 \times 25.89) - 26.98 - (3 \times 29.07) = -62.41$$
$$\Delta b = (2 \times 33.00 - 5.912 + 3 \times 0.837) \times 10^{-3} = 62.60 \times 10^{-3}$$
$$\Delta c = [-(2 \times 30.46) + 3.376 - 3 \times 20.12] \times 10^{-7} = -117.9 \times 10^{-7}$$
$$\Delta_r H_m^{\ominus}(398K) = -92.22 \times 10^3 + [-62.41 \times (398-298) + 31.30 \times 10^{-3}(398^2 - 298^2)$$
$$- 39.3 \times 10^{-7}(398^3 - 298^3)]$$
$$= -92.22 \times 10^3 - 4.21 \times 10^3$$
$$= -96.43 kJ\cdot mol^{-1}$$

重点小结

　　热力学是研究热与其他形式能量相互转化所遵循规律的一门学科。本章主要介绍热力学的基本概念,热力学能与焓两个状态函数以及热与功的计算,盖斯定律的应用及生成热、燃烧热的概念与计算。其中热力学第一定律的数学表达式是本章的核心,掌握状态函数的特征是学好本章的关键。

Object detection

I. Select the correct option for the following problems (one option for each problem).

1. When the first law of thermodynamics is applied to chemical reactions, which problem is mainly solved?

    A. reaction direction   B. reaction limit   C. thermal effect

    D. reaction rate   E. chemical equilibrium

2. The first law of thermodynamics $\Delta U = Q + W$ only applies to

    A. simple state change   B. phase change   C. chemical change

    D. any change of isolated system   E. any change of closed system

3. For changes in isolated systems, what range are the values of ΔU and ΔH

    A. $\Delta U > 0, \Delta H > 0$ B. $\Delta U = 0, \Delta H = 0$

    C. $\Delta U < 0, \Delta H < 0$ D. $\Delta U = 0, \Delta H$ cannot be determined

    E. neither ΔU nor ΔH can be determined

4. Under the condition of constant volume, for a certain amount of ideal gas, when the temperature rises, the thermodynamic energy will

    A. decrease   B. increase   C. not change

    D. not be determined   E. be related to the ideal gas type

5. For the following four gases with 1mol of substance, if they are heated from T_1 to T_2 under constant volume, which gas absorbs the most heat?

    A. helium   B. hydrogen   C. oxygen

    D. sulfur dioxide   E. chlorine

6. When the ideal gas expands adiabatically against a constant external pressure, then

    A. $\Delta U < 0$ B. $\Delta U = 0$ C. $\Delta H > 0$

    D. $\Delta H = 0$ E. unable to determine

7. Hess's law contains two important problems, namely

    A. the first law of thermodynamics and the third law of thermodynamics

    B. the first law of thermodynamics and the basic properties of heat

    C. the third law of thermodynamics and the basic properties of heat

    D. the first law of thermodynamics and the basic characteristics of state function

    E. direction and limit of chemical reaction

8. The standard molar reaction enthalpy of known reaction $H_2(g) + 1/2 O_2(g) = H_2O(g)$ is $\Delta_r H_m^\ominus(T)$, and the incorrect answer is

    A. $\Delta_r H_m^\ominus(T)$ is the standard molar enthalpy of formation of $H_2O(g)$

    B. $\Delta_r H_m^\ominus(T)$ is the standard molar enthalpy of combustion of $H_2(g)$

    C. $\Delta_r H_m^\ominus(T)$ is negative

    D. the values of $\Delta_r H_m^\ominus(T)$ and $\Delta_r H_m^\ominus(T)$ are not equal

    E. $\Delta_r H_m^\ominus(T)$ isn't the standard molar enthalpy of combustion of $H_2(g)$

9. Heat of combustion of graphite

    A. equal to the heat of formation of CO

    B. equal to the heat of formation of CO_2

    C. equal to the heat of combustion of diamond

    D. equal to zero

    E. positive

10. Which of the following relationships does not require the assumption of an ideal gas?

    A. $C_p - C_V = nR$

    B. $\mathrm{d}\ln p/\mathrm{d}T = \Delta H/RT^2$

    C. $\Delta H = \Delta U + p\Delta V$ (constant pressure process)

    D. adiabatic reversible process, $pV^\gamma = $ constant

    E. $W = -nRT\ln\dfrac{v_2}{v_1}$

II. Select the correct options for the following problem (at least two options for each problem).

1. Which of the following properties belongs to extensive properties?

A. Density	B. U	C. H_m
D. C_p	E. $C_{p,m}$	F. p
G. molar mass	H. T	

2. Which of the following physical quantities are state functions?

A. U_m	B. H	C. Q
D. ΔU	E. W	

III. Try to answer the following problem.

Someone said: the higher the temperature of the system, the greater the heat. Is that right?

Reference answers

I . 1. C；2. E；3. D；4. B；5. D；6. A；7. D；8. B；9. B；10. C.

II. 1. BD；2. AB.

III. It isn't right, because temperature is a function of state and heat is a function of path.

Chapter 2 The Second Law of Thermodynamics and Chemical Equilibrium

知识要求

1. 掌握

(1) 熵的定义。

(2) 亥姆霍兹能和吉布斯自由能的定义。

(3) 克劳修斯不等式。

(4) 简单状态变化、相变和化学变化的 ΔS、ΔF、ΔG 计算。

2. 熟悉

(1) 自发变化的定义。

(2) 熵变和熵的物理意义。

(3) 热力学基本关系式和其应用范围。

(4) 化学势及其应用。

(5) 稀溶液的依数性。

(6) 化学平衡常数、化学反应等温方程式。

3. 了解

(1) 自发过程的特征。

(2) 热机效率。

(3) 卡诺定理和其与热力学之间的关系。

能力要求

1. 能够通过设计可逆过程计算不可逆过程的 ΔS、ΔG。

2. 更够利用熵判据、亥姆霍兹自由能判据和吉布斯自由能判据判断热力学过程的方向。

Section 1   The Second Law of Thermodynamics

1.1   Common characteristics of the spontaneous process——irreversibility

<u>**Spontaneous process**(自发过程)</u> is a process that happens naturally with no extra work to bring it about. e.g. a gas expands to fill the available volume, a hot body cools to the temperature of its surroundings, an object in the high place automatically falls on the ground, and a chemical reaction runs in one direction rather than another. The contrary process is referred to as non-spontaneous process. For instance, a gas is confined to a smaller volume, an object is cooled by using a refrigerator, and some reactions are driven in reverse (as in the electrolysis of water). However, none of these processes is spontaneous: each one must be brought about by doing work.

The common feature of spontaneous process is irreversibility. The so-called "irreversibility" is not that it cannot be reversed, but that if, with the help of external forces, the system is completely restored to its initial state when it is reversed, the environment, however, cannot be restored, and there must be traces that cannot be eliminated in the environment. For example, heat can be automatically transferred from high-temperature object to low-temperature one. On the other hand, if the heat is transferred from the low-temperature object to the high-temperature one, it cannot be released automatically. External work must be done by surroundings like a refrigerator or an air conditioner. The surroundings do the electric work, and cannot be restored.

Another example is the expansion of gas to vacuum, a spontaneous process, in which $Q = 0$, $W = 0$, $\Delta U = 0$ and $\Delta T = 0$. The expanded gas is to be restored to its original state with an isothermal reversible compression process. However, during the compression process, the environment must work on the gas (e.g. 100kJ), and at the same time, the environment obtains the heat that releases from the gas (100kJ, according to the first law). That is, when the system is restored to its original state, the environment loses work, and gets equivalent heat. We know the positive of reaction $Cd(s) + PbCl_2(aq) \rightarrow CdCl_2(s) + Pb(s)$ is a spontaneous process with reaction heat ($|Q|$) releasing to the surroundings. In order to restore the system to its original state, it is necessary to electrolyze the system. During electrolysis, the electric work ($|W|$) is done and the heat $|Q'|$ is released. When the system is restored to its original state, the environmental cannot restored because work ($|W|$) is lost, and obtains the heat ($|Q| + |Q'|$, the value of which equals to $|W|$ according to the energy conservation obtained. Similarly, if the environment is restored to its original state, it depends on whether the heat $|Q| + |Q'|$ obtained in the environment can be transformed into work $|W|$ unconditionally. The same as the upper example, it is impossible.

Numerous experiments show that when the spontaneous process returns to its original state, the environment have to pay the price without exception. That is, the environment cannot be completely restored. Because the transformation of heat and work also has direction: work can be spontaneously all transformed into heat, while heat cannot spontaneously all transformed into work.

1.2　Empirical description of the second law of thermodynamics

The recognition of two classes of process, spontaneous and non-spontaneous, is summarized by the second law of thermodynamics. This law may be expressed in a variety of equivalent ways. One statement was formulated by Clausius (Clausius R.): it is impossible to transfer heat from a cold to a hot reservoir without at the same time converting a certain amount of work to heat. Another statement was formulated by Kelvin (Kelvin L.): It is impossible by a cyclic process to take heat from a reservoir and convert it into work without at the same time transferring heat from a hot to a cold reservoir. In other words, it is impossible for a system to undergo a cyclic process that turns heat completely into work done on the surroundings. The heat engine that takes heat from a single source and converts it completely into work is called the second type of perpetual motion machine, which does not contrary to the first law of thermodynamics. Consequently, statement of Kelvin can be simplified as "The second type of perpetual motion machine can never be manufactured".

Although the forms of the above two statements are different, the rules expounded are consistent. If the heat energy is automatically transferred from the cold reservoir to the hot reservoir, the heat taken from the hot reservoir is transmitted to the cold reservoir and do work at the same time. Then the heat obtained from the cold reservoir can be automatically transmitted to the hot reservoir again, resulting in the recovery of the cold reservoir. As a result, the heat from the single hot reservoir completely convert to work without any other change, so that the second type of perpetual motion machine can be designed, with which heat can be transformed into work continuously from the huge heat source such as the sea, air or the earth. In practice, it has proved that the second type of perpetual motion machine never be manufactured.

In principle, the second law of thermodynamics can be directly applied to determine the direction of a process, but in fact it is very difficult to apply it. Can we find some thermodynamic functions, with which we can judge the direction and limit of the process conveniently, like the change of internal energy and enthalpy in the first law of thermodynamics? Therefore, using the analysis of the thermal work transformation relationship in the Carnot cycle, Clausius solved the problem of transformation efficiency of heat into work, found the most basic state function, entropy, in the second law of thermodynamics, and finally obtained the entropy criterion with which the direction and limit of the process can be judged quantitatively.

Section 2　Carnot Cycle and Carnot Theorem

2.1　Carnot Engine（卡诺热机）

In the early 19th century, the steam engine was invented and applied to industry and transportation. In view of the low efficiency of steam engine converting heat into work, many people raced to study how to improve the efficiency of heat engine. In 1824, a 28-year-old french young engineer Carnot wrote in a

PPT

微课

医药大学堂
WWW.YIYAODXT.COM

paper entitled "Reflections on the Motive Power of Fire" that the heat engine, ideally, cannot convert all the heat absorbed from the high-temperature heat source into work, and the efficiency of the heat engine cannot be improved indefinitely, but there is a limit.

The Carnot heat engine is an imaginary model machine that Carnot devised in 1824 to represent a steam engine. A simple steam engine is depicted schematically in Fig. 2–1a. It has a cylinder with a piston connected to a crankshaft by a connecting rod. There is an intake valve through which a boiler can inject high-pressure steam into the cylinder and an exhaust valve through which spent steam can be exhausted into the atmosphere. This steam engine operates with a two-stroke cycle. The cycle begins with the piston at top dead center (the position of minimum volume in the cylinder) and with the intake valve open. High-pressure steam from the boiler enters the cylinder through the intake valve and pushes on the piston, which turns the crankshaft. When the piston reaches bottom dead center (the position of maximum volume in the cylinder) the intake valve closes and the exhaust valve opens. The inertia of the crankshaft and flywheel pushes the piston back toward top dead center, expelling the spent steam through the exhaust valve. The exhaust valve closes and the intake valve opens when top dead center is reached, and the engine is ready to repeat its cycle.

The Carnot engine is depicted in Fig. 2–1b. It operates reversibly, so there can be no friction. The cylinder contains a gaseous "working fluid" which we define to be the system. The Carnot engine has no valves and the system is closed. To simulate passing steam into and out of the cylinder the Carnot engine allows heat to flow from a "hot reservoir" into its working fluid and exhausts heat into a "cold reservoir" by conduction through the cylinder walls or cylinder head. Assume that the working fluid of a Carnot engine is an ideal gas with a constant heat capacity.

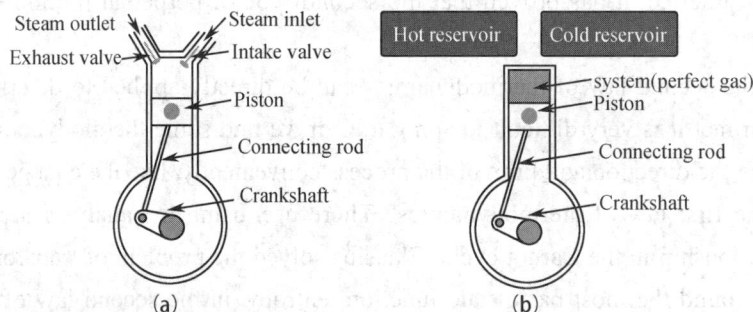

Fig. 2–1   The theories of steam engine(a) and Carnot engine(b)

The Carnot engine operates on a two-stroke cycle that is called the **Carnot cycle(卡诺循环)**. We begin the cycle with the piston at top dead center and with the hot reservoir in contact with the cylinder. We break the expansion stroke into two steps. Fig. 2–2 shows the Carnot cycle using p and V as the state variables. The first step (A → B) is an isothermal reversible expansion of the system at the temperature of the hot reservoir. The final volume of the first step is chosen so that the second step (B → C), which is an adiabatic reversible expansion, ends with the system at the temperature of the cold reservoir and with the piston at bottom dead center. The compression stroke is also broken into two steps. The third step of the cyclic process (C → D) is a reversible isothermal compression with the cylinder in contact with the cold reservoir. This step ends at a volume such that the fourth step (D → A), a reversible adiabatic compression, ends with the piston at top dead center and the system at the temperature of the hot reservoir. The engine is now ready to repeat the cycle. Now let derive the heat and work of each steps respectively.

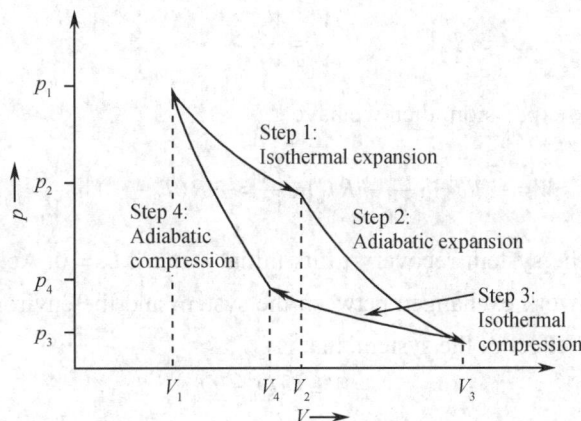

Fig. 2-2   Carnot cycle

(1) A $(p_1, V_1, T_h) \rightarrow$ B (p_2, V_2, T_h) Isothermal reversible expansion: The ideal gas in the cylinder of the Carnot engine is in contact with the hot reservoir (T_h). From the state A to the state B, the system (ideal gas) absorbs heat Q_h from the hot reservoir, and do work W_1 to the environment.

$$Q_h = -W_1 = \int_{V_1}^{V_2} p dV = nRT_h \ln \frac{V_2}{V_1}$$

(2) B $(p_2, V_2, T_h) \rightarrow$ C (p_3, V_3, T_c) Reversible adiabatic expansion: In this step, no heat change between system and environment. The system's temperature falls from T_h to T_c, and do work W_1 to the environment.

$$W_2 = \Delta U_2 = \int_{T_h}^{T_c} C_V dT$$

(3) C $(p_3, V_3, T_c) \rightarrow$ D (p_4, V_4, T_c) Isothermal reversible compression: The ideal gas in the cylinder of the Carnot engine is in contact with the cold reservoir (T_c). From the state C to the state D, the system (ideal gas) exhausts heat Q_c to the cold reservoir, and get work W_3 from the environment.

$$Q_c = -W_3 = \int_{V_3}^{V_4} p dV = nRT_c \ln \frac{V_4}{V_3}$$

(4) D $(p_4, V_4, T_c) \rightarrow$ A (p_1, V_1, T_h) Reversible adiabatic compression: In this step, no heat exchange between system and environment. The system's temperature rises from T_c to T_h, and get work W_4 from the environment.

$$W_4 = \Delta U_4 = \int_{T_c}^{T_h} C_V dT$$

For the entire cycle, the total work is

$$W = W_1 + W_2 + W_3 + W_4 = -nRT_h \ln \frac{V_2}{V_1} + \int_{T_h}^{T_c} C_V dT - nRT_c \ln \frac{V_4}{V_3} + \int_{T_c}^{T_h} C_V dT$$

$$= -nRT_h \ln \frac{V_2}{V_1} - nRT_c \ln \frac{V_4}{V_3}$$

Since the step 2 and step 4 are both adiabatic, according to the equation (1-44)

$$T_h V_2^{\gamma-1} = T_c V_3^{\gamma-1}$$
$$T_c V_4^{\gamma-1} = T_h V_1^{\gamma-1}$$

So
$$\frac{V_2}{V_1} = \frac{V_3}{V_4}$$

Replace the total work expression, then we have

$$W = -nRT_h \ln\frac{V_2}{V_1} - nRT_c \ln\frac{V_4}{V_3} = -nR(T_h - T_c)\ln\frac{V_2}{V_1}$$

In the Carnot cycle, the system recovery to its initial state, $\Delta U = 0$. According to the first law of thermodynamics, the total work exchanged between the system and the environment in the Carnot cycle is equal to the total thermal effect of the system, that is

$$W = -(Q_h + Q_c)$$

For any heat engine, its efficiency η(eta), is expressed by the ratio of work and heat absorbing from the hot reservoir

$$\eta = \frac{-W}{Q_h} = \frac{Q_h + Q_c}{Q_h} \tag{2-1}$$

Note: On account of $W<0$, to ensure η is positive, $-W$ is used.

For Carnot engine, its efficiency is

$$\eta = \frac{-W}{Q_h} = \frac{Q_h + Q_c}{Q_h} = \frac{-nR(T_h - T_c)\ln\dfrac{V_2}{V_1}}{nRT_h \ln\dfrac{V_2}{V_1}} = \frac{T_h - T_c}{T_h} = 1 - \frac{T_c}{T_h} \tag{2-2}$$

Now we see the efficiency of Carnot engine is related to the temperatures of two reservoirs. The greater the temperature difference between the two reservoirs, the greater the efficiency of the heat engine. Since T cannot be 0K, the efficiency is always smaller than 1. The formula (2–2) points a clear way improving the efficiency of the heat engine.

2.2　Carnot's theorem（卡诺定理）

On the basis of the fact that Carnot's engine is a reversible one, Carnot advanced famous **Carnot's theorem**: ① An engine working in a reversible cycle is at least as efficient as any other engine working between the same limits of temperature; ② the efficiency of such an engine being a function of the two limiting temperatures and not dependent on the mechanical design or the working substance of the engine.

Firstly, we are ready to generalize conclusion ①. Suppose there are two heat engine A and B work in between a hot reservoir and a cold sink, A is an arbitrary (maybe reversible or irreversible), and B is reversible. Both of them can absorb heat from the hot reservoir and do work, accompany with releasing heat to the cold sink. Now adjust the two heat engines to do the same work, but heats absorbed and released are permitted be different, as shown in Fig. 2–3(a). We know

$$\eta_A = \frac{-W}{Q_h}$$

$$\eta_B = \frac{-W}{Q_h'}$$

Since heat engine B is reversible, now we let the two engineers operate jointly, and reverse heat engine B, which becomes a refrigerator. The work needed is just supplied from heat engine A, as shown in Fig. 2–3(b).

Here, suppose $\eta_A > \eta_B$, that is $\dfrac{-W}{Q_h} > \dfrac{-W}{Q'_h}$, then $Q'_h > Q_h$. When the cycle finished, heat engine A and B recover their initial state, while cold sink lost heat $Q_h - Q'_h$ and hot reservoir gains heat $Q_h - Q'_h$. It means that without external interference, if the two engines are operated together, the heat $Q_h - Q'_h$ can be transferred from the cold sink to the high-temperature heat source without any other change, indicating that the combined heat engine is a second type of perpetual motion machine. Because the conclusion is contrary to experience, the initial assumption is wrong and $\eta_A \leqslant \eta_B$.

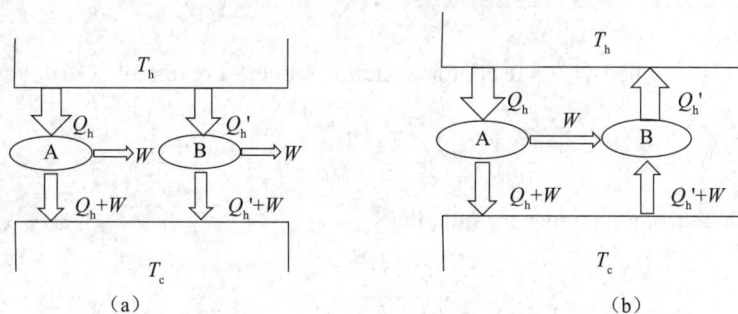

Fig. 2–3   The proving of the first conclusion of Carnot's theorem

Now we are ready to generalize conclusion ②. Suppose two reversible engines are coupled together and run between the same two reservoirs (Fig. 2–4). The working substances and details of construction of the two engines are entirely arbitrary. Initially, suppose that engine A is more efficient than engine B, and that we choose a setting of the controls that causes engine B to acquire energy as heat Q_c from the cold reservoir and to release a certain quantity of energy as heat into the hot reservoir. However, because engine A is more efficient than engine B, not all the work that A produces is needed for this process, and the difference can be used to do work. The net result is that the cold reservoir is unchanged,

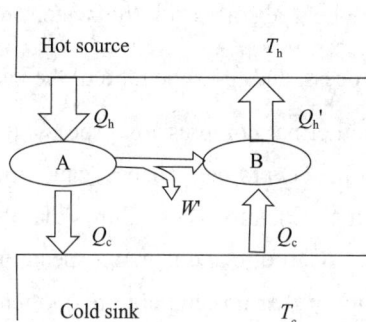

Fig. 2–4   The proving of the second conclusion of Carnot's theorem

work has been done, and the hot reservoir has lost a certain amount of energy. This outcome is contrary to the Kelvin statement of the second law, because some heat has been converted directly into work. Because the conclusion is contrary to experience, the initial assumption that engines A and B can have different efficiencies must be false. It follows that the relation between the heat transfers and the temperatures must alike be independent of the working material, and therefore that equation (2–2) is always true for any substance involved in a Carnot cycle.

Based on Carnot theorem, $\eta_A \leqslant \eta_B$, it follows

$$\frac{T_h - T_c}{T_h} \geqslant \frac{Q_h + Q_c}{Q_h} \tag{2-3}$$

In the formula, ">" is used for the irreversible heat engine, "=" is used for the reversible heat engine. The Carnot theorem distinguishes the reversible cycle process from the irreversible cycle process quantitatively, which lays the foundation for the discovery of another new state function, entropy.

Section 3　Concept of Entropy——Entropy and Entropy Increase Principle

3.1　Heat-temperature quotient of reversible cyclic processes and reversible processes——entropy function(熵函数)

From equation (2–3), when "=" is used, the system conducts a reversible Carnot cycle, then

$$\frac{T_h-T_c}{T_h}=\frac{Q_h+Q_c}{Q_h}$$

It is easy to deduce from the upper formula that

$$\frac{Q_c}{T_c}+\frac{Q_h}{T_h}=0 \tag{2-4}$$

The formula $\frac{Q}{T}$ is called the **heat-temperature quotient(热温商)** of the process. $\frac{Q_h}{T_h}$ is the ratio of the heat absorbed by the system to the heat source temperature in the reversible isothermal expansion process, and $\frac{Q_c}{T_c}$ is the ratio of the heat released by the system to the heat source temperature in the reversible isothermal compression process. it should be noted that the T is the temperature of heat source, and only in the reversible process, can it be regarded as the temperature of the system, in which case they are equal. Equation (2–4) shows that the sum of heat-temperature quotient in a Carnot cycle is zero.

Carnot cycle is just a special reversible process, what about the other any reversible process? Is the sum of thermo-temperature quotient also zero? We can prove it is true indeed as follows.

Any reversible cycle can be approximated as a collection of Carnot cycles (Fig. 2–4). The dashed part of the figure is canceled as a result of doing equal work in the adjacent Carnot cycle. The integral around an arbitrary path is the sum of the integrals around each of the Carnot cycles. This approximation becomes exact as the individual cycles are allowed to become infinitesimal. For each small Carnot cycle, the sum of hermo-temperature quotient in a Carnot cycle is zero, then

$$\frac{(\delta Q_{h1})_R}{T_{h1}}+\frac{(\delta Q_{c2})_R}{T_{c2}}=0,\ \ \frac{(\delta Q_{h3})_R}{T_{h3}}+\frac{(\delta Q_{c4})_R}{T_{c4}}=0\cdots$$

The sum of the upper equations is

$$\frac{(\delta Q_{h1})_R}{T_{h1}}+\frac{(\delta Q_{c1})_R}{T_{c1}}+\frac{(\delta Q_{h2})_R}{T_{h2}}+\frac{(\delta Q_{c2})_R}{T_{c2}}+\cdots+\frac{(\delta Q_{hi})_R}{T_{hi}}+\frac{(\delta Q_{ci})_R}{T_{ci}}=0$$

Or

$$\sum\frac{(\delta Q_i)_R}{T_i}=0$$

In the limit of infinitesimal cycles, the non-cancelling edges of the Carnot cycles match the overall cycle exactly, and the sum becomes an integral, so

$$\oint \frac{(\delta Q)_R}{T} = 0 \tag{2-5}$$

If the arbitrary reversible cycle process A → B → A is considered be composed of two reversible processes (I) and (II), equation (2-5) can be regarded as the sum of the two integrals (Fig. 2-5), that is

$$\int_A^B \left(\frac{\delta Q_R}{T}\right)_I + \int_B^A \left(\frac{\delta Q_R}{T}\right)_{II} = 0$$

Or

$$\int_A^B \left(\frac{\delta Q_R}{T}\right)_I = \int_A^B \left(\frac{\delta Q_R}{T}\right)_{II}$$

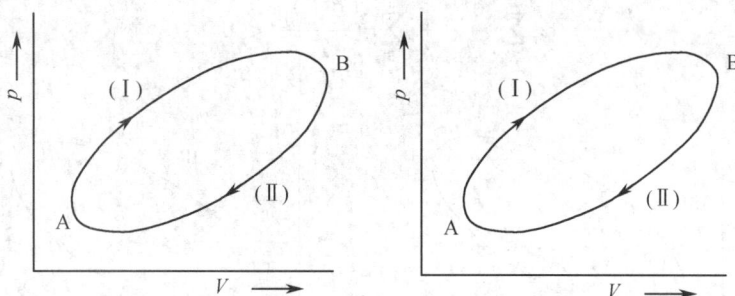

Fig. 2-5   The arbitrary reversible cycle process

This expression indicates from A to B, that the integral of the path (I) is equal to that of the path (II). It is seen that the integral value depends only on the states of the system, but is independent of the path, which suggests that the integral value reflects the change of a certain state property of the system and is related to that property closely. Accordingly, Clausius defines a new thermodynamic function, entropy, which is represented by S.

When the state of the system changes from A to B, the entropy change is

$$\Delta S_{A \to B} = \int_A^B \frac{\delta Q_R}{T} \tag{2-6}$$

For a infinitesimal change, the entropy change is

$$dS = \frac{\delta Q_R}{T} \tag{2-7}$$

Entropy is a state function, which has the characteristics of extensive property, and the units of it is joule per kelvin ($J \cdot K^{-1}$).

3.2   Heat-temperature quotient of irreversible cyclic processes and irreversible processes

From equation (2-3), when ">" is used, the system conducts an irreversible cycle, then

$$\frac{T_{\mathrm{h}}-T_{\mathrm{c}}}{T_{\mathrm{h}}}>\frac{Q_{\mathrm{h}}+Q_{\mathrm{c}}}{Q_{\mathrm{h}}}$$

Corresponding inequality can be easily conducted

$$\frac{Q_{\mathrm{c}}}{T_{\mathrm{c}}}+\frac{Q_{\mathrm{h}}}{T_{\mathrm{h}}}<0 \tag{2-8}$$

So for any irreversible cycle, there must be

$$\sum \frac{\delta Q_i}{T_i}=0 \tag{2-9}$$

Equation (2–9) shows that the sum of thermo-temperature quotient in any irreversible cycle is smaller than zero.

Suppose the system reaches state B from state A through an irreversible process (IR) and returns to state A through a reversible process (R). Obviously, the whole cycle is an irreversible cycle (Fig. 2–6), so

$$\sum_{\mathrm{A}}^{\mathrm{B}}\frac{\delta Q_i}{T_i}+\sum_{\mathrm{B}}^{\mathrm{A}}\frac{(\delta Q_i)_{\mathrm{R}}}{T_i}<0$$

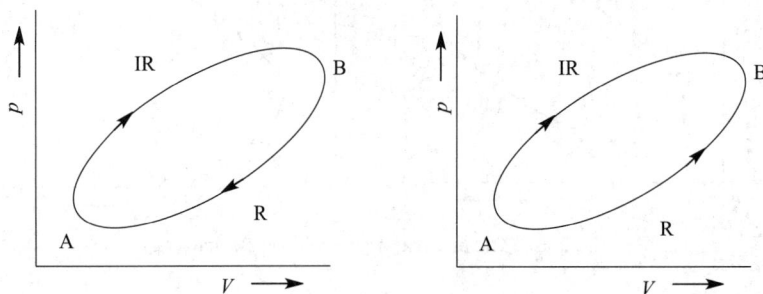

Fig. 2–6 The reversible process

For a reversible process, we've known

$$\sum_{\mathrm{B}}^{\mathrm{A}}\frac{(\delta Q_i)_{\mathrm{R}}}{T_i}=S_{\mathrm{A}}-S_{\mathrm{B}}$$

Then

$$\Delta S_{\mathrm{A}\rightarrow\mathrm{B}}=S_{\mathrm{B}}-S_{\mathrm{A}}>\sum_{\mathrm{A}}^{\mathrm{B}}\frac{\delta Q_i}{T_i} \tag{2-10}$$

Inequality (2–10) shows that the sum of thermo-temperature quotient in any irreversible process(IR) is smaller than the entropy change of the system (Fig. 2–6).

Combine equation (2–6) with inequality (2–10) to get

$$\Delta S_{\mathrm{A}\rightarrow\mathrm{B}}=S_{\mathrm{B}}-S_{\mathrm{A}}>\sum_{\mathrm{A}}^{\mathrm{B}}\frac{\delta Q_i}{T_i} \tag{2-11}$$

or

$$\mathrm{d}S\geqslant\frac{\delta Q}{T} \tag{2-12}$$

Inequality (2–12) shows that between the same inital state and the same final state, if a reversible process is performed, the sum of its heat-temperature quotient is equal to the entropy change of the system; if an irreversible process is performed, the sum of its heat-temperature quotient is less than the entropy change of the system.

Inequality (2–12) is called the **Clausius inequality(克劳修斯不等式)**, which is also the mathematical expression of the second law of thermodynamics. dS is the entropy change of the system, δQ is the heat exchanged in the process, T is the temperature of the heat source, and $\dfrac{\delta Q}{T}$ is the heat-temperature quotient of the process. The equality sign is used for reversible processes and the unequal sign is used for irreversible processes. By comparing dS with $\dfrac{\delta Q}{T}$ of the process, we can judge whether the process is reversible. Moreover, the Clausius inequality, as a criterion of reversibility, is a measure of the degree of irreversibility. If the heat-temperature quotient of the process is much smaller than the entropy changes of the system, the degree of irreversibility of the process is the greater.

3.3   The principle of entropy increase（熵增原理）

For any process occurring in an adiabatic system, $\delta Q_i = 0$, so

$$\Delta S_{adi} \geqslant 0 \tag{2–13}$$

Therefore, an important conclusion can be drawn: if a reversible process occurs in an adiabatic system, the entropy of the system will remain constant; if an irreversible process occurs, the entropy of the system will inevitably increase. That is, the entropy of the adiabatic system will never decrease, which is the famous principle of increase of entropy.

3.4   Entropy criterion（熵判据）

For an isolated system, because neither heat nor work exchanges between the system and the environment, that is to say, the system does not interact with the environment, and the driving force of the process is from the system itself. Any irreversible process occurring in the isolated system must be spontaneous process. Likewise, the entropy of the isolated system will never decrease. when the entropy value does not increase again, the system is in equilibrium state. That is

$$\Delta S_{iso} \geqslant 0 \tag{2–14}$$

There is no perfect isolated system due to the unavoidable relationships between the system and the surrounding. Generally, we consider the combination of the system and its closet surroundings as isolated system. On the basis of the addictivity of entropy, there is

$$\Delta S_{iso} = \Delta S_{sys} + \Delta S_{sur} \geqslant 0 \tag{2–15}$$

It can be seen that the direction of the spontaneous process in the isolated system is always in the direction of increasing the entropy value until the system entropy value reaches the maximum. That is, the limit of the process in the isolated system is that its entropy value reaches the maximum. This is the extension of the principle of entropy increase in isolated systems. Inequality (2–14) is called **entropy criterion**. It is often used to judge the direction and limits of the process, and also, it is another form of the second law of thermodynamics.

Section 4   Essence of the Second Law: Statistical Significance of Entropy

In section 3, we've known that entropy is a state function, whose change value is only related to the states of the system, but independent of the path of change, and that the value of entropy change is fixed value, which is measured by the thermal temperature quotient measure of the reversible process, however, we never know what is entropy. In this section, we will introduce the statistical view of entropy.

4.1   Entropy and thermodynamic probability——Boltzmann formula

Since molecules can occupy various states without changing the macroscopic state of the system of which they are a part, it is apparent that many microstates of a macroscopic system correspond to one macroscopic state. We denote the number of microstates corresponding to a given macrostate by Ω. The quantity Ω is sometimes called the thermodynamic probability of the macrostate. The thermodynamic probability is a measure of lack of information about the microstate of the system for a particular macrostate. A large value corresponds to a small amount of information, and a value of unity corresponds to knowledge that the system is in a specific microstate. For instance, four different molecules (A, B, C, D) is placed in closed containers which is divided into two equal parts with a separator. When the two containers are connected, the microstate, thermodynamic probability and mathematical odds are shown in Table 2–1.

Table 2–1   The microstate, thermodynamic probability of molecules in an equal container

Distribution mode	Microstate		Thermodynamic probability / Ω	Mathematical odds
	Left	Right		
4,0	ABCD	/	1	1/16
3,1	ABC	D	4	4/16
	ABD	C		
	ACD	B		
	BCD	A		
2,2	AB	CD	6	6/16
	AC	BD		
	AD	BC		
	BC	AD		
	BD	AC		
	CD	AB		
1,3	A	BCD	4	4/16
	B	ACD		
	C	ACD		
	D	ABC		
0,4	/	ABCD	1	1/16

In the same closed containers, if a perfect gas is put in the left, and the right is vacuum. When the separator is removed, the gas fills the container spontaneously. In the final state, the mathematical odds that all molecules are concentrated on one side are almost zero, while the mathematical odds that all molecules are distributed throughout the whole system are greatest, at the same time, the thermodynamic probability is also greatest. Consequently, the more Thermodynamic probability corresponding to microstates, the greater the likelihood that microstate will appear, which is precisely the view of statistical mechanics that the equilibrium state is the most evenly distributed.

Generally, in an isolated system, the spontaneous process is always changed from a state with low thermodynamic probability to a state with high thermodynamic probability. Thermodynamic probability Ω of the system has the same change direction as entropy of the system. Then there must be a kind of function relation between S and Ω of the system, that is $S=f(\Omega)$.

Assumed that a system is composed with two different parts A and B, the thermodynamic probabilities of them are Ω_A and Ω_B, the corresponding entropies are $S_A=f(\Omega_A)$ and $S_B=f(\Omega_B)$. For the whole system, the according to the probability theorem, the total probability is equal to the product of the probability of each part, that is $\Omega=\Omega_A \cdot \Omega_B$, so

$$S = S_A + S_B = f(\Omega_A) + f(\Omega_B) = f(\Omega_A\Omega_B)$$

Only the logarithmic function is in accordance with the upper function, that is only the logarithmic function, that is, the relationship of S and Ω can be wrote

$$S = k_B\ln\Omega = (\text{definition of statistical entropy}) \tag{2-16}$$

where k_B is Boltzmann's constant, equal to R/N_{Av}, the value is $1.38 \times 10^{-23}\text{J} \cdot \text{K}^{-1}$.

To sum up, from the microcosmic point of view, entropy is a statistical property, which is a measure of the number of microstates of a system which composed with a large number of particles. The smaller the entropy of the system is, the lower of the number of micro-states in the state, and the lower of the degree of disorder. The bigger the entropy of the system is, the higher of the number of micro-states in the state, and the higher of the degree of disorder. The direction of the spontaneous process in an isolated system is from a state with a small entropy (small degree of confusion) to a state with a large entropy (large degree of disorder), until to the state with the largest entropy.

4.2   Essence of the second law of thermodynamics

The second law of thermodynamics states that all spontaneous processes are irreversible and that all irreversible processes can be attributed to irreversibility of thermal and work (that is, it is impossible for a system to undergo a process that turns heat completely into work done on the surroundings). People always want to get more work, and hope that the heat can be completely turned into work, but failed time and again. Heat is a manifestation of the disorder motion of molecules, and the collision of molecules can only lead to the increase of the degree of disorder, while the work is related to the directed motion, which is an orderly motion, so the transformation of work into heat is the transformation of regular motion into irregular motion, and is also the dispersal of energy. The direction is to the increasing the degree of disorder. All irreversible processes proceed in the direction of increasing the degree of disorder, which is the essence of the irreversible process as recited in the second law of thermodynamics.

Section 5　Calculation of Entropy Change

The entropy changes on going from initial state to final state is given by equation (2–6) as

$$\Delta S_{sys} = \int_{ini}^{fin} \frac{\delta Q_R}{T}$$

(2–17)

where T is the absolute temperature. For a reversible process, we can apply equation (2–17) directly to calculate ΔS. For an irreversible process, we cannot integrate $\dfrac{\delta Q_{IR}}{T}$ to obtain ΔS because dS equal dQ/T only for reversible processes. However, S is a state function, and therefore S depends only on the initial and final states. We can therefore find ΔS for an irreversible process that goes from initial state to final state if we can conceive of a reversible process that goes from the initial state to final state. We then calculate ΔS for this reversible change from the initial state to final state with equation (2–17), and this is the same as ΔS for the irreversible change from the initial state to final state.

In summary, to calculate ΔS for any process, the following steps should be used: (a) Identify the initial and final states. (b) Devise a or some convenient reversible paths from the initial state and final state. (c) Calculate ΔS with equation (2–17).

Since entropy criterion can merely be used in isolated system, the environment and system are often combined to form an isolated system, so we need to calculate the entropy change of the environment. We can use the definition in equation (2–7) to formulate an expression for the change in entropy of the surroundings, ΔS_{sur}. Consider an infinitesimal transfer of heat the surroundings. The surroundings consist of a reservoir of constant volume, so the energy supplied to them by heating can be identified with the change in the internal energy of the surroundings, dU_{sur}. The internal energy is a state function, and dU_{sur} is an exact differential. As we have seen, these properties imply that dU_{sur} is independent of how the change is brought about and in particular is independent of whether the process is reversible or irreversible. The same remarks therefore apply to dU_{sur} to which dU_{sur} is equal. Therefore, we can adapt the definition in equation (2–7), delete the constraint "R", and write

$$dS_{sur} = \frac{\delta Q_{sur,R}}{T_{sur}} = \frac{\delta Q_{sur}}{T_{sur}}$$

Furthermore, because the temperature of the surroundings is constant whatever the change, and the Q_{sur} equals the negative of the heat releasing from the system, for a measurable change,

$$\Delta S_{sur} = \frac{Q_{sur}}{T_{sur}} = -\frac{Q_{sys}}{T_{sur}}$$

(2–18)

Let us calculate ΔS for some typical processes.

5.1　Entropy change in the process of simple state change

Here, we provide four processes including: ① isothermal process of perfect gas; ② heating process (under constant pressure and constant volume, respectively); ③ the process of ideal gas where p, V, T change simultaneously; ④ mixing of perfect gases.

5.1.1　Entropy change of isothermal process of perfect gas

In isothermal process of perfect gas, $\Delta U = 0$, $\Delta H = 0$, $Q_R = -W_R$

Then
$$\Delta S_{iso} = \frac{Q_R}{T} = \frac{-W_{max}}{T} = nR\ln\frac{V_2}{V_1} = nR\ln\frac{p_1}{p_2}$$

[Example 2-1] For 1.0mol ideal gas with a pressure of 101.325kPa and a temperature of 600K, after the following process: (Ⅰ) isothermal reversible expansion; (Ⅱ) expansion to vacuum, respectively, the state changes to 10.1325kPa. Calculate the entropy change of the two processes, and judge whether the process Ⅱ is reversible.

Solution: Process Ⅰ is an isothermal reversible expansion $Q_R = W_{max}$, so

$$\Delta S_{Ⅰ} = nR\ln\frac{p_1}{p_2} = 1.0\times8.314\times\ln\frac{101325}{10132.5} = 19.14\text{J}\cdot\text{K}^{-1}$$

Since the final state of process Ⅱ is the same as the one of process Ⅰ, so

$$\Delta S_{Ⅱ} = \Delta S_{Ⅰ} = 19.14\text{J}\cdot\text{K}^{-1}$$

And because $p_{su} = 0$, $Q = -W = 0$, then $\Delta S_{sur} = -\dfrac{Q_{sys}}{T_{sur}} = 0$

$$\Delta S_{iso} = \Delta S_{Ⅰ} + \Delta S_{sur} = 19.14\text{J}\cdot\text{K}^{-1} > 0$$

So, process Ⅱ is irreversible.

5.1.2　Entropy change of heating process

We shall be particularly interested in the entropy change when the system is subjected to constant pressure (such as from the atmosphere) during the heating (here, when heating, provided no phase change, chemical change and non-expansion work). Then, from the definition of constant-pressure heat capacity ($\delta Q_p = C_p dT$) and equation (2-7).

$$dS = \frac{C_p dT}{T} \tag{2-19a}$$

For a measurable heating process:

$$\Delta S = \int_{T_1}^{T_2} C_p \frac{dT}{T} \tag{2-19b}$$

The same expression applies at constant volume, but with replaced by C_V, and write:

$$\Delta S = \int_{T_1}^{T_2} C_V \frac{dT}{T} \tag{2-19c}$$

When C_p or C_V is independent of temperature in the temperature range of interest, it can be taken outside the integral and we obtain

$$\Delta S = C_p \ln\frac{T_2}{T_1} \tag{2-19d}$$

Or
$$\Delta S = C_V \ln\frac{T_2}{T_1} \tag{2-19e}$$

Note: The equation (2-19) can used for any heating process with no phase change, chemical change and non-expansion work, including any gas, solid and liquid.

[Example 2–2] Calculate the ΔS when 1mol $H_2O(l)$ is heated from 25℃ to 50℃ under a pressure of 100kPa. Given from 25℃ to 50℃, $\overline{C}_{p,m}(H_2O, l) = 73.4 J \cdot mol^{-1} \cdot K^{-1}$.

Solution:

$$\Delta S = \overline{C}_p \ln \frac{T_2}{T_1} = n\overline{C}_{p,m} \ln \frac{T_2}{T_1} = 1 \times 73.4 \times \ln \frac{323}{298} = 5.91 J \cdot K^{-1}$$

5.1.3 The process of ideal gas where p, V, T change simultaneously

For calculating the ΔS when 1mol perfect gas changes from inital state $A(p_1, V_1, T_1)$ to final statre $D(p_2, V_2, T_2)$, two different reversible paths can be designed, as shown in Fig. 2–7.

Path one: First go from the initial state A to the intermediate state C through an isothermal change, then to the final state D through a constant volume path.

Path two: First go from the initial state A to the intermediate state B through an isothermal change, then to the final state D through a constant pressure path.

Evidently, ΔS of the two paths are equal.

Furthermore, according to the first law of thermodynamics, when $\delta W'=0$, the heat of the reversible process of the ideal gas is

$$\delta Q_R = dU + pdV = nC_{V,m}dT + pdV$$

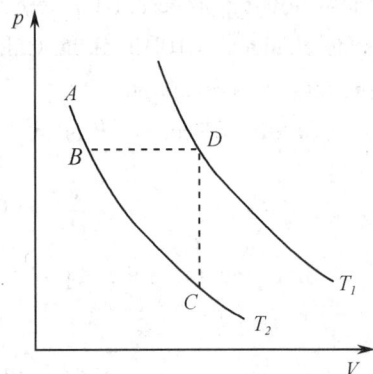

Fig. 2–7 Two different reversible paths from A to D

Substituting this equation into equation (2–7), then

$$dS = \frac{\delta Q_R}{T} = \frac{nC_{V,m}}{T}dT + \frac{nRdV}{V}$$

When $C_{V,m}$ is considered a constant, integration of the upper formula gives:

$$\Delta S = nC_{V,m}\ln \frac{T_2}{T_1} + nR\ln \frac{V_2}{V_1} \tag{2-20}$$

When the state equation of perfect gas $pV=nRT$ was substituted into equation (2–20), it becomes

$$\Delta S = nC_{p,m}\ln \frac{T_2}{T_1} - nR\ln \frac{p_2}{p_1} \tag{2-21}$$

$$\Delta S = nC_{V,m}\ln \frac{p_2}{p_1} + nC_{p,m}\ln \frac{V_2}{V_1} \tag{2-22}$$

Anyone of the equation (2–20, 2–21 and 2–22) can be used for the calculation of ΔS of the process of ideal gas where p, V, T change simultaneously with the same results.

[Example 2–3] Calculate the ΔS of the following process: 2mol He perfect gas heated from inital state with the temperature of 300K and pressure of 3.0×10^5Pa to final state with the temperature of 500K and pressure of 6.0×10^5Pa.

Solution:
$$\Delta S = nC_{p,m}\ln \frac{T_2}{T_1} - nR\ln \frac{p_2}{p_1}$$
$$= 2 \times 2.5 \times 8.314\ln \frac{500}{300} - 2 \times 8.314\ln \frac{6.0 \times 10^5}{3.0 \times 10^5}$$
$$= 9.7 J \cdot K^{-1}$$

5.1.4 The process of mixing of perfect gases

There is no force between molecules of ideal gas, and the existence of one gas does not affect the behavior of another gas. When the temperature and pressure of the surrounding are constant, the mixing process of ideal gas is irreversible, so a reversible process can be designed for the calculation of the entropy change of this process. Therefore, the mixture of two ideal gases with same temperature and pressure can be regarded as two adiabatic free expansion processes simultaneously. That is, n_A mol A expands from V_A to V_{A+B}, and n_B mol B expands from V_B to V_{A+B} adiabaticly. ΔS of the mixing process is the sum of the entropy changes of two adiabatic free expansions:

$$\Delta S = nR\ln\frac{V_A+V_B}{V_A} + nR\ln\frac{V_A+V_B}{V_B} = -nR\ln x_A - nR\ln x_B \tag{2-23}$$

[**Example 2–4**] At 298K, an adiabatic rigid container is divided into two parts with a separator. The left side of the partition is 1mol O_2 with the pressure of 200kPa, and the right side is 1mol N_2 with the pressure of 200kPa. After removing the separator, the two gases diffuse each other to the uniform state. Calculate the entropy change of the system in this mixing process, and judge whether the process is reversible. (O_2 and N_2 are considered perfect gases)

Solution:
$$\Delta S_{sys} = n_{O_2}R\ln\frac{V_{O_2}+V_{N_2}}{V_{O_2}} + n_{N_2}R\ln\frac{V_{O_2}+V_{N_2}}{V_{N_2}}$$

$$= -n_{O_2}R\ln x_{O_2} - n_{N_2}R\ln x_{N_2}$$
$$= -1\times8.314\times\ln0.5 - 1\times8.314\times\ln0.5$$
$$= 11.53\,\text{J}\cdot\text{K}^{-1}$$

There is no heat during the mixing process, so $\Delta S_{sur}=0$
$$\Delta S_{iso} = \Delta S_{sys} + \Delta S_{sur} = 11.53\,\text{J}\cdot\text{K}^{-1}$$

It suggests that the mixing process is spontaneous.

5.2 Entropy change of phase change

The phase transition process could be reversible or irreversible. The phase transition under the condition of phase equilibrium is reversible, such as gas-liquid transition at normal boiling point and solid-liquid transition at normal melting point. If the phase transition is not carried out under the condition of phase equilibrium, it is irreversible, such as the process of supercooled liquid condensation into solids at atmospheric pressure and below the melting point (freezing point), the process of liquid evaporation below the pressure of liquid saturated vapor and at a certain temperature; and the process of supersaturated vapor condensation into liquid at a certain temperature and above the pressure of liquid saturated vapor.

5.2.1 Calculation of Entropy Change in Reversible Phase transition

Reversible phase change carries out at constant temperature and constant pressure,
So $Q_R = Q_p = \Delta H_{trs}$, then

$$\Delta S = \frac{Q_R}{T} = \frac{Q_p}{T} = \frac{\Delta_{trs}H}{T_{trs}} \tag{2-24}$$

[**Example 2–5**] Calculate the entropy change when 1mol ice melts into water at normal melting point 0℃. The melting heat is 6.008kJ·mol^{-1}.

Solution:
$$\Delta S = \frac{\Delta_{trs}H}{T_{trs}} = \frac{6008}{273.15} = 21.99\,\text{J}\cdot\text{K}^{-1}$$

5.2.2 Calculation of Entropy Change in Irreversible Phase transition

To calculate the entropy change of an irreversible process, it is usually necessary to design a reversible pathway including the reversible phase change, the entropy change of which is also the entropy change of the irreversible phase change process.

[**Example 2–6**] 1mol $H_2O(l)$ Condensed into $H_2O(s)$ at standard pressure through the following two processes: (1) at normal freezing point 273.15K;(2)at 263.15K. Calculate the ΔS of the two process, and charge their reversibility. Given that the solidification heat of water is –6008J · mol^{-1} at 273.15K, and the average molar constant pressure heat capacity of water and ice is 75.3J · K^{-1} · mol^{-1} and 37.1J · K^{-1} · mol^{-1}, respectively.

Solution: Water condensation into ice at 263.15K and 101.325kPa is an abnormal phase transition, so it is an irreversible process. To calculate the entropy of the process, we need to design a reversible process as follows (Fig. 2–8).

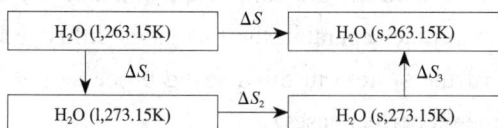

Fig. 2–8 Solution of entropy change in irreversible phase change process

$$\Delta S_1 = nC_{p,m}(l)\ln\frac{T_2}{T_1} = 1\times75.3\times\ln\frac{273.15}{263.15} = 2.81\text{J} \cdot \text{K}^{-1}$$

$$\Delta S_2 = \frac{\Delta_{trs}H}{T_2} = \frac{-6008}{273.15} = -22\text{J} \cdot \text{K}^{-1}$$

$$\Delta S_3 = nC_{p,m}(s)\ln\frac{T_1}{T_2} = 1\times37.1\times\ln\frac{263.15}{273.15} = -1.38\text{J} \cdot \text{K}^{-1}$$

$$\Delta S = \Delta S_1 + \Delta S_2 + \Delta S_3 = 2.81 - 21.99 - 1.38 = -20.56\text{J} \cdot \text{K}^{-1}$$

To judge whether the process is reversible, the entropy change of the environment should be calculated at the same time.

For constant pressure process, $Q_p = \Delta H$. Enthalpy is a state function, so

$$\Delta H = \Delta H_1 + \Delta H_2 + \Delta H_3$$
$$= \int_{263.15}^{273.15} nC_{p,m}(l)\,dT + \Delta_{trs}H + \int_{273.15}^{263.15} nC_{p,m}(s)\,dT$$
$$= 1\times75.3\times(273.15-263.15) - 1\times6008 + 1\times37.1\times(263.15-273.15)$$
$$= -5626\text{J}$$

$$\Delta S_{sur} = -\frac{Q_{sys}}{T_{sur}} = -\frac{\Delta_{trs}H}{T_{sur}} = \frac{5626}{263.15} = 21.38\text{J} \cdot \text{K}^{-1}$$

$$\Delta S_{iso} = \Delta S_{sys} + \Delta S_{sur} = -20.57 + 21.38 = 0.81\text{J} \cdot \text{K}^{-1} > 0$$

It shows that at conditions of 263.15K and 101325Pa, water becomes ice spontaneously.

5.3 Calculation of molar entropy

The entropy of a system at a temperature T is related to its entropy at $T=0$ by measuring its heat capacity C_p, at different temperatures and evaluating the integral in equation (2–19b), taking care to add the entropy of transition ($\Delta_{trs} H/T_{trs}$) for each phase transition between $T = 0$ and the temperature of interest. For example, if a substance melts at T_f and boils at T_b, then its molar entropy above its boiling temperature is given by

$$S_m(T) = S_m(0) + \int_0^{T_f} \frac{C_{p,m}(s,T)}{T} dT + \frac{\Delta_{fus}H}{T_f} + \int_{T_f}^{T_b} \frac{C_{p,m}(l,T)}{T} dT + \frac{\Delta_{vap}H}{T_b} + \int_{T_b}^{T} \frac{C_{p,m}(g,T)}{T} dT \quad (2\text{–}25)$$

All the properties required, except $S_m(0)$, can be measured calorimetrically, and the integrals can be evaluated either graphically or, as is now more usual, by fitting a polynomial to the data and integrating the polynomial analytically. The former procedure is illustrated in Fig. 2–9: the area under the curve of $C_{p,m}/T$ against T is the integral required.

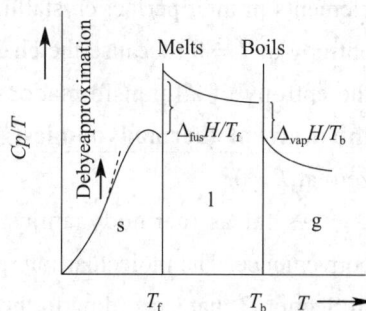

Fig. 2–9   Graphical integration method for determination of entropy

One problem with the determination of entropy is the difficulty of measuring heat capacities near $T=0$. There are good theoretical grounds for assuming that the heat capacity is proportional to T^3 when T is low, and this dependence is the basis of the Debye extrapolation. In this method, C_p is measured down to as low a temperature as possible, and a curve of the form aT^3 is fitted to the data. That fit determines the value of a, and the expression $C_{p,m} = aT^3$ is assumed valid down to $T = 0$.

For example, the standard molar entropy of nitrogen gas at 25°C has been calculated from the following data:

	$S_m^\ominus /(\text{J} \cdot \text{K}^{-1} \cdot \text{mol}^{-1})$
Debye extrapolation	1.92
Integration, from 10K to 35.61K	25.25
Phase transition at 35.61K	6.43
Integration, from 35.61K to 63.14K	23.38
Fusion at 63.14K	11.42
Integration, from 63.14K to 77.32K	11.41
Vaporization at 77.32K	72.13
Integration, from 77.32K to 298.15K	39.20
Correction for gas imperfection	0.92
Total	192.06

Therefore

$$S_m^\ominus(298.15K) = S_m(0) + 192.1 \text{J} \cdot \text{K}^{-1} \cdot \text{mol}^{-1}$$

5.4   The third law of thermodynamics

At $T = 0$, all energy of thermal motion has been quenched, and in a perfect crystal all the atoms or ions are in a regular, uniform array. The localization of matter and the absence of thermal motion suggest that such materials also have zero entropy. This conclusion is consistent with the molecular interpretation of entropy, because $S = 0$ if there is only one way of arranging the molecules and only one microstate is accessible (see Section 5).

The experimental observation that turns out to be consistent with the view that the entropy of a regular array of molecules is zero at $T = 0$ is summarized by the Nernst heat theorem.

The entropy change accompanying any physical or chemical transformation approaches zero as the temperature approaches zero: $\Delta S \to 0$ as $T \to 0$ provided all the substances involved are perfectly ordered.

It follows from the Nernst theorem that, if we arbitrarily ascribe the value zero to the entropies of elements in their perfect crystalline form at $T = 0$, then all perfect crystalline compounds also have zero entropy at $T = 0$ (because the change in entropy that accompanies the formation of the compounds, like the entropy of all transformations at that temperature, is zero). This conclusion is summarized by **the third law of thermodynamics(热力学第三定律)**: The entropy of all perfect crystalline substances is zero at $T = 0$.

As far as thermodynamics is concerned, choosing this common value as zero is a matter of convenience. The molecular interpretation of entropy, however, justifies the value $S = 0$ at $T = 0$. We saw in Section 3 that, according to the Boltzmann formula, the entropy is zero if there is only one accessible microstate ($\Omega = 1$). In most cases, $\Omega = 1$ at $T = 0$ because there is only one way of achieving the lowest total energy: put all the molecules into the same, lowest state. Therefore, $S = 0$ at $T = 0$, in accord with the Third Law of thermodynamics. In certain cases, though, Ω may differ from 1 at $T = 0$. This is the case if there is no energy advantage in adopting a particular orientation even at absolute zero. For instance, for a diatomic molecule AB there may be almost no energy difference between the arrangements . . . AB AB AB . . . and . . . BA AB BA . . ., so $\Omega > 1$ even at $T = 0$. If $S > 0$ at $T = 0$ we say that the substance has a residual entropy. Ice has a residual entropy of $3.4 J \cdot K^{-1} \cdot mol^{-1}$. It stems from the arrangement of the hydrogen bonds between neighbouring water molecules: a given O atom has two short O–H bonds and two long O · · · H bonds to its neighbours, but there is a degree of randomness in which two bonds are short and which two are long.

Entropies reported on the basis that $S(0)=0$ are called Third-Law entropies (and often just "entropies"). When the substance is in its standard state at the temperature T, the standard (Third-Law) entropy is denoted as $S_m^\ominus (T)$. A list of values of some substances at 298K is given in Appendix 1.

The standard reaction entropy, $\Delta_r S_m^\ominus (T)$, is defined, like the standard reaction enthalpy, as the difference between the molar entropies of the pure, separated products and the pure, separated reactants, all substances being in their standard states at the specified temperature.

$$\Delta_r S_m^\ominus (T) = \sum_{Products} \nu S_m^\ominus - \sum_{Reactants} \nu S_m^\ominus \tag{2-26a}$$

In this expression, each term is weighted by the appropriate stoichiometric coefficient. A more sophisticated approach is to adopt the notation introduced in Chapter 1 and to write

$$\Delta_r S_m^\ominus (T) = \sum_B \nu_B S_m^\ominus (B) \tag{2-26b}$$

For $\Delta_r S_m^\ominus (T)$ at other temperatures except for 298.15K, the following formula used:

$$\Delta_r S_m^\ominus (T) = \Delta_r S_m^\ominus (298.15K) + \int_{298.15}^{T} \frac{\sum \nu_B C_{p,m} dT}{T} \tag{2-27}$$

[Example 2–7] Calculate the $\Delta_r S_m^\ominus$ of reaction of synthesis of methanol, at 298.15K and standard pressure. $CO(g) + 2H_2(g) \rightarrow CH_3OH(g)$.

Solution: From the data in appendix,

$$S_m^{\ominus}(CO,g) = 197.7J \cdot K^{-1} \cdot mol^{-1}$$

$$S_m^{\ominus}(H_2,g) = 130.7J \cdot K^{-1} \cdot mol^{-1}$$

$$S_m^{\ominus}(CH_3OH,g) = 239.7J \cdot K^{-1} \cdot mol^{-1}$$

$$\Delta_r S_m^{\ominus}(298.15K) = \sum \nu_B S_m^{\ominus}(B)(298.15K)$$

$$= (1 \times 239.7 - 1 \times 197.7 - 2 \times 130.7) = -219.4J \cdot K^{-1} \cdot mol^{-1}$$

Section 6   Helmholtz Function and Gibbs Function

PPT

The general criterion for spontaneous processes is that the entropy of the isolated system must increase. Entropy is the basic concept for discussing the direction of natural change, but to use it we have to analyse changes in both the system and its surroundings. We have seen that it is always very simple to calculate the entropy change in the surroundings, and we shall now see that it is possible to devise a simple method for taking that contribution into account automatically. This approach focuses our attention on the system and simplifies discussions. Moreover, it is the foundation of all the applications of chemical thermody that follow.

6.1   Helmholtz function (work function)

Consider a closed system in thermal equilibrium with its surroundings at a temperature T. When a change in the system occurs and there is a transfer of energy as heat between the system and the surroundings, the Clausius inequality reads

$$dS \geqslant \frac{\delta Q}{T}$$

Or

$$TdS \geqslant \delta Q$$

Substituting δQ with the first law of thermodynamics, obtaining

$$TdS \geqslant dU - \delta W \tag{2-28}$$

That is

$$-d(U - TS) \geqslant -\delta W \tag{2-29}$$

U, T, and S are all state functions, so their combination is also a state function. The Helmholtz function, also named **Helmholtz free energy**(亥姆霍兹自由能), F, is defined as

$$F = U - TS \tag{2-30}$$

Substituting equation (2–30) into Inequality (2–29), we get

$$-dF \geqslant -\delta W \tag{2-31}$$

Inequality (2–31) shows that at constant temperature, if a process is reversible, the work that the system does (maximum work) is equal to the reduction of Helmholtz free energy, and if a process is irreversible, the work that the system does is less than the reduction of Helmholtz free energy. The reduction of Helmholtz free energy stands for the ability of the system doing work under the condition of constant temperature, as a result, it was called the "maximum work function" or the "work function". Helmholtz free energy is the property of the system and is a state function.

If the volume of the system is constant and no expansion work done at the same time, the Inequality (2–31) can be written as

$$-\mathrm{d}F_{T,V,W'=0} \geqslant 0 \tag{2-32a}$$

For a macroscopic change, Inequality (2–32a) becomes

$$\Delta F_{T,V,W'=0} \leqslant 0 \tag{2-32b}$$

Inequality (2–32) suggests that under the condition of constant temperature, constant volume and without expansion work, the Hemholtz free energy of the closed system will only decrease spontaneously, and decrease to the minimum allowed under this condition, and at minimum point, the system reaches the equilibrium state. the process of $\Delta F>0$ cannot occur automatically under the condition of constant temperature, constant volume and without expansion work. therefore, formula (2–31) is the criterion of spontaneous process under the condition of constant temperature constant volume and without expansion work, which is called **Helmholtz free energy criterion(亥姆霍兹自由能判据)**.

6.2 Gibbs function (free energy)

Another and important isothermal process is the case that the pressure of the system is constant. In this case, $T_1 = T_2 = T_{su}$, $p_1 = p_2 = p_{su}$, then, inequality (2–28) becomes

$$T\mathrm{d}S - \mathrm{d}U \geqslant -(-p\mathrm{d}V + \delta W')$$

That is

$$-\mathrm{d}(U + pV - TS) \geqslant -\delta W'$$

Or

$$-\mathrm{d}(H - TS) \geqslant -\delta W' \tag{2-33}$$

The **Gibbs free energy(吉布斯自由能)**, or Gibbs function, is defined by

$$G = H - TS \tag{2-34}$$

Substituting equation (2–34) into inequality (2–33), we get

$$-\mathrm{d}G_{T,p} \geqslant -\delta W' \tag{2-35a}$$

For a macroscopic change

$$-\Delta G_{T,p} \geqslant -W' \tag{2-35b}$$

Inequality (2–35) shows that at constant temperature and constant pressure, if a process is reversible, the additional work (non-expansion work) that the system does (maximum work) is equal to the reduction of Gibbs free energy, that is

$$\Delta G_{T,p} \geqslant W'_R \tag{2-36}$$

And if a process is irreversible, the additional work that the system does is less than the reduction of Gibbs free energy. The reduction of Gibbs free energy stands for the ability of the system doing additional work under the condition of constant temperature and constant pressure. This is the physical significance of Gibbs free energy.

If no expansion work is done($\delta W' = 0$), inequality (2–35a) becomes

$$-\mathrm{d}G_{T,p,W'=0} \leqslant 0 \tag{2-37a}$$

For a macroscopic change, inequality (2–35b) becomes

$$\Delta G_{T,p,W'=0} \leqslant 0 \tag{2-37b}$$

Inequation (2–37) indicates that for the closed system under the condition of constant temperature, constant pressure and zero non-volume work, only the process of reducing the system Gibbs function can carry out until the minimum value allowed under this condition, and when Gibbs function reduces to the value, the system reaches the equilibrium state. The process of dG>0 cannot occur automatically under the above condition. Therefore, inequation (2–37) is the criterion of spontaneous process at constant temperature, constant pressure and zero non-volume work, which is called **Gibbs free energy criterion(吉布斯自由能判据)**.

We summarize the three criterions for the direction of themodynamics process:

1. If a system is isolated, its entropy S cannot decrease ($\Delta S_{U,V} \geqslant 0$).

2. If a closed system is at constant T,V and zero non-volume work, F cannot increase ($\Delta F_{T,V,W'=0} \leqslant 0$).

3. If a closed system is at constant T, p and zero non-volume work, G cannot increase ($\Delta G_{T,p,W'=0} \leqslant 0$).

6.3　Calculation of Gibbs function

The Gibbs function is the most widely used thermodynamic function in chemistry because most actual process occurs at constant temperature and pressure. Because G is a state function and the Gibbs free energy change is a definite value between the same initial and final states, a reversible process with the same initial and final states, generally, a reversible process is always designed for the calculate of ΔG.

6.3.1　Gibbs energy Change in the Process of Simple State Change

For a reversible change with no expansion work,

$$\mathrm{d}U = \delta Q_R - p\mathrm{d}V = T\mathrm{d}S - p\mathrm{d}V$$

Because of $G = H - TS$ and $H = U + pV$, the change of Gibbs energy is:

$$\begin{aligned}
\mathrm{d}G &= \mathrm{d}H - T\mathrm{d}S - S\mathrm{d}T = \mathrm{d}U + p\mathrm{d}V + V\mathrm{d}p - T\mathrm{d}S - S\mathrm{d}T \\
&= T\mathrm{d}S - p\mathrm{d}V + p\mathrm{d}V + V\mathrm{d}p - T\mathrm{d}S - S\mathrm{d}T \\
&= -S\mathrm{d}T + V\mathrm{d}p
\end{aligned} \tag{2-38}$$

For a reversible process at constant temperature with no expansion work,

$$\mathrm{d}G = V\mathrm{d}p \tag{2-39}$$

The corresponding expression of ΔG of an isothermal changes of perfect gas is

$$\Delta G = \int_{p_1}^{p_2} V\mathrm{d}p = \int_{p_1}^{p_2} \frac{nRT}{p}\mathrm{d}p = nRT\ln\frac{p_2}{p_1} \tag{2-40}$$

The value of the isothermal compressibility of a typical solid or liquid is roughly equal to $10^{-9}\mathrm{Pa}^{-1}$, so that a change in pressure of 10atm (roughly $10^6\mathrm{Pa}$) changes the volume by only a tenth of a percent. So for condensed matte, the volume is considered not to change with pressure and keep constant, so ΔG of an isothermal changes of liquid or solid is

$$\Delta G = \int_{p_1}^{p_2} V\mathrm{d}p = V(p_2 - p_1) \tag{2-41}$$

[**Example 2–8**] At 301.2K, 1mol perfect gas expanse from 1000kPa to 100kPa by:(1)reversible isothermal expansion;(2)expansion to vacuum. Calculate the Q, W, ΔU, ΔH, ΔS, ΔF and ΔG of the two processes.

Solution: (1) For perfect gas, in isothermal change, $\Delta U = \Delta H = 0$

$$\Delta G = \int_{p_1}^{p_2} V \mathrm{d}p = \int_{p_1}^{p_2} \frac{nRT}{p} \mathrm{d}p = nRT \ln \frac{p_2}{p_1}$$

$$= 1 \times 8.314 \times 301.2 \times \ln \frac{100}{1000} = -5766 \text{J}$$

$$Q_R = -W_R = \int_{V_1}^{V_2} p \mathrm{d}V = \int_{V_1}^{V_2} \frac{nRT}{V} \mathrm{d}V = nRT \ln \frac{V_2}{V_1}$$

$$= nRT \ln \frac{p_1}{p_2} = 8.314 \times 301.2 \times \ln \frac{1000}{100} = 5766 \text{J}$$

$$\Delta S = \frac{Q_R}{T} = \frac{5766.1}{301.2} = 19.14 \text{J} \cdot \text{K}^{-1}$$

$$\Delta F = \Delta U - T\Delta S = -5766 \text{J}$$

(2)Expansion to vacuum, $Q = W = 0$

All state function change is equal to process (1), since they have the same initial and final states, so

$$\Delta U = 0, \Delta H = 0, \Delta G = -5766 \text{J}, \Delta F = 5766 \text{J}, Q = W = 5766 \text{J}, \Delta S = 19.14 \text{J} \cdot \text{K}^{-1}$$

6.3.2 The Temperature Dependence of the Gibbs Energy

From equation (2–38), if the pressure is constant and the system is closed

$$\mathrm{d}G = -S\mathrm{d}T \tag{2–42}$$

Integration of this equation at constant pressure would give a relation for ΔG for a constant pressure and temperature change

$$G(T_2, p) - G(T_1, p) = \int_{T_1}^{T_2} -S(T, p) \mathrm{d}T \tag{2–43}$$

We cannot use this relation, because a constant can be added to the value of the entropy without any physical effect. The most we can do is to consider an isothermal process that can be carried out once at temperature T_1 and a fixed pressure p and again at temperature T_2 and pressure p. We write equation (2–43) once for the initial state and once for the final state. The difference of these equations gives

$$\Delta G(T_2, p) - \Delta G(T_1, p) = \int_{T_1}^{T_2} -\Delta S(T, p) \mathrm{d}T \tag{2–44}$$

Equation (2–44) does not mean that we are considering a nonisothermal process. It gives the difference between ΔG for an isothermal process carried out at T_2 and ΔG for the same isothermal process carried out at T_1.

If ΔS is nearly independent of temperature between T_1 and T_2, equation (2–44) becomes

$$\Delta G(T_2, p) - \Delta G(T_1, p) \approx -\Delta S(T_2 - T_1) \tag{2–45}$$

An alternate to equation (2–44) is known as the Gibbs-Helmholtz equation

$$\frac{\Delta G(T_2, p)}{T_2} - \frac{\Delta G(T_2, p)}{T_1} = -\int_{T_2}^{T_1} \frac{\Delta H}{T^2} \mathrm{d}T \tag{2–46}$$

If ΔH is nearly independent of temperature,

$$\frac{\Delta G(T_2, p)}{T_2} - \frac{\Delta G(T_2, p)}{T_1} = \Delta H \left(\frac{1}{T_2} - \frac{1}{T_1} \right) \tag{2–47}$$

The Gibbs-Helmholtz equation can be derived as follow

$$\left(\frac{\partial \frac{\Delta G}{T}}{\partial T}\right)_p = \frac{1}{T}\left(\frac{\partial \Delta G}{\partial T}\right)_p - \frac{\Delta G}{T^2} = -\frac{\Delta S}{T} - \frac{\Delta G}{T^2} = -\frac{T\Delta S}{T^2} - \frac{\Delta G}{T^2} = -\frac{\Delta H}{T^2}$$

Integration of the upper equation from T_1 to T_2

$$\int_{T_1}^{T_2}\left(\frac{\partial \frac{\Delta G}{T}}{\partial T}\right)_p dT = \frac{\Delta G(T_2,p)}{T_2} - \frac{\Delta G(T_1,p)}{T_1} = -\int_{T_2}^{T_1}\frac{\Delta H}{T^2}dT$$

6.3.3   Calculation of Gibbs energy change in phase transition

The common phase transition processes maybe reversible, and maybe irreversible. The reversible phase transition is at constant temperature, constant pressure and without expansion work. Therefore, according to the Gibbs function criterion, $\Delta G = 0$. To calculate the value of ΔG of an irreversible phase transition, a reversible process is supposed to be designed.

[Example 2–9] Calculate ΔG of when 1mol water is vaporized to steam under the following conditions: (1)373.15K, 101325Pa; (2)373.15K, 26664Pa

Solution: (1) for the reversible phase transition, $\Delta G = 0$;

(2) when the pressure is 26664Pa, 373.15K is not a normal phase temperature, so the process is irreversible, we are supposed to design reversible processes as follows (Fig. 2–10).

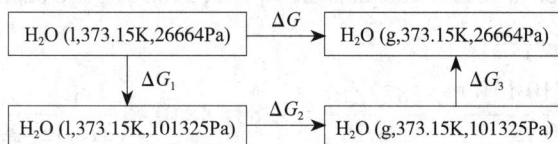

Fig. 2–10   Solution of Gibbs free energy change in irreversible phase change process

$$\Delta G_1 = V_1(p_2-p_1) = nV_m(p_2-p_1) = 1\times1.8\times10^{-5}\times(101325-26664) = 1.34J$$

$$\Delta G_2 = 0\ (\text{reversible phase transition})$$

$$\Delta G_3 = \int_{p_1}^{p_2} V_g dp = nRT\ln\frac{p_2}{p_1} = 1\times8.314\times373.15\times\ln\frac{26664}{101325}$$
$$= -4141\ J\ (\text{the vapour is treated as perfect gas})$$

$$\Delta G = \Delta G_1 + \Delta G_2 + \Delta G_3 = 1.34 + 0 + (-4141.72) = -4140J$$

$\Delta G < 0$, Hence, the process is spontaneous.

6.3.4   Calculation of Gibbs energy change in chemistry reaction

According to the definition of Gibbs free energy, $G = H - ST$, at constant temperature,

$$\Delta G = \Delta H - T\Delta S \tag{2-48}$$

And if the pressure is at standard pressure, for a chemical reaction, the standard Gibbs energy of reaction (or standard reaction Gibbs energy),

$$\Delta_r G^\ominus = \Delta_r H^\ominus - T\Delta_r S^\ominus \tag{2-49}$$

Or

$$\Delta_r G_m^\ominus = \Delta_r H_m^\ominus - T\Delta_r S_m^\ominus \tag{2-50}$$

$\Delta_r G_m^\ominus$ is the standard molar Gibbs energy of reaction. $\Delta_r G_m^\ominus$ is also the maximum non-expansion work of a reaction (equation 2–36).

[Example 2–10] How much energy is available for sustaining muscular and nervous activity from the combustion of 1.00mol of glucose molecules under standard conditions at 37℃ (blood temperature)? The relevant data at 298.15K is as follows.

	$O_2(g)$	$C_6H_{12}O_6(s)$	$CO_2(g)$	$H_2O(l)$
$\Delta_f H_m/(kJ \cdot mol^{-1})$	0	−1274	−393.5	−285.8
$S_m/(J \cdot K^{-1} \cdot mol^{-1})$	205.2	212	213.6	70.0

Solution:

$$\Delta_r H_m(298.15K) = \sum \nu_B \Delta_f H_{m,B}^{\ominus}(298.15K)$$

$$= 6\Delta_f H_{m,H_2O(l)}^{\ominus} + 6\Delta_f H_{m,CO_2(g)}^{\ominus} - \Delta_f H_{m,C_6H_{12}O_6(s)}^{\ominus} - 6\Delta_f H_{m,O_2(g)}^{\ominus}$$

$$= 6\times(-285.8) + 6\times(-393.5) - (-1274) - 6\times0 = -2801.8 kJ \cdot mol^{-1}$$

$$\Delta_r S_m(298.15K) = \sum \nu_B S_{m,B}(298.15K)$$

$$= 6S_{m,H_2O(l)}^{\ominus} + 6S_{m,CO_2(g)}^{\ominus} - S_{m,C_6H_{12}O_6(s)}^{\ominus} - 6S_{m,O_2(g)}^{\ominus}$$

$$= 6\times70.0 + 6\times213.6 - 212 - 6\times205.2 = 258.4 J \cdot K^{-1} \cdot mol^{-1}$$

$$\Delta_r G_m(298.15K) = \Delta_r H_m^{\ominus}(298.15K) - T\Delta_r S_m^{\ominus}(298.15K)$$

$$= -2801.8 - 298.15\times258.4\times10^{-3}$$

$$= -2879 kJ \cdot mol^{-1}$$

Gibbs-Helmholtz equation is used to calculate the $\Delta_r G_m^{\ominus}$ at 310.15K, and suppose $\Delta_r G_m^{\ominus}$ is independent of the above temperature range, then

$$\frac{\Delta_r G_m(310.15K)}{310.15} - \frac{-2879\times10^3}{298.15} = -2801.8\times10^3\times\left(\frac{1}{310.15} - \frac{1}{298.15}\right)$$

$$\Delta_r G_m^{\ominus}(310.15K) = 2882 kJ \cdot mol^{-1}$$

Therefore, for the combustion of 1mol glucose molecules, the reaction can be used to do up to 2882kJ of non-expansion work. To place this result in perspective, consider that a person of mass 70kg needs to do 2.1kJ of work to climb vertically through 3.0m; therefore, at least 0.13g of glucose is needed to complete the task (and in practice significantly more).

If there is no additional work, since $\Delta_r G_m^{\ominus} < 0$, the reaction is spontaneous at the given conditions.

Section 7   the Relationship between Thermodynamic State Functions

In the previous sections, five different state functions, including U, H, S, F, G are introduced. U and S have the definite physical significance, and only under specific conditions, have H, F, G the definite physical significance. From the definitions of H, F, G, we've known that

$$H = U + pV$$

$$F = U - TS$$

$$G = H - TS = U + pV - TS$$

The relationship between these thermodynamic functions can be

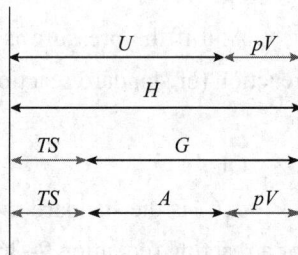

Fig. 2–11 The relationship of the thermodynamic functions

clearly expressed in Fig. 2–11.

7.1   Fundamental relations of thermodynamics

The first and second laws of thermodynamics are both relevant to the behaviour of matter, and we can bring the whole force of thermodynamics to bear on a problem by setting up a formulation that combines them.

We have seen that the first law of thermodynamics may be written $dU = \delta Q + \delta W$. For a reversible change in a closed system of constant composition, and in the absence of any additional (non-expansion) work, we may set $\delta W_R = -pdV$ and $\delta Q_R = TdS$, where p is the pressure of the system and T its temperature.

Therefore, for a reversible change in a closed system,

$$dU = TdS - pdV \tag{2-51}$$

From $H=U+pV$, We can get

$$dH = dU + pdV + Vdp = TdS - pdV + pdV + Vdp$$

Then

$$dH = TdS + Vdp \tag{2-52}$$

Similarly, from $F=U - TS$, we have

$$dF = -SdT - pdV \tag{2-53}$$

From $G=H - TS$, we have

$$dG = -SdT + Vdp \tag{2-54}$$

Equations (2–51)~(2–54) are called the Gibbs equation or the fundamental relation of chemical thermodynamics. They can only be used in a closed system without expansion work. Equation (2–51) can be written down from the first law and knowledge of the expressions for δW_R and δQ_R. Equation (2–51 and 2–53) can be quickly derived from the first by use of the definitions of H, F. Thus they need not be memorized sedulously. The expression for dG is used so often, however, that it needs to be memorized.

Many useful relations can be derived from these four basic thermodynamic formulas, such as:

$$T = \left(\frac{\partial U}{\partial S}\right)_V = \left(\frac{\partial H}{\partial S}\right)_p \tag{2-55}$$

$$V = \left(\frac{\partial H}{\partial p}\right)_S = \left(\frac{\partial G}{\partial p}\right)_T \tag{2-56}$$

$$p = -\left(\frac{\partial U}{\partial V}\right)_S = -\left(\frac{\partial F}{\partial V}\right)_T \tag{2-57}$$

$$S = -\left(\frac{\partial F}{\partial T}\right)_V = -\left(\frac{\partial G}{\partial T}\right)_p \tag{2-58}$$

7.2   Maxwell relations（麦克斯韦关系式）

An infinitesimal change in a function $f(x,y)$ can be written $df = gdx + hdy$ where g and h are functions of x and y. The mathematical criterion for df being an exact differential (in the sense that its integral is independent of path) is that

$$\left(\frac{\partial g}{\partial y}\right)_x = -\left(\frac{\partial h}{\partial x}\right)_y$$

From (2–51), obtain

$$\left(\frac{\partial T}{\partial V}\right)_S = -\left(\frac{\partial p}{\partial S}\right)_V \tag{2–59}$$

From (2–52), (2–53) and (2–54), we can obtain

$$\left(\frac{\partial S}{\partial p}\right)_T = -\left(\frac{\partial V}{\partial T}\right)_p \tag{2–60}$$

$$\left(\frac{\partial V}{\partial S}\right)_p = \left(\frac{\partial T}{\partial p}\right)_S \tag{2–61}$$

$$\left(\frac{\partial S}{\partial V}\right)_T = \left(\frac{\partial p}{\partial T}\right)_V \tag{2–62}$$

These are the Maxwell relations. Maxwell relations (2–59) to (2–61) are little used. However, (2–60) and (2–62) are extremely valuable, since they relate the isothermal pressure and volume variations of entropy to measurable properties.

Section 8　Partial Molar Quantity and Chemical Potential

The thermodynamic system discussed previously is pure matter or multicomponent homogeneous system with constant components. For this case, the function X (e.g. V, U, F, S, and G) can be determined by only two independent variables, temperature (T) and pressure (p), then X can be expressed as follows:

$$X = f(T,p)$$

However, for multicomponent system or the the system whose composition changes due to chemical reaction, if only the temperature and pressure of the system are specified, the state of the system cannot be determined. Because in homogeneous mixtures, a certain thermodynamic property of a system is not equal to the sum of those of each substance in its pure state. For example, When 1mol of water (18.06cm^{-3} at 20℃) at 1 atm was mixed with 1mol of ethanol (58.39cm^{-3} at 20℃), the total volume V is NOT 76.45cm^{-3}, but 74.40cm^{-3}. For the mixture of ethanol and water, the certain temperature and pressure cannot determine the volume of the system, that is, unless the concentration of ethanol in water is determined. Here is another example: if a 50cm^{-3} solution containing 20% ethanol is mixed with another 50ml solution containing 20% ethanol, the total volumn must be 100ml. Therefore, for the multicomponent single-phase system, to determine the thermodynamic equilibrium state, the amount of each substance in the system must be additionally specified, except for the temperature and pressure. Two new concepts will be introduced in this section: partial molar quantities and chemical potentials.

8.1   Partial molar quantity

In this part, we firstly begin with the easiest partial molar property, partial molar volume, then generalize it to define the partial molar quantity.

Imagine a huge volume of pure water at 25℃. When a further 1mol H_2O is added, the volume increases by 18cm^3 and we say that 18cm$^3 \cdot$ mol^{-1} is the molar volume of pure water, and write it as $V_{H_2O,m} = 18$cm$^3 \cdot$ ml^{-1}. However, when 1mol H_2O is added to a huge volume of pure ethanol, the volume increases by only 14cm^3. The reason for the different increase in volume is that the volume occupied by a given number of water molecules depends on the identity of the molecules that surround them. In the latter case there is so much ethanol present that each H_2O molecule is surrounded by ethanol molecules. The network of hydrogen bonds that normally hold H_2O molecules at certain distances from each other in pure water does not form. The packing of the molecules in the mixture results in the H_2O molecules increasing the volume by only 14cm^3. The quantity 14cm$^3 \cdot$ mol^{-1} is the partial molar volume of water in pure ethanol, which can be written as $V_{m,H_2O} = $ 14cm$^3 \cdot$ ml^{-1}. In general, the partial molar volume of a substance A in a mixture is the change in volume per mole of A added to a large volume of the mixture.

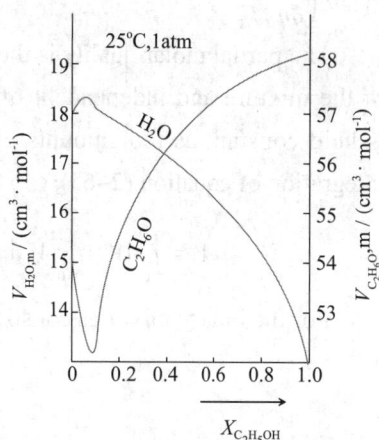

Fig. 2–12   The partial molar volumes of water and ethanol across the full composition range at 25℃

The partial molar volumes of the components of a mixture vary with composition because the environment of each type of molecule changes as the composition changes from pure A to pure B. It is this changing molecular environment, and the consequential modification of the forces acting between molecules, that results in the variation of the thermodynamic properties of a mixture as its composition is changed. The partial molar volumes of water and ethanol across the full composition range at 25℃ are shown in Fig. 2–12.

Now, provided that the volume V is the function of T, p and amount of substance of each component $n_1, n_2, \cdots$, that is

$$V = f(T, p, n_1, n_2, n_3 \ldots)$$

The total differential of V is

$$\mathrm{d}V = \left(\frac{\partial V}{\partial T}\right)_{p,n_i} \mathrm{d}T + \left(\frac{\partial V}{\partial p}\right)_{T,n_i} \mathrm{d}p + \left(\frac{\partial V}{\partial n_1}\right)_{T,p,n_{i(i \neq 1)}} \mathrm{d}n_1 + \cdots + \left(\frac{\partial V}{\partial n_B}\right)_{T,p,n_{i(i \neq B)}} \mathrm{d}n_B \qquad (2\text{–}63)$$

Note: In the equation, n_i represents the amount of all components keep constant, $n_{i(i \neq B)}$ represents the amount of all components keep constant but B.

In equation (2–63), we order

$$V_{B,m} = \left(\frac{\partial V}{\partial n_B}\right)_{T,p,n_{i(i \neq B)}}$$

$V_{B,m}$ is called the partial molar volume of a substance B in a multicomponents system.

Then, equation (2–63) becomes

$$dV=\left(\frac{\partial V}{\partial T}\right)_{p,n_i}dT+\left(\frac{\partial V}{\partial p}\right)_{T,n_i}dp+\sum_B V_{B,m}dn_B \tag{2-64}$$

At constant temperature and pressure, equation (2–64) then becomes

$$dV=\sum_B V_{B,m}dn_B \tag{2-65}$$

Similarly, if any extensive property of a system X can be specified by the variables of T, p and n_1, $n_2,\cdots$, that is $X=f(T,p,n_1,n_2,n_3...)$, the partial molar quantity of X is

$$X_{B,m}=\left(\frac{\partial X}{\partial n_B}\right)_{T,p,n_i(i\neq B)} \tag{2-66}$$

For example, $S_{B,m}=\left(\frac{\partial S}{\partial n_B}\right)_{T,p,n_i}$, $U_{B,m}=\left(\frac{\partial U}{\partial n_B}\right)_{T,p,n_i}$, $H_{B,m}=\left(\frac{\partial H}{\partial n_B}\right)_{T,p,n_i}$, $H_{B,m}=\left(\frac{\partial H}{\partial n_B}\right)_{T,p,n_i}$ and $G_{B,m}=\left(\frac{\partial G}{\partial n_B}\right)_{T,p,n_i}$.

The partial molar quality is the intensive property, which is related to the amount of each component of the mixture and independent of the total amount of the mixture. Provided the relative composition is held constant as the amounts of each component are changed, we can obtain the final volume by integration of equation (2–65).

$$V=\int_0^V dV=\int_0^{n_1}V_1 dn_1+\int_0^{n_2}V_2 dn_2+...=n_1V_{1,m}+n_2V_{2,m}+...=\sum_i n_i V_{i,m} \tag{2-67}$$

For the binary mixtures consisted of water and ethanol, the total volume of the system is

$$V=n_{H_2O}V_{H_2O,m}+n_{C_2H_6O}V_{C_2H_6O,m} \tag{2-68}$$

8.2 Chemical potential

8.2.1 Definition of chemical potential

For a substance in a multicomponent system, the chemical potential is defined as the partial molar Gibbs energy, and denoted by the symbol μ_B

$$\mu_B=G_{B,m}=\left(\frac{\partial G}{\partial n_B}\right)_{T,p,n_i(i\neq B)} \tag{2-69}$$

In an equilibrium one-phase system containing i components, we can describe Gibbs function as

$$G=f(T,p,n_1,n_2,n_3...)$$

The differential of G is

$$dG=\left(\frac{\partial G}{\partial T}\right)_{p,n_i}dT+\left(\frac{\partial G}{\partial p}\right)_{T,n_i}dp+\left(\frac{\partial G}{\partial n_1}\right)_{T,p,n_i(i\neq 1)}dn_1+\cdots+\left(\frac{\partial G}{\partial n_B}\right)_{T,p,n_i(i\neq B)}dn_B \tag{2-70a}$$

From equation (2–56 and 2–58), when the composition keeps constant, we know

$$\left(\frac{\partial G}{\partial T}\right)_{p,n_i}=-S, \left(\frac{\partial G}{\partial p}\right)_{T,n_i}=V$$

So

$$dG = -SdT + Vdp + \sum_B \mu_B dn_B \tag{2-70b}$$

Equation (2–70) is one of the basic thermodynamics equation of multicomponent. The extra terms $\sum_B \mu_B dn_B$ allow for the effect of the composition changes on the state functions G.

From the definition of $H=U+pV$ and equation (2–71), we can obtain

$$dU = dH - pdV - Vdp = d(G-TS) - pdV - Vdp = dG - TdS - SdT - pdV - Vdp$$

$$= -SdT + Vdp + \sum_B \mu_B dn_B - TdS - SdT - pdV - Vdp$$

$$dU = TdS - pdV + \sum_B \mu_B dn_B \tag{2-71}$$

Similarly, From the definition of $H=U+pV$ and equation (2–71), we can obtain

$$dH = TdS + Vdp + \sum_B \mu_B dn_B \tag{2-72}$$

From the definition of $F=U-TS$ and equation (2–71), we can get

$$dF = -SdT - pdV + \sum_B \mu_B dn_B \tag{2-73}$$

Equations (2–70~2–73) are the extensions of the Gibbs equations (2–51)~(2–54) to processes involving exchange of matter with the surroundings or irreversible composition changes. They are the thermodynamics basic equations (or Gibbs equations) of multicomponent, multiphase systems.

From $U = f(T,p,n_1,n_2,n_3...)$, we can obtain

$$dU = TdS - pdV + \sum_B \left(\frac{\partial U}{\partial n_B}\right)_{S,V,n_i(i \neq B)} dn_B \tag{2-74}$$

From $H = f(S,p,n_1,n_2,n_3...)$, we can obtain

$$dH = TdS + Vdp + \sum_B \left(\frac{\partial H}{\partial n_B}\right)_{S,p,n_i(i \neq B)} dn_B \tag{2-75}$$

From $F = f(T,V,n_1,n_2,n_3...)$, we can obtain

$$dF = -SdT - pdV + \sum_B \left(\frac{\partial F}{\partial n_B}\right)_{T,V,n_i(i \neq B)} dn_B \tag{2-76}$$

Comparing the above three formulas with equation (2–71~2–73), we can obtain three other expression of chemical potentials.

$$\mu_B = \left(\frac{\partial G}{\partial n_B}\right)_{T,p,n_i(i\neq B)} = \left(\frac{\partial U}{\partial n_B}\right)_{S,V,n_i(i\neq B)} = \left(\frac{\partial H}{\partial n_B}\right)_{S,p,n_i(i\neq B)} = \left(\frac{\partial F}{\partial n_B}\right)_{T,V,n_i(i\neq B)}$$

The above equations are all chemical potentials, but the last three chemical potentials are seldom used.

8.2.2　Chemical potential criterion and its application

Based on chemical potential, the condition for material equilibrium, including both phase equilibrium and reaction equilibrium, can be derived.

In a closed system under condition of constant T and p and no expansion work, dG can be used to judge the direction of a chemical reaction or interphase transport of matter, and the criteria is:

$$dG_{T,p,W'} \leqslant 0$$

At constant T and p, $dT = 0$ $dp=0$, from equation (2–70), the criteria dG becomes

$$dG_{T,p,W'=0} = \sum_B \mu_B dn_B \qquad (2\text{–}77)$$

Combine two formulas, obtain

$$\sum_B \mu_B dn_B \leqslant 0 \qquad (2\text{–}78)$$

The equation (2–78) is called **chemical potential criteria(化学势判据)**, which indicates that in a closed system at constant temperature and pressure and with expansion work only, the direction of any process is always spontaneously from the state with high chemical potential to the state with low chemical potential, and the limit of the process is the minimum of chemical potential (equilibrium state). The chemical potential criteria is widely used in studying both phase equilibrium and reaction equilibrium.

(1) The usage of chemical potential criteria in reaction equilibrium Chemical potential criteria is mainly used in reaction to judge a reaction's reaction. For example, for the reaction

$$C_2H_4 + 3O_2 \rightleftharpoons 2\,CO_2 + 2H_2O$$

Suppose that at constant temperature and pressure, when dn mol C_2H_4 disappears, there must be $3dn$ mol O_2 disappears, accompanied with the generation of $2dn$ mol CO_2 and 2mol H_2O. The Gibbs energy change of the process is:

$$dG = \sum_B \mu_B dn_B = 2\mu_{CO_2} dn + 2\mu_{H_2O} dn - \mu_{C_2H_4} dn - \mu_{O_2} dn$$

If the reaction process is spontaneous, $dG < 0$, that is

$$2\mu_{CO_2} + 2\mu_{H_2O} < \mu_{C_2H_4} + \mu_{O_2}$$

If the reaction process is in equilibrium, $dG = 0$, that is

$$2\mu_{CO_2} + 2\mu_{H_2O} < \mu_{C_2H_4} + \mu_{O_2}$$

Generalized to any reaction $aA + dD \rightleftharpoons gG + hH$, the chemical potential criteria is:

$$\left. \begin{aligned} \sum p_B\mu_B &= \sum r_B\mu_B \text{ equlibrilium} \\ \sum p_B\mu_B &< \sum r_B\mu_B \text{ spontaneous forward} \\ \sum p_B\mu_B &> \sum r_B\mu_B \text{ spontaneous backward} \end{aligned} \right\} \qquad (2\text{–}79)$$

(2) The usage of chemical potential criteria in phase equilibrium Consider a biphase system consist of substance $1, 2, \cdots, i$, that is in equilibrium, and suppose that dn_B moles of substance B were to flow from phase α to phase β (Fig. 2–13). The Gibbs energy change is

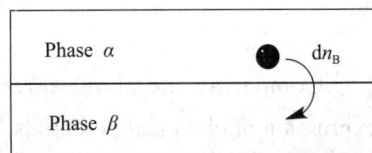

Fig. 2–13 **The usage of chemical potential criteria in phase equilibrium**

$$dG = \mu_B^\alpha dn_B^\alpha + \mu_B^\beta dn_B^\beta$$

Obviously, $dn_B^\alpha = -dn_B$, $dn_B^\beta = dn_B$, so

$$dG = (\mu_B^\beta - n_B^\alpha) + dn_B$$

If the flowing process is spontaneous, $dG = (\mu_B^\beta - n_B^\alpha) + dn_B^\beta < 0$, that is

$$\mu_B^\beta < \mu_B^\alpha$$

If the two phases is in equilibrium, $dG = (\mu_B^\beta - n_B^\alpha) + dn_B^\beta = 0$, that is

$$\mu_B^\beta = \mu_B^\alpha$$

We have thus shown that for a system in thermal and mechanical equilibrium: each substance can flow spontaneously from a phase with higher chemical potential to a phase with lower chemical potential. This flow will continue until the chemical potential of the substance has been equalized in two phases.

Generally, in a multi-phase system, when it is in equilibrium, except T and P, the chemical potential of each substance equals to each other, that is

$$\mu_B^\alpha = \mu_B^\beta = \cdots \mu_B^\varphi$$

(3) Expression of chemical potential   Chemical potential is an important state function, with which we can judge the direction of thermodynamics. Like Gibbs free energy, its absolute value cannot be determined precisely, however, we just need to concern with its variation. For substance in different state, such as gas, liquid, or a component of solution, a standard state can be chosen as a relative starting point, the chemical potential of which is called standard chemistry potential. With standard chemistry potential, the chemistry potential of a substance at other condition can be expressed as its relationship. Then the problem of chemical potential criteria as the direction of spontaneous change can be easily solved.

8.3   Chemical potential of gas

The chemical potential of a one-component perfect gas is equal to the molar Gibbs energy, $\mu = G_m$, when temperature is constant,

$$\left(\frac{\partial \mu}{\partial p}\right)_T = \left(\frac{\partial G_m}{\partial p}\right)_T = V_m = \frac{RT}{p}$$

$$d\mu = \frac{RT}{p}dp$$

If the gas undergoes an isothermal change of state from pressure $p^\ominus$ to p_2, Integration of the equation gives

$$\mu(T, p) = \mu^\ominus(T) + RT\ln\frac{p}{p^\ominus} \tag{2-80}$$

Because chemical potential is the function of temperature and pressure for a pure substance, so at standard pressure and temperature T, $\mu^\ominus(T)$, which equals $\mu(T,p^\ominus)$ is a constant. $\mu^\ominus(T)$ here is the standard chemistry potential of perfect gas. Since at a certain T and standard pressure, $\mu^\ominus(T)$, R,T, and $p^\ominus$ are all constant, $\mu(T,p)$ is only a function of pressure.

For perfect gas mixture, since there is no other interaction force between perfect gas molecules except elastic collisions, a certain component B in perfect gas mixture behaves exactly the same as pure B that occupies the same volume. Therefore, the chemical potential expression of component B in perfect gas mixture should be the same as that of pure perfect gas:

$$\mu_B = \mu_B^\ominus(T) + RT\ln\frac{p_B}{p^\ominus} \tag{2-81}$$

where p_B is the partial pressure of component B of the perfect gas mixture, rather than the total pressure of the mixed gas, $\mu_B^\ominus(T)$ is the standard chemistry potential of perfect gas mixture.

For a pure actual gas, according to $\left(\frac{\partial \mu}{\partial p}\right)_T = \left(\frac{\partial G_m}{\partial p}\right)_T = V_m$, if the relationship between V_m and p is substituted into the integral $\mu(T,p) = \mu^\ominus(T) + \int_{p^\ominus}^{p} V_m dp$, it can be obtained the results. Unfortunately, because the state equation of the actual gas is very complex and vary from one kind of gas to another kind, it is difficult to get a general simple chemical potential expression. To keep the chemical potential expression of the real gas in a simple form similar to that of the ideal gas, Lewis replaces the pressure p with a new thermodynamic function f, then the expression of chemical potential of the real gas is:

$$\mu(T,p)=\mu^{\ominus}(T)+RT\ln\frac{f}{p^{\ominus}} \tag{2-82}$$

where f is fugacity, whose relation to the pressure is

$$f=\gamma p \tag{2-83}$$

And at the same time, f must approach p in the limit as the gas's pressure p goes to zero and the gas becomes ideal:

$$\lim_{p\to0}\frac{f}{p}=1 \tag{2-84}$$

where γ is fugacity coefficient, whose value is not only related to the characteristics of the gas, but also to the temperature and pressure of the gas. Generally speaking, when the temperature is fixed, the pressure is small, and the fugacity coefficient $\gamma<1$; when the pressure is very large, the fugacity coefficient $\gamma>1$, when the pressure tends to zero, the behavior of the real gas is close to the behavior of the ideal gas, and the value of the fugacity is close to the value of the pressure, so $\gamma\to1$. Obviously, the fugacity is equivalent to a "correction pressure" and the fugacity coefficient is equivalent to a "correction factor".

When the pressure $p^{\ominus}=100\text{kPa}$, any actual gas has a deviation to the perfect gas, then the standard states of each actual gas are also different. For unification, the ideal gas with a specified temperature of T and $p^{\ominus}$ is selected as the standard state of the actual gas.

8.4 Chemical potential of solution components

A solution is a homogeneous mixture of two or more components (substances whose amounts can be independently varied). The discussion is divided into ideal solutions and non-ideal solution.

8.4.1 Chemical potential of component of the ideal liquid mixture

(1) **Raoult's Law(拉乌尔定律)** In 1887, Raoult, a French chemist, concluded an empirical law nearly obeyed by some solutions from the experimental results that the vapor pressure of the solvent in the dilute solution was lower than that of the pure solvent. The Raoult law was depicted as follow: At a specified temperature and pressure, the vapor pressure p_A of the solvent in the solution equals to the saturated vapor pressure p_A^* of the pure solvent multiplied by its molar fraction of x_A in the solution, that is

$$p_A=p_A^*x_A \tag{2-85}$$

The law is applicable not only to binary solution, but also to the solution composed of many substances. For a binary solution, because $1-x_A=x_B$, Raoult law can also be expressed as

$$p_A=p_A^*(1-x_B) \tag{2-86}$$

Actually, only an ideal liquid mixture fits this rule. Because there is no difference of the interaction force between the various molecules in the ideal liquid mixture. There is no thermal effect ($\Delta H=0$) or volume change ($\Delta V=0$) when a mixture of several pure substances constitutes an ideal liquid mixture. In this case, the situation of any molecule in an ideal liquid mixture is exactly the same as that in a pure substance, therefore the solution in which any component of the solution conform to Raoult law in all range of concentrations is called an **ideal liquid mixture(理想液态混合物)**.

The ideal liquid mixture, like the ideal gas, is also a limit concept, which summarize the general law of solution in extremely simple form. No gas can obey the perfect gas law at any temperature or pressure, however, there are solutions that are very similar to the ideal liquid mixture at any concentration. If the chemical structure and properties of the two substances are very similar, there is a basis for meeting the ideal solution conditions, e.g. mixtures of benzene and toluene, hexane and n-heptane.

(2) Chemical potential of component of the ideal liquid mixture   If the ideal liquid solution is at equilibrium with an ideal gas mixture at the constant temperature and pressure, from the fundamental fact of phase equilibrium, the chemical potential of component B has the same value in the solution and in the vapor:

$$\mu_B(l,T,p) = \mu_B(g,T,p)$$

Provide that the partial pressure of component B is p_B, from equation (2-81),

$$\mu_B(l,T,p) = \mu_B(g,T,p) = \mu_B^\ominus(g,T) + RT\ln\frac{p_B}{p^\ominus}$$

Substituting p_B with Raoult's Law to get

$$\mu_B(l,T,p) = \mu_B^\ominus(g,T) + RT\ln\frac{p_B^* x_B}{p^\ominus} = \mu_B^\ominus(g,T) + RT\ln\frac{p_B^*}{p} + RT\ln x_B$$

As a result of T, p and p_B^* being the fixed values, $\mu_B^\ominus(g,T) + RT\ln\frac{p_B^*}{p^\ominus}$ is also a constant. In fact, its value is equivalent to the chemical potential of pure gas B when the temperature is T and the pressure is saturated vapor pressure of gas B, p_B^*, $\mu_B^*(g,T)$, that is

$$\mu_B^\ominus(g,T) + RT\ln\frac{p_B^*}{p^\ominus} = \mu_B^*(g,T) = \mu_B^*(l,T)$$

Thus, the chemical potential of each component of the ideal liquid mixture is

$$\mu_B(l,T,p) = \mu_B^*(l,T) + RT\ln x_B \qquad (2-87)$$

where $\mu_B^*(l,T)$ is the standard chemistry potential of component B. Equation (2-87) also gives the function relationship between $\mu_B(l,T,p)$ and x_B.

8.4.2   Chemical potential of component of dilute solution

(1) **Henry's Law(亨利定律)**   Most solutions are not well described by Raoult's law for all compositions. Fig. 2-14 shows the relationship of pressure of component B p_B and x_B. The partial vapor pressure of component B is greater than the prediction value of Raoult's law, which is represented by broken lines. In Fig. 2-14, we find that when x_B is small, p_B is still in proportion to x_B with a different slope and the relationship is called Henry's Law.

In 1803, an English chemist, William Henry, studied dilute solutions with volatile solutes, such as water-soluble solutions for gases (O_2, N_2, etc.) and dilute solutions for volatile liquids such as methanol, and found that the partial pressure in the equilibrium gas phase of the volatile solutes was related to the solubility of solutes in dilute solutions (that is concentrations) . Henry concluded from a large number of experimental results that in the sufficiently dilute solution, when temperature is constant, the equilibrium partial

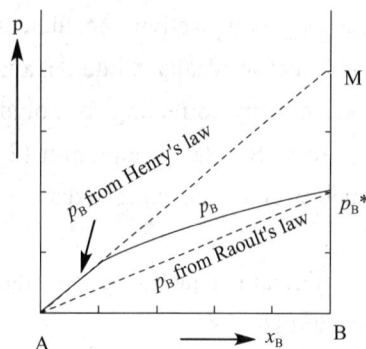

Fig. 2-14   The relationship of pressure of component B p_B and x_B in solution

pressure of the volatile nonionic solute p_B is proportional to the concentration of the solute in the solution. If the concentration of solute B is expressed as the molar fraction x_B, then the mathematical formula of Henry's law is

$$p_B = k_{B,x} x_B \tag{2-88}$$

where $k_{B,x}$ is is called the Henry's law constant for substance B.

(2) Chemical potential of component of dilute solution   Consider a dilute solution in which the solvent A and the solute B are volatile. We equilibrate the solution with a vapor phase, which we assume to be an ideal gas mixture. Since the solvent A of dilute solution obeys Raoul's law, the chemical potential of solvent in dilute solution is

$$\mu_A(1,T,p) = \mu_A^*(1,T) + RT\ln x_A \tag{2-89}$$

When the solution are equilibrium with its vapor phase, for solute B,

$$\mu_B(1,T,p) = \mu_B(g,T,p) = \mu_B^\ominus(g,T) + RT\ln \frac{p_B}{p^\ominus}$$

$$= \mu_B^\ominus(g,T) + RT\ln \frac{k_x}{p^\ominus} + RT\ln x_B$$

Let $\mu_{B,x}^*(T,p) = \mu_B^\ominus(g,T) + RT\ln \frac{k_x}{p^\ominus}$, (all physical quantity is constant), then

$$\mu_B(1,T,p) = \mu_{B,x}^*(T,p) + RT\ln x_B \tag{2-90}$$

where, $\mu_{B,x}^*(T,p)$ is the standard chemical potential of the solute, the value of which is equal to that of the state whose pressure is inferred from the Henry's Law when $x_A \to 1$. In fact, Henry's Law can only used in a sufficiently dilute solution, when $x_B \to 1$, the solution is not a dilute solution any more and the pressure of solute B can not figured out from Henry's Law any more, as a result, the standard state is a imaginary state, which correspond to point M in Fig. 2–14.

8.4.3 Chemical potential of component of nonideal liquid mixture

A nonideal solution is defined as one that is neither ideal nor ideally dilute, in which the solvent A doesn't obey the Raoult's Law and solute B doesn't obey the Henry's Law. For convenience and simplicity, Lewis introduced the concept of activity. He concentrates the departure of nonideal solution on the correction of concentration of the non-ideal liquid mixture. Activity is defined as:

$$a_{x,B} = \gamma_{x,B} x_B \tag{2-91}$$

where $\gamma_{x,B}$ is the activity coefficient, which measures the degree of departure of substance B's behavior from ideal or ideally dilute behavior. The activity $a_{x,B}$ can be viewed as being obtained from the mole fraction x_B by correcting for nonideality. In an ideal or ideally dilute solution, the activity coefficients $\gamma_{x,B}$ are 1. Similar to equation (2–89), the chemical potentials of solvent in a nonideal solution of nonelectrolytes are expressed as

$$\mu_A(1,T,p) = \mu_A^*(T,p) + RT\ln a_{A,x} \tag{2-92}$$

Similar to equation (2–90), the chemical potentials of solute in a nonideal solution of nonelectrolytes are expressed as

$$\mu_B(1,T,p) = \mu_{B,x}^*(T,p) + RT\ln a_{B,x} \tag{2-93}$$

In all, the chemical potentials of various forms of matter have similar forms, which can be uniformly expressed as

$$\mu_B(1,T,p) = \mu_B^*(T,p) + RT\ln a_{B,x} \tag{2-94}$$

Section 9   Application Examples of Chemical Potential

9.1   Colligative properties of dilute solution

When a solute is dissolved in a solvent to form a solution, if the solute is nonvolatile and insoluble in a solid solvent, a colligative properties will be happened. Colligative properties（依数性）of dilute solution are properties that depend on the concentration of a solute but not on its identity. The name comes from a Latin word colligatus, meaning "tied together" and is used because of the common dependence that these properties have on solute concentration. The four principal colligative properties are freezing point depression, boiling point elevation, vapor pressure lowering, and osmotic pressure.

All the colligative properties stem from the reduction of the chemical potential of the liquid solvent as a result of the presence of solute. For an ideal-dilute solution, the chemical potential of solvent is

$$\mu_A = \mu_A^* + RT\ln x_A$$

When there is only pure A in the system, $x_A = 1$ so $\mu_A = \mu_A^*$, and when a certain amount of solute is added to pure A to form a solution, then $x_A < 1$, so $\mu_A < \mu_A^*$, that is, addition of a solute at constant T and p lowers the solvent chemical potential μ_A below μ_A^*. There is no direct influence of the solute on the chemical potential of the solvent vapour and the solid solvent because the solute appears in neither the vapour nor the solid. The reduction in chemical potential of the solvent implies that the liquid–vapour equilibrium occurs at a higher temperature (the boiling point is raised) and the solid–liquid equilibrium occurs at a lower temperature (the freezing point is lowered), as shown in Fig. 2–15.

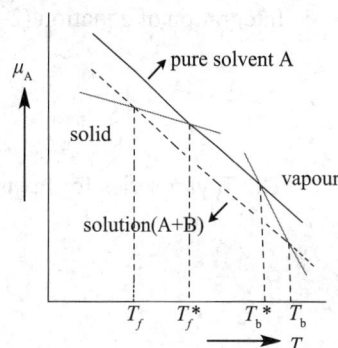

Fig. 2–15   Colligative properties of solution

9.1.1   Vapor pressure lowering

The vapor pressure p_A of the solvent in the solution is lower than the saturated vapor pressure p_A^* of the pure solvent at the same temperature. This phenomenon is called vapor pressure lowering. From Rault's Law, in the dilute solution, the change in vapor pressure is

$$\Delta p_A = p_A^* - p_A = p_A^* - p x_A = p_A^* - p_A^*(1 - x_B)$$
$$\Delta p_A = p_A^* x_B \tag{2-95}$$

Equation (2–95) indicates that the value of vapor pressure lowering of dilute solution is proportional to the molar fraction of the solute in the solution, but independent of the type of the solute.

9.1.2   Freezing–point Depression

Given a heterogeneous equilibrium between pure solid solvent A and the solution with solute present at a mole fraction x_B. At the freezing point T_f, the chemical potential of A in the liquid phase are equal to that in solid phase:

$$\mu_A^*(s, T_f, p) = \mu_A(1, T_f, p) = \mu_A^*(1, T_f, p) + RT_f \ln x_A \tag{2-96}$$

where p is standard pressure, * represents a pure substance, μ_A^* of a pure substance equals its molar Gibbs energy G_m, so

$$\ln x_{\mathrm{A}} = \frac{G_{\mathrm{m,A}}^{*}(\mathrm{s}, T_{\mathrm{f}}) - G_{\mathrm{A}}^{*}(1, T_{\mathrm{f}})}{RT_{\mathrm{f}}} = -\frac{\Delta_{\mathrm{fus}} G_{\mathrm{m,A}}(T_{\mathrm{f}})}{RT_{\mathrm{f}}} \tag{2-97}$$

The solution's freezing point T_{f} is a function of the mole fraction x_{A} of A in solution. Alternatively, we can consider T_{f} to be the independent variable and view x_{A} as a function of T_{f}. Differentiate the equation with respect to T_{f} at constant p

$$\frac{\mathrm{d}}{\mathrm{d}T_{\mathrm{f}}}\left(\frac{\Delta_{\mathrm{fus}} G_{\mathrm{m,A}}(T_{\mathrm{f}})}{RT_{\mathrm{f}}}\right) = \frac{1}{R}\frac{\mathrm{d}\left(\frac{\Delta_{\mathrm{fus}} G_{\mathrm{m,A}}(T_{\mathrm{f}})}{T_{\mathrm{f}}}\right)}{\mathrm{d}T_{\mathrm{f}}} \tag{2-98}$$

Based on Gibbs-Helmholtz equation

$$\frac{\mathrm{d}\left(\frac{\Delta_{\mathrm{fus}} G_{\mathrm{m,A}}(T_{\mathrm{f}})}{T_{\mathrm{f}}}\right)}{\mathrm{d}T_{\mathrm{f}}} = -\frac{\Delta_{\mathrm{fus}} H_{\mathrm{m,A}}(T_{\mathrm{f}})}{T_{\mathrm{f}}^{2}} \tag{2-99}$$

Finally, combination of equation (2–97, 2–98 and 2–99), obtain

$$\left(\frac{\partial \ln x_{\mathrm{A}}}{\partial T_{\mathrm{f}}}\right)_{p} = \frac{\Delta_{\mathrm{fus}} H_{\mathrm{m,A}}(T_{\mathrm{f}})}{RT_{\mathrm{f}}^{2}} \tag{2-100}$$

Integration of equation (2–100) from state 1 (x_{A}=1, T_{f}^{*}, pure A) to state 2 (x_{A}, T_{f}, solution), gives

$$\ln x_{\mathrm{A}} = \int_{T_{\mathrm{f}}^{*}}^{T_{\mathrm{f}}} \frac{\Delta_{\mathrm{fus}} H_{\mathrm{m,A}}(T_{\mathrm{f}})}{RT_{\mathrm{f}}^{2}} \tag{2-101}$$

The Taylor series for $\ln x$ is $\ln x = (x-1) - \frac{(x-1)^{2}}{2} - \frac{(x-1)^{3}}{3} - \cdots$, with $x_{\mathrm{A}} = 1 - x_{\mathrm{B}}$,

$$\ln x_{\mathrm{A}} = \ln(1 - x_{\mathrm{B}}) = -x_{\mathrm{B}} - \frac{x_{\mathrm{B}}^{2}}{2} - \frac{x_{\mathrm{B}}^{3}}{3} \cdots$$

For dilute solution, x_{B} is very small, and terms in $-\frac{x_{\mathrm{B}}^{2}}{2}$ and higher powers can be negligible compared with the $-x_{\mathrm{B}}$ term. Thus

$$\ln x_{\mathrm{A}} = \ln(1 - x_{\mathrm{B}}) \approx -x_{\mathrm{B}}$$

So

$$-x_{\mathrm{B}} = \int_{T_{\mathrm{f}}^{*}}^{T_{\mathrm{f}}} \frac{\Delta_{\mathrm{fus}} H_{\mathrm{m,A}}(T_{\mathrm{f}})}{RT_{\mathrm{f}}^{2}} = \frac{\Delta_{\mathrm{fus}} H_{\mathrm{m,A}}}{R}\left(\frac{1}{T_{\mathrm{f}}^{*}} - \frac{1}{T_{\mathrm{f}}}\right) = \frac{\Delta_{\mathrm{fus}} H_{\mathrm{m,A}}}{R}\left(\frac{T_{\mathrm{f}} - T_{\mathrm{f}}^{*}}{T_{\mathrm{f}}^{*} T_{\mathrm{f}}}\right) \tag{2-102}$$

Since T_{f} is close to T_{f}^{*}, the quantity $T_{\mathrm{f}}^{*} T_{\mathrm{f}}$ can be replaced with T_{f}^{*2} with negligible error for dilute solutions. The quantity $T_{\mathrm{f}}^{*} - T_{\mathrm{f}}$ is the freezing-point depression ΔT_{f}, equation (2–102) becomes

$$\Delta T_{\mathrm{f}} = \frac{RT_{\mathrm{f}}^{*2} x_{\mathrm{B}}}{\Delta_{\mathrm{fus}} H_{\mathrm{m,A}}(T_{\mathrm{f}}^{*})} \tag{2-103}$$

Equation (2–103) indicates that the value of freezing-point depression of dilute solution is proportional to the molar fraction of the solute in the solution, but independent of the type of solute.

In dilute solution,

$$x_{\mathrm{B}} = \frac{n_{\mathrm{B}}}{n_{\mathrm{A}} + n_{\mathrm{B}}} \approx \frac{n_{\mathrm{B}}}{n_{\mathrm{A}}} = M_{\mathrm{A}} \frac{n_{\mathrm{B}}}{W_{\mathrm{A}}} = M_{\mathrm{A}} m_{\mathrm{B}} \, (m_{\mathrm{B}} \text{ is molal concentration})$$

Substituting equation (2-103) with it, and let $k_f = \dfrac{RT_f^{*2}M_A}{\Delta_{fus}H_{m,A}(T_f^*)}$

$$\Delta T_f = k_f m_B \qquad (2-104)$$

where k_f is the solvent's molar freezing-point-depression constant, which is only related to the nature of solvent itself, and its Units is $kg \cdot K \cdot mol^{-1}$. For example, $k_f(H_2O) = 1.86 kg \cdot K \cdot mol^{-1}$.

An application of freezing-point-depression data is to find molecular weights of nonelectrolytes. If ΔT_f is measured by experiments, the molar mass of the solute can be calculated from

$$M_B = \frac{K_f}{\Delta T_f} \cdot \frac{m_B}{m_A} \qquad (2-105)$$

9.1.3　Boiling-point Elevation

Boiling point refers to the temperature when the saturated vapor pressure of the liquid is equal to the external pressure. The decrease of the vapor pressure results in the elevation of boiling point. The boiling-point-elevation formula is found the same way as for freezing-point depression. Going through the same steps as for freezing-point depression, one derives equations that correspond to equation (2-103 and 2-104).

$$\Delta T_b = \frac{RT_b^{*2}x_B}{\Delta_{vap}H_{m,A}(T_b^*)} \qquad (2-106)$$

$$\Delta T_b = k_b m_B \qquad (2-107)$$

where, k_b is solvent's molar Boiling-point elevation, whose value is

$$k_b = \frac{RT_b^{*2}M_A}{\Delta_l^g H_m(T_b^*)}$$

Boiling-point elevation can also be used to find molecular weights but is less accurate than freezing-point depression. The equation is similar as equation (2-105).

$$M_B = \frac{K_b}{\Delta T_b} \cdot \frac{m_B}{m_A} \qquad (2-108)$$

9.1.4　Osmotic Pressure(渗透压)

This colligative property, osmotic pressure, involves the equilibrium between a solution and the pure solvent on the opposite side of a semipermeable membrane which allows only the solvent to equilibrate, but not the solute, as a result, when the equilibrium is achieved, the pressures in the two phases are different, the pressure in the pure solvent is lower than that in the pure solution. A simple osmometer is shown in Fig. 2-16.

We denote the pressure on the pure solvent by p, and the pressure on the solution by $p+\Pi$. The difference Π is called the osmotic pressure (from the Greek word for "push").

The generation of osmotic pressure can be explained by the thermodynamic principle. At a certain temperature, when the two pure solvents are separated by a semipermeable membrane, the two are in equilibrium state, and their chemical potential is equal. If the solute is added to the pure solvent on one side of the membrane to

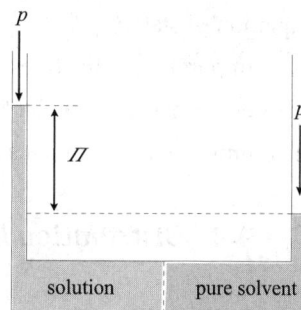

Fig. 2-16　Osmotic Pressure

form the solution, the chemical potential of the solvent in the solution is reduced because of the disorder distribution of the solute. According to the principle of phase equilibrium, the phase with high chemical potential must be automatically transferred to the phase with low chemical potential, so the pure solvent has the tendency to enter the solution automatically, which is the cause of the osmotic phenomenon.

The chemical potential increases with the pressure. when the solution reaches the equilibrium from the beginning of osmosis and the pressure increases from p to $p + \Pi$, the chemical potential of the solvent in the solution $\mu_A(1, p + \Pi, x_A)$ gradually increases, and finally reaches the chemical potential of the pure solvent $\mu_A^*(1, p)$. The macroscopic osmosis phenomenon stops at that time. Using chemical potential, the relationship between osmotic pressure and concentration of the solution can be deduced.

If the solvent obeys Raoult's law, the chemical potential of the dilute solution is

$$\mu_A(1, T, p + \Pi) = \mu_A^*(1, T, p + \Pi) + RT\ln x_A = \mu_A^*(1, T, p) + \int_p^{p+\Pi} V_m^* \, dp + RT\ln x_A$$

For pure solvent, $\mu_A^*(1, p) = G_{m,}^*$ according the relationship of G and p

$$\left(\frac{\partial G_m}{\partial p}\right)_T = V_m$$

So

$$\mu_A^*(1, T, p + \Pi) = \mu_A^*(1, T, p) + \int_p^{p+\Pi} V_m^* \, dp$$

When it is in the osmosi quilibrium

$$\mu_A(1, T, p+\Pi) = \mu_A^*(1, T, p)$$

Therefore

$$\int_p^{p+\Pi} V_m^* \, dp = - RT\ln x_A$$

For the dilute solution, we have known that $\ln x_A = \ln(1-x_B) \approx -x_B$, and V_m^* can be regarded as a constant, so the integration becomes

$$\Pi V_m^* = RTx_B$$

For the dilute solution, $x_B \approx \frac{n_B}{n_A}$, $V \approx n_A V_m^*$, $c_B = \frac{n_B}{V}$, then

$$\Pi = c_B RT \tag{2-109}$$

Equation (2-109) is known as the van't Hoff equation. It is remarkably similar to the ideal gas equation of state.

Important applications of osmosis include transport of fluids through cell membranes, dialysis, and the determination of molar mass by the measurement of osmotic pressure. Osmometry is widely used to determine the molar masses of macromolecules especially.

9.2 Distribution law and its application

9.2.1 Distribution law（分配定律）

Consider the equilibration of two solutions containing the same solute but with different solvents that are almost insoluble in each other. For example, if I_2 is dissolved in water most of the I_2 can be extracted from the water by equilibrating this phase with carbon tetrachloride. For dilute solutions, it is found experimentally that the equilibrium mole fraction of I_2 in the water phase is proportional to the mole fraction of I_2 in the carbon tetrachloride phase. This fact is called Nernst's distribution law. For a solute i and two phases denoted by A and B, this empirical law is given by

$$K_d = \frac{x_{i,eq}(B)}{x_{i,eq}(A)} \tag{2-110}$$

where $x_{i,eq}(A)$ is the equilibrium mole fraction of the solute in phase A and $x_{i,eq}(B)$ is the equilibrium mole fraction of the solute in phase B. The constant K_d is called the *distribution constant* or *distribution coefficient*. For a given solute, the value of K_d depends on temperature and on the identities of the two solvents.

Nernst's distribution law is valid for solutions that obey Henry's law. Its rightness can be proved by chemical potential.

The chemical potential of the solute in the two phases is given by

$$\mu_i(A) = \mu_i^\ominus(A) + RT_f \ln x_{i,eq}(A) \tag{2-111a}$$

And

$$\mu_i(B) = \mu_i^\ominus(B) + RT_f \ln x_{i,eq}(B) \tag{2-111b}$$

When distribution get to equilibrium, from knowledge of phase equilibrium,

$$\mu_i(A) = \mu_i(B)$$

$$\mu_i^\ominus(A) + RT_f \ln x_{i,eq}(A) = \mu_i^\ominus(B) + RT_f \ln x_{i,eq}(B)$$

$$\mu_i^\ominus(A) - \mu_i^\ominus(B) = RT_f \ln \frac{x_{i,eq}(B)}{x_{i,eq}(A)}$$

$$\frac{x_{i,eq}(B)}{x_{i,eq}(A)} = \exp\left(\frac{\mu_i^\ominus(A) - \mu_i^\ominus(B)}{RT_f}\right) = K_d$$

That is right equation (2-110).

If the concentrations of i in two phases are not very large, c_A and c_B can replace $x_{i,eq}(A)$ and $x_{i,eq}(A)$, then

$$K_d = \frac{c_B}{c_A} \tag{2-111}$$

In some solution systems, due to molecular association or dissociation, the average size of the particle is different, resulting in formula (2-111) being not applicable; if the particle of the solute in solvent A is half smaller than in solvent B, the following formula can be used:

$$K_d = \frac{\sqrt{c_B}}{c_A}$$

For example, the distribution of benzoic acid between water and benzene, benzoic acid is partially ionized in water. As shown in Table 2-2.

Table 2-2   Distribution of benzoic acid between water and benzene

$c_W/(10^{-2}kg \cdot dm^{-3})$	$c_B/(10^{-2}kg \cdot dm^{-3})$	c_B/c_W	$\sqrt{c_B}/c_A$
0.0150	0.242	16.133	32.796
0.0195	0.412	21.128	32.916
0.0298	0.970	32.550	33.050

Note: B represents benzene and W represents water.

9.2.2 Application of distribution law-extraction(萃取)

Extraction is an important application of distribution law. It means the separation of a certain solute from another solution that is insoluble by using a solvent. Extraction can be used used in separation the productions.

It is assumed that there is no association, dissociation, chemical action, and so on between solute and the two solvents.

Provide that the solution with a volume of V_1 contains a solute $m$kg, if the solute is extracted with a solvent (volume V_2) each time, the remaining amount of solute in the original solution after the first equilibrium is m_1, then

$$\frac{m_1/V_1}{(m-m_1)/V_2}$$

So

$$m_1 = m\frac{KV_1}{KV_1+V_2}$$

If the same volume of extractant is used for the second extraction, the remaining amount of solute in the original solution m_2 is

$$m_2 = m_1\left(\frac{KV_1}{KV_1+V_2}\right) = m\left(\frac{KV_1}{KV_1+V_2}\right)^2$$

Each time, if it is extracted with a solvent (volume V_2), after n times extraction, the mass of the remaining solute in the original solution is

$$m_n = m\left(\frac{KV_1}{KV_1+V_2}\right)^n$$

So the efficiency of the extraction is $\frac{m_0-m_n}{m_0}\times100\%$.

For a certain amount of extractant, it is more efficient that using the extractant with multiple times than using with all the extractant only once.

Section 10   Chemical Equilibrium

All chemical reactions can occur either forward or reverse. For example, for the synthesis of

$NH_3(g)$ using $N_2(g)$ and $H_2(g)$. Under certain conditions, at the beginning of the reaction, the forward reaction rate is much larger than the reverse reaction rate; with the progress of time, the positive reaction rate decreases, while the inverse reaction rate increases. Finally, two rates are equal, and the system reaches the equilibrium state. The so-called chemical equilibrium refers to the state in which the forward and reverse rates of the reversible reaction are equal and the concentration or partial pressure of each substance is constant. As long as the external conditions (such as temperature, pressure, concentration, etc.) remain unchanged, and the type and quantity of substances in the system do not change with time, the equilibrium state will remain unchanged; When the external conditions change, the equilibrium state will also change with it until a new equilibrium is reached. Macroscopically, the chemical equilibrium behaves as static, and the concentration of the substances involved in the reaction does not change with the time; Microscopically, when the chemical reacations are in equilibrium, the positive and inverse reactions are still going on, only their rates are equal.

In this section, the chemical potential and Gibbs free energy introduced previously are used to calculate the chemical equilibrium constant, to judge the direction and equilibrium conditions of the chemical reaction, to derive the isothermal formula of the chemical reaction, and to discuss the effects of temperature, pressure and inert gas on the equilibrium constant.

10.1　Direction and equilibrium conditions of chemical reaction

For a chemical reaction

$$a\text{A} + d\text{D} \rightleftharpoons g\text{G} + h\text{H}$$

Its stoichiometric equation can be wrote as

$$\sum_{\text{B}} v_{\text{B}}\text{B} = 0$$

where B represents any substance in the reaction, v_{B} is the stoichiometric coefficients, the value of which is negative for reactant A and D, and positive for product G and H.

We define the extent of reaction ξ by

$$\xi = \frac{n_{\text{B}} - n_{\text{initial}}}{v_{\text{B}}}$$

The extent of reaction has the dimensions of moles, If ξ changes in value from 0 to 1mol, we say that 1mol of reaction has occurred. If 1mol of reaction occurs, v_{B} moles of B have appeared if B is a product, and $|v_{\text{B}}|$ moles of B have disappeared if B is a reactant. Think of a stoichiometric coefficient as representing moles of substance per mole of reaction, so that the stoichiometric coefficients are dimensionless.

For an infinitesimal extent of reaction,

$$d\xi = \frac{dn_{\text{B}}}{v_{\text{B}}} \tag{2-112}$$

Under constant temperature and pressure and no expansion work, if the reaction occurs infinitely small step to the right, the Gibbs free energy of the system changes

$$dG(T,p) = \sum_{\text{B}} \mu_{\text{B}} dn_{\text{B}} \tag{2-113}$$

From equation (2–112)

$$dG_{T,p} = \sum_B \mu_B dn_B = \sum_B \nu_B \mu_B d\xi = \left(\sum_B \nu_B \mu_B \right) d\xi$$

Then

$$\left(\frac{\partial G}{\partial \xi} \right)_{T,p} = \sum_B \nu_B \mu_B \qquad (2\text{–}114a)$$

If ξ is 1mol, the Gibbs free energy change of the system is

$$\Delta_r G_m = \left(\frac{\partial G}{\partial \xi} \right)_{T,p} = \sum_B \nu_B \mu_B \qquad (2\text{–}114b)$$

where, $\left(\frac{\partial G}{\partial \xi} \right)_{T,p}$ is the rate of change of Gibbs energy per mole of reaction. $\Delta_r G_m$ means that the Gibbs free energy of changes when 1mol reaction (μ_B is approximately invariant) occurs in an infinitely large number of systems at constant temperature constant pressure; In other words, in a finite system, when the temperature and pressure keep constant, and the extent of reaction is ξ, if a further dξ mol reaction occurs(μ_B can also be regarded as invariant), $\left(\frac{\partial G}{\partial \xi} \right)_{T,p}$ is $\Delta_r G_m$.

According to the Gibbs free energy criterion

$\Delta_r G_m = \left(\frac{\partial G}{\partial \xi} \right)_{T,p} < 0$ or $\sum_B \nu_B \mu_B < 0$, the forward reaction is spontaneous,

$\Delta_r G_m = \left(\frac{\partial G}{\partial \xi} \right)_{T,p} > 0$ or $\sum_B \nu_B \mu_B > 0$, the reverse reaction is spontaneous,

$\Delta_r G_m = \left(\frac{\partial G}{\partial \xi} \right)_{T,p} = 0$ or $\sum_B \nu_B \mu_B = 0$, the reaction is at equilibrium.

The situation is as represented in Fig. 2–17, with a smooth minimum in G at the equilibrium value of ξ. A system in any nonequilibrium state will spontaneously react to approach the equilibrium state at the minimum in the curve representing G as a function of ξ, beginning from either side of the minimum. So The essence of chemical equilibrium, from the kinetic point of view, is that the rate of positive and inverse reactions is equal, and from the thermodynamic point of view, the sum of the chemical potential of the product is equal to the sum of the chemical potential of the reaction.

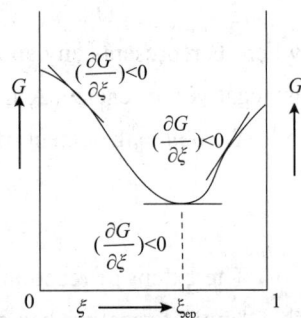

Fig. 2–17 Relation of G and ξ in the chemistry reaction

Why do chemical reactions always reach chemical equilibrium, but cannot be carried out to the end (the reactants cannot become products thoroughly)? Because at isothermal and constant pressure, the chemical reaction always spontaneously occurs to direction of decreasing of Gibbs function. When the reaction occurs, once the product is generated, the mixing of the product with the reactant must cause the mixing entropy, whose value is $\Delta S_{mix} > 0$. from $\Delta G_m = \Delta H_m - T\Delta S_m$, the presence of mixed entropy leads to a further decrease of G. when G decreases to the minimum and the reaction reaches equilibrium, there are more or less reactants in the system. This means that the reaction can only be carried out to a certain extent, and not all the reactants become products.

10.2　Isothermal equation of chemical reaction

Suppose a chemical reaction carries out at constant temperature and pressure, all reactants and products are perfect gas

$$aA + dD \rightleftharpoons gG + hH$$

The Gibbs free energy change of the system is

$$\Delta_r G_m = \sum_B \nu_B \mu_B$$

From equation (2–94), for any substance B in the reaction, the chemical potential is expressed as

$$\mu_B(T,p) = \mu_B^\ominus(T) + RT\ln\frac{p_B}{p}$$

Substituting μ_B with the its expression to get

$$\Delta_r G_m = \sum_B \nu_B \mu_B^\ominus(T) + RT \sum_B \nu_B \ln\left(\frac{p_B}{p^\ominus}\right)$$

That is

$$\Delta_r G_m = \Delta_r G_m^\ominus(T) + RT \sum_B \ln\left(\frac{p_B}{p^\ominus}\right)^{\nu_B}$$

Or

$$\Delta_r G_m = \Delta_r G_m^\ominus(T) + RT\ln\Pi\left(\frac{p_B}{p^\ominus}\right)^{\nu_B} \tag{2–115}$$

The notation Π denotes a product of factors, just as Σ denotes a sum of terms. For example, $\prod_{i=1}^{5} i = 1 \times 2 \times 3 \times 4 \times 5$.

We define pressure quotient below

$$Q_p = \Pi\left(\frac{p_B}{p^\ominus}\right)^{\nu_B} \tag{2–116}$$

Then obtain

$$\Delta_r G_m = \Delta_r G_m^\ominus(T) + RT\ln Q_p \tag{2–117}$$

When it reaches equilibrium, the Gibbs free energy change is zero, so

$$\Delta_r G_m^\ominus(T) = -RT\ln\Pi\left(\frac{p_B}{p^\ominus}\right)^{\nu_B}_{eq} \tag{2–118}$$

$\Delta_r G_m^\ominus(T)$ is a function of T, when T is a constant, the right term of the equation is also a constant. Here, let

$$K^\ominus = \Pi\left(\frac{p_B}{p^\ominus}\right)^{\nu_B}_{eq} \tag{2–119}$$

$K^\ominus$ is called standard equilibrium constant, or thermodynamics equilibrium constant.
Equation (2–118) now can be wrote as

$$\Delta_r G_m^\ominus(T) = -RT\ln K^\ominus \tag{2–120}$$

From equation (2–120), equation (2–117) now can be wrote as

$$\Delta_r G_m = -RT\ln K^\ominus + RT\ln Q_p \tag{2–121}$$

Equation (2–121) is the reaction isotherm of the chemical reaction.

Equation (2–121) is a reaction between perfect gas, if it was extended to a more general chemical reactions, equation (2–121) then becomes

$$\Delta_r G_m = -RT\ln K^\ominus + RT\ln Q_a \tag{2–122}$$

For general none-perfect ga*s*, a_B denotes $\dfrac{f_B}{p^\ominus}$, for ideal liquid mixture, it denotes x_B.

It can be concluded from equation (2–122) that

If $K^\ominus > Q_a$, then $\Delta_r G_m < 0$, the forward reaction is spontaneously;

If $K^\ominus < Q_a$, then $\Delta_r G_m > 0$, the reverse reaction is spontaneously;

If $K^\ominus = Q_a$, then $\Delta_r G_m = 0$, the reaction is in equilibrium.

[**Example 2–11**] At 2000K, the $\Delta_r G_m^\ominus$ of $2H_2(g) + O_2(g) \rightleftharpoons 2H_2O(g)$ is -275.62kJ $\cdot$ mol^{-1},

(1) Calculate $K_p^\ominus$ at 2000K.

(2) When 100kPa H_2 and O_2 are mixed with 100kPa H_2O, is the reaction spontaneous?

(3) If the partial pressure of H_2 is 0.09 $p^\ominus$ and 0.009 $p^\ominus$ of O_2, To prevent the forward reaction spontaneously, how much of the minimum water vapor pressure should be controlled?

Solution：

(1) From

$$\Delta_r G_m^\ominus = -RT\ln K^\ominus$$
$$-275.62 \times 10^3 = -8.314 \times 2000\ln K^\ominus$$
$$K^\ominus = 1.58 \times 10^7$$

(2)

$$Q_p = \frac{\left(\dfrac{p_{H_2O}}{p^\ominus}\right)^2}{\left(\dfrac{p_{H_2}}{p^\ominus}\right)^2 \left(\dfrac{p_{O_2}}{p^\ominus}\right)} = \frac{1^2}{1^2 \times 1} = 1 \ll K_p^\ominus$$

The forward reaction can process spontaneously.

(3) To prevent the forward reaction, it is supposed to let $K_p^\ominus < Q_p$

$$1.58 \times 10^7 < \frac{\left(\dfrac{p_{H_2O}}{p^\ominus}\right)^2}{0.09^2 \times 0.009}$$

So

$$p_{H_2O} > 33.9\, p^\ominus$$

10.3 Calculations of standard molar Gibbs function and equilibrium constant of reaction

As we have said before, the equilibrium constant is required to determine the direction and limits of the reaction. It is rather cumbersome that the concentration (or partial pressure) of each substance in the system is determined by direct measure of the equilibrium system, and what is more, some reactions are sometimes cannot be directly determined. Usually, it can be calculated by using thermodynamic data.

10.3.1　Calculation of the free energy change of the standard Molar Gibbs reaction

at constant temperature and standard pressure, for reaction in a closed system,

$$aA + dD \rightleftharpoons gG + hH$$

Its standard molar Gibbs energy change is

$$\Delta_r G_m^{\ominus} = \sum_B \nu_B \mu_B^{\ominus} = \sum_B \nu_B G_{m,B}^{\ominus}$$

where, $G_{m,B}^{\ominus}$ is standard molar Gibbs energy of B, which cannot be measured precisely up to now. Similar to the method of computing reaction heat $\Delta_r H_m^{\ominus}$ with enthalpy of formation $\Delta_r H_m^{\ominus}$, the $G_{m,B}^{\ominus}$ of simple substance is set zero, at temperature T and pressure $p^{\ominus}$, the Gibbs free energy change of the reaction from the stable simple substances to 1mol compound B is defined as the standard mole Gibbs free energy of formation of compound B, which is denotes as $\Delta_r G_m^{\ominus}$ (B). According to the definition, $\Delta_r G_m^{\ominus}$ of simple substance is zero, and other substances' $\Delta_r G_m^{\ominus}$ (B) is equal to $G_{m,B}^{\ominus}$ of themselves. The appendix lists $\Delta_r G_m^{\ominus}$ (B) of some substances at 298.15K. For example,

$$H_2(g) + \frac{1}{2}O_2(g) = H_2O(l) \qquad \Delta_r G_m^{\ominus} = -237.1 kJ \cdot mol^{-1}$$

Then

$$\Delta_f G_m^{\ominus}(H_2O) = -237.1 kJ \cdot mol^{-1}$$

So, at 298.15K, $\Delta_r G_m^{\ominus}$ of a reaction is given by

$$\Delta_r G_m^{\ominus} = \sum_B \nu_B G_{f,m}^{\ominus}(B) \tag{2-123}$$

At other temperature, $\Delta_r G_m^{\ominus}$ (T) can be calculated by Gibbs-Helmholtz equation.

$\Delta_r G_m^{\ominus}$ is important and can be used in many aspects:

(1) Estimate the possibility of a reaction

At a constant T and p, according to equation (2-121), the reaction isotherm of the chemical reaction

$$\Delta_r G_m = \Delta_r G_m^{\ominus} + RT \ln Q_a$$

If absolute value of $\Delta_r G_m^{\ominus}$ is very big, while Q_a not, $\Delta_r G_m^{\ominus}$ can determine whether $\Delta_r G_m^{\ominus}$ is positive or negative, and whether a chemical reaction can proceed spontaneously. According to the empirical rough estimation, when $\Delta_r G_m^{\ominus} < -42 kJ \cdot mol^{-1}$, the reaction is considered to process forward spontaneously; when $\Delta_r G_m^{\ominus} > -42 kJ \cdot mol^{-1}$, the reaction cannot process forward spontaneously.

[**Example 2-12**]　Three synthetic routes of Benzenamine from benzene are designed as follows steps:

① Firstly Nitrified to nitrobenzene, then reduced to benzenamine;

② Firstly chloridized to Chlorobenzene, then substituted with ammonia;

③ Substituted with ammonia directly.

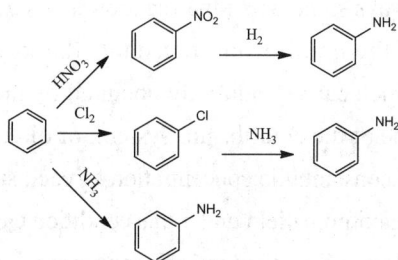

Which route is applicable?

Solution:

①
	$C_6H_6(l)$	+	$HNO_3(aq)$	→	$H_2O(l)$	+	$C_6H_5NO_2(l)$
$\Delta_f G_m^{\ominus}(kJ \cdot mol^{-1})$	124.45		-80.71		-237.13		146.2

$\Delta_r G_m^{\ominus} = -134.67 kJ \cdot mol^{-1}$

	$C_6H_5NO_2(l)$	+	$3H_2(g)$	→	$2H_2O(l)$	+	$C_6H_5NH_2(l)$
$\Delta_f G_m^{\ominus}(kJ \cdot mol^{-1})$	146.2		0		23.7.13		153.2

$\Delta_r G_m^{\ominus} = -476.26 kJ \cdot mol^{-1}$

②
	$C_6H_6(l)$	+	$Cl_2(aq)$	→	$HCl(g)$	+	$C_6H_5Cl(l)$
$\Delta_f G_m^{\ominus}(kJ \cdot mol^{-1})$	124.45		0		-95.3		116.3

$\Delta_r G_m^{\ominus} = -103.45 kJ \cdot mol^{-1}$

	$C_6H_5Cl(l)$	+	$NH_3(g)$	→	$HCl(l)$	+	$C_6H_5NH_2(l)$
$\Delta_f G_m^{\ominus}(kJ \cdot mol^{-1})$	116.3		-16.45		-95.3		153.2

$\Delta_r G_m^{\ominus} = -41.95 kJ \cdot mol^{-1}$

③
	$C_6H_6(l)$	+	$NH_3(aq)$	→	$H_2(g)$	+	$C_6H_5NH_3(l)$
$\Delta_f G_m^{\ominus}(kJ \cdot mol^{-1})$	124.45		-16.45		0		153.2

$\Delta_r G_m^{\ominus} = 45.2 \ kJ \cdot mol^{-1}$

The results of each $\Delta_r G_m^{\ominus}$ shows that route ③ has a more positive value, suggesting an impossible synthetic route at the given condition, route ① and route ② have negative value of $\Delta_r G_m^{\ominus}$, suggesting better routes, which were already applied in industry.

(2) Calculate $\Delta_r G_m^{\ominus}$ of an unknown reaction from $\Delta_r G_m^{\ominus}$ of the known reactions

Some reactions' $\Delta_r G_m^{\ominus}$ are not easily obtained by experiments. Due to G being a state function, $\Delta_r G_m^{\ominus}$ can be calculated by a method similar to calculation of reaction heat by Hess Law.

(3) Calculate $K^{\ominus}$ of the chemical reaction by $\Delta_r G_m^{\ominus} = -RT \ln K^{\ominus}$

10.3.2 Calculation of equilibrium constant

The equilibrium constant is a characteristic of a chemical equilibrium, and also a measure of the limits of a chemical reaction. The following methods are usually used to determine whether a reaction has actually reached equilibrium:

① If the system has reached equilibrium, the concentration of each substance in the system will no longer change no matter how long it takes, unless the external conditions changed;

② The equilibrium constant shall be always equal no matter the chemical equilibrium is obtained from the reactant or from the product；

③ When the initial concentration of the reactants changed optionally at constant temperature, and the equilibrium constant will be always same when the reaction is in equilibrium.

According the definition of the equilibrium constant, the key point is the calculation of the concentration of each substance, which can be indirectly obtained by the refractive index, optical rotation, electrical conductivity or absorbance of the equilibrium system, or directly obtained by chemical analysis.

Similarly, from the equilibrium constant, the concentration of each substance in the reaction equilibrium can also be calculated, and then the maximum yield under this condition can be calculated as well.

Equilibrium conversion is also called theoretical conversion or highest conversion (degree of

dissociation), which is defined as

$$\alpha = \frac{\text{Amount of reactant consumed}}{\text{Original amount of the reactant}} \times 100\% \tag{2-124}$$

If a side reaction occurs, only part of the reactant becomes the product and the other part becomes the by-product. So the concept of "yield" is commonly used in industry, that is

$$\text{Yield}(\%) = \frac{\text{Amount of a reactant converted to a specified product}}{\text{Original amount of the reactant}} \times 100\% \tag{2-125}$$

[Example 2-13] Calculate the equilibrium constant $K_p^\ominus$

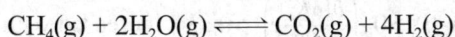

$$CH_4(g) + 2H_2O(g) \rightleftharpoons CO_2(g) + 4H_2(g)$$

The thermodynamic data of the related substances at 298.15K list below (Table 2-3).

Table 2-3   The thermodynamic data of the related substances

Substances	CH$_4$/g	H$_2$O/g	CO$_2$/g	H$_2$/g
$\Delta_f H_m^\ominus(B) / (\text{kJ} \cdot \text{mol}^{-1})$	−74.8	−241.8	−393.5	0
$S_{m,B}^\ominus / (\text{J} \cdot \text{K}^{-1} \cdot \text{mol}^{-1})$	187.9	188.8	213.8	130.7

Solution: $\Delta_r H_m^\ominus = \sum\limits_B \nu_B \Delta_f H_m^\ominus(B) = -393.5 - (-74.8) - 2 \times (-241.8) = 164.9 \text{kJ} \cdot \text{mol}^{-1}$

$$\Delta_r S_m^\ominus = \sum\limits_B \nu_B S_{m,B}^\ominus = 213.8 + 4 \times 130.7 - 187.9 - 2 \times 188.85 = 171.1 \text{J} \cdot \text{K}^{-1} \cdot \text{mol}^{-1}$$

$$\Delta_r G_m^\ominus = \Delta_r H_m^\ominus - T\Delta_r S_m^\ominus = 164.9 - 298.15 \times 171.1 \times 10^{-3} = 113.9 \text{kJ} \cdot \text{mol}^{-1}$$

From the relationship $\Delta_r G_m^\ominus = -RT \ln K^\ominus$

$$K_p^\ominus = \exp\left(-\frac{\Delta_r G_m^\ominus}{RT}\right) = \exp\left(-\frac{113.9 \times 10^3}{8.314 \times 298.15}\right) = 1.11 \times 10^{-20}$$

[Example 2-14] At 400K, 0.0163mol PCl$_5$ is put in a 1.0L container, when the reaction

$$PCl_5(g) \rightleftharpoons PCl_3(g) + Cl_2(g)$$

is in equilibrium, the system's pressure is 100kPa, calculate the equilibrium constant $K_p^\ominus$, and degree of dissociation α. Perfect gas is supposed.

Solution: $\qquad\qquad PCl_5(g) \rightleftharpoons PCl_3(g) + Cl_2(g)$

The amount in equilibrium $\qquad$ 0.0163(1−α) $\quad$ 0.0163α $\quad$ 0.0163α

The total amount in equilibrium $\qquad n_{total} = 0.0163(1-\alpha) + 0.0163\alpha + 0.0163\alpha = 0.0163(1+\alpha)$

For the perfect gas, according to $pV = n_{total}RT$,

$$100000 \times 1 \times 10^{-3} = 0.0163(1+\alpha) \times 8.314 \times 400$$

So $\qquad\qquad\qquad\qquad\qquad\qquad \alpha = 0.8844$

$$K_p^\ominus = \Pi\left(\frac{p^B}{p^\ominus}\right)_{eq}^{\nu_B} = \Pi\left(\frac{px_B}{p^\ominus}\right)_{eq}^{\nu_B} = \frac{x_{Cl_2} x_{PCl_3}}{x_{PCl_5}}\left(\frac{p}{p^\ominus}\right)_{eq}^{\Sigma\nu_B} = \frac{\alpha^2}{1-\alpha^2} \cdot \frac{p}{p^\ominus} = \frac{0.844^2}{1-0.844^2} = 2.48$$

10.4   Effect of temperature on the chemical equilibrium constant

Substituting $\Delta_r G_m^\ominus = -RT \ln K^\ominus$ into Gibbs-Helmholtz equation

$$\left[\frac{\partial\left(\frac{\Delta_r G_m^{\ominus}(T)}{T}\right)}{\partial T}\right]_p = -\frac{\Delta_r H_m^{\ominus}(T)}{T^2}$$

We can write

$$\left(\frac{\partial \ln K^{\ominus}}{\partial T}\right)_p = \frac{\Delta_r H_m^{\ominus}(T)}{T^2} \tag{2-126}$$

Equation (2–126) is called reaction isobar, which is also knows as *Van't Hoff equation*. It indicates that:

For endothermic reaction, $\Delta_r H_m^{\ominus} > 0$, $\left(\frac{\partial \ln K^{\ominus}}{\partial T}\right)_p > 0$, $K^{\ominus}$ Increased with temperature.

For exothermic reaction, $\Delta_r H_m^{\ominus} < 0$, $\left(\frac{\partial \ln K^{\ominus}}{\partial T}\right)_p < 0$, $K^{\ominus}$ decreased with temperature.

Therefore, rising temperature is beneficial to endothermic reaction and unfavorable to exothermic reaction. For the reversible reaction in equilibrium, heating can make the equilibrium move towards endothermic direction, while cooling can make the equilibrium move towards exothermic direction.

The value of $\Delta_r H_m^{\ominus}$ is known as a function of temperature, equation (2–126) can be integrated to obtain the value of K at one temperature from the value at another temperature:

$$\ln \frac{K_2^{\ominus}}{K_1} = \frac{1}{R} \int_{T_1}^{T_2} \frac{\Delta_r H_m}{T_2} dT \tag{2-127}$$

If $\Delta_r H_m^{\ominus}$ is temperature-independent in a certain temperature range, integral of equation (2–126) is

$$\ln K = -\frac{\Delta_r H_m^{\ominus}}{RT} + C \tag{2-128}$$

The indefinite integral of equation (2–126) is given by

$$\ln K = -\frac{\Delta_r H_m^{\ominus}}{RT} + C \tag{2-129}$$

where C is an integral constant. A straight can be obtained when plotting $\ln K^{\ominus}$ with $\frac{1}{T}$, with the slope of $\frac{-\Delta_r H_m^{\ominus}}{R}$ and intercept of C, and the reaction heat $\Delta_r H_m^{\ominus}$ can be obtained from the slope at the same time.

重 点 小 结

　　人类在对热机效率的探索过程中总结出一切自发过程的不可逆性来自于功热转变的不可逆,并总结出热力学第二定律, 同时根据卡诺对热机效率的研究结果, 总结出来热力学第二定律的数学表达式, 并把热力学第二定律应用到孤立系统得到熵判据 $\Delta S \geq 0$, 利用熵判据判断过程的方向时,必须要求系统是孤立体系, 现实中一般把系统和密切相关的环境组合在一起成为一个孤立体系, 利用 $\Delta S_{iso} = \Delta S_{sys} + \Delta S_{sur}$ 判断系统的自发性, 这样稍显麻烦, 于是又引入了亥姆霍兹函数和吉布斯函数,并导出了定温、定容、不做非体积功的过程的亥姆霍兹自由能判据 $\Delta F \leq 0$ 和定温、定压、不做非体积功的过程的吉布斯自由能靠判据 $\Delta G \leq 0$, 该两个判据只需计算系统的 F 和 G 的变化量就可判定过程的方向。

　　对于多组分热力学平衡系统, 热力学容量性质不仅取决于 T 和 p, 还和每个组分的量相关,因此引入了偏摩尔量和化学势(偏摩尔吉布斯自由能),重点引入在定温定压非体积功为零的条件下化学反应和相变化的方向和限度的判据即化学势判据,在该条件下,不论是化学变化还是相变化,系统均总是自发地从化学势高的状态转变到化学势低的状态,直到化学势达到相等,此时系统达到了热力学平衡。

在化学平衡系统,利用化学势判据推导出标准状态下的吉布斯自由能变化量和平衡常数的关系,$\Delta_r H_m^{\ominus} = -RT \ln K^{\ominus}$,并推导出化学反应等温方程式,并利用该公式,利用反应前后各物质的可观测的物理量压强或浓度的大小判断化学变化的方向和限度。

热力学第二定律是热力学的基础定律,也是化学四大平衡的理论基础,定律中引入的S、G等函数是评价药物和靶点之间作用力的重要参数。

Object detection

I. Select the correct option for the following problems (one option for each problem).

1. The maximum efficiency of heat engine working between 100℃ hot reservoir and 25℃ cold sink is

    A. 100%　　　　　B. 75%　　　　　C. 25%　　　　　D. 20%

2. There are two paths for the system to change from state A to state B: Ⅰ is reversible and Ⅱ is irreversible. Which of the following is false?

    A. $\Delta S_I = \Delta S_{II}$　　　　　　　　B. $\Delta S_{II} = \int_A^B \left(\frac{\delta Q}{T}\right)_I$

    C. $\Delta S_I = \int_A^B \left(\frac{\delta Q}{T}\right)_I$　　　　　D. $\sum_A^B \left(\frac{\delta Q}{T}\right)_I = \sum_A^B \left(\frac{\delta Q}{T}\right)_{II}$

3. Suppose a perfect gas expands to the same volume V_2 from the same initial state, respectively by (1) adiabatic reversible expansion, and (2) adiabatic irreversible expansion. The relationship between the entropy change $\Delta S(1)$ of process (1) and $\Delta S(2)$ of process (2) is

    A. $\Delta S(1) > \Delta S(2)$

    B. $\Delta S(1) < \Delta S(2)$

    C. $\Delta S(1) = \Delta S(2)$

    D. no definite relationship due to their different final state reached

4. Which of the following answers is correct for an adiabatic reversible expansion of an non-perfect gas ?

    A. $\Delta S>0$　　　　B. $\Delta S<0$　　　　C. $\Delta S=0$　　　　D. $\Delta S \geqslant 0$

5. 1mol perfect gas irreversibly expands to twice volume of the initial state at the room temperature($Q=0$). The entropy changes of the system and that of the environment, respectively, is

    A. 5.76J · K^{-1} · mol^{-1}, −5.76J · K^{-1} · mol^{-1}

    B. 5.76J · K^{-1} · mol^{-1}, 0J · K^{-1} · mol^{-1}

    C. 0J · K^{-1} · mol^{-1}, 0J · K^{-1} · mol^{-1}

    D. 0J · K^{-1} · mol^{-1}, 5.76J · K^{-1} · mol^{-1}

6. If the volume of 1mol ideal gas increases to five times at constant temperature and constant

external pressure, the entropy of the system changes is

    A. $13.38J \cdot K^{-1}$ B. $19.15J \cdot K^{-1}$ C. $8.314J \cdot K^{-1}$ D. $-8.314J \cdot K^{-1}$

7. Under pressure of 101325kPa, 1.5mol H_2O (l) was heated from $10^{\circ}C$ to $50^{\circ}C$, and its average molar constant pressure heat capacity is $75.295J \cdot K^{-1} \cdot mol^{-1}$. The entropy change of the system is

    A. $6.48J \cdot K^{-1}$ B. $1.8225kJ \cdot K^{-1}$ C. $78.94J \cdot K^{-1}$ D. $14.93J \cdot K^{-1}$

8. 1mol Water condenses into ice at 101.3kPa and 260K. which of the following is true for the process?

    A. $\Delta S_{sys}+\Delta S_{cir} \geqslant 0$ B. $\Delta S_{sys}+\Delta S_{cir} > 0$

    C. $\Delta S_{sys}+\Delta S_{cir} = 0$ D. $\Delta S_{sys}+\Delta S_{cir} < 0$

9. At 298.2K, 100kPa, the difference of $\Delta_r G_m$ and $\Delta_r F_m$ of the reaction $H_2(g)+1/2O_2=H_2O(l)$ is

    A. $1239J \cdot mol^{-1}$ B. $-3719J \cdot mol^{-1}$

    C. $2477J \cdot mol^{-1}$ D. $3719J \cdot mol^{-1}$

    E. $0J \cdot mol^{-1}$

10. The ΔG of which following process does not equal zero?

    A. Any substance goes through a cycle process

    B. Irreversible process at constant temperature and volume with $W'=0$

    C. Irreversible process at constant temperature and pressure with $W'=0$

    D. Normal phase transition of any pure substance

11. 1mol perfect gas isothermally expands to five times the initial volume at 300K and 100kPa, then the ΔG of the process is

    A. 4014J   B. $-$ 4014J   C. 13.4J   D. $-$13.4J   E. 0

12. An ideal gas expands adiabaticly to a vacuum, then

    A. $dS = 0$, $dW = 0$ B. $dH = 0$, $dU = 0$ C. $dG = 0$, $dH = 0$ D. $dU = 0$, $dG = 0$

13. Under $-10^{\circ}C$ and 101.325kPa, 1mol water condensed to ice, which of the following formula can be applied in the process?

    A. $\Delta U = T\Delta S$ B. $\Delta S = \dfrac{\Delta H - \Delta G}{T}$ C. $\Delta H = T\Delta S + V\Delta p$ D. $\Delta G_{T,p} = 0$

14. Which of the following statement is accurate for the basic equations of thermodynamics $dU=TdS-pdV$

    A. TdS is the heat of the process.

    B. pdV is expansion work.

    C. pdV is expansion work and TdS is the heat of the process at reversible process.

    D. None of the above is accurate.

15. (1) The standard combustion enthalpy of $CO_2(g)$ and O_2 (g) in the standard state is zero.

    (2) $\Delta_r G_m^{\ominus} = -RT \ln K_p^{\ominus}$, and $K_p^{\ominus}$ is represented by the composition at equilibrium, as a result, $\Delta_r G_m^{\ominus}$ is the difference between the Gibbs free energy of the products at equilibrium and that of the reactants at equilibrium.

    (3) When water evaporates at $25^{\circ}C$ and $p^{\ominus}$, $\Delta S_m^{\ominus}$ can be calculated with $\Delta S_m^{\ominus} = (\Delta H_m^{\ominus} - \Delta G_m^{\ominus})/T$.

    (4) The formula for calculating entropy change is $\Delta_r S_m = \Delta_r H_m/T$ for reversible cell reaction at constant temperature and pressure.

    Which of the above statements are true?

    A. (1), (2)   B. (2), (3)   C. (1), (3)   D. (3), (4)

16. Which of the following is partial molar quantities?

A. $\left(\frac{\partial U}{\partial n_i}\right)_{T,p,n_j}$ B. $\left(\frac{\partial H}{\partial n_i}\right)_{T,V,n_j}$ C. $\left(\frac{\partial F}{\partial n_i}\right)_{T,V,n_j}$ D. $\left(\frac{\partial \mu_i}{\partial n_i}\right)_{T,p,n_j}$

17. The relation of chemical potential of N_2 at 298K, $p^{\ominus}$ (state I) and N_2 at 323K, $p^{\ominus}$ (state II)

A. $\mu(\mathrm{I}) > \mu(\mathrm{II})$ B. $\mu(\mathrm{I}) < \mu(\mathrm{II})$ C. $\mu(\mathrm{I}) = \mu(\mathrm{II})$ D. uncomparable

18. Both Substance A and B are in phase α and β, when equilibrium is reached, which of the following is right?

A. $\mu_A^{\alpha} = \mu_B^{\alpha}$ B. $\mu_A^{\alpha} = \mu_A^{\beta}$ C. $\mu_B^{\alpha} = \mu_A^{\beta}$ D. $\mu_B^{\alpha} = \mu_B^{\beta} = \mu_A^{\alpha} = \mu_A^{\beta}$

19. The saturated vapor pressures of the two liquids A and B are p_A^* and p_B^*, respectively, when they are mixed to form an ideal solution, supposed the composition of the liquid phase is x, gas phase y, if $p_B^* > p_B^*$, then

A. $y_A > x_A$ B. $y_A > y_B$ C. $x_A > y_A$ D. $y_B > y_A$ E. $x_A = y_A$

20. The main factors affecting the boiling-point-depression constant and the freezing-point-depression constant is

A. nature of solvent

B. temperature and pressure

C. nature of solute

D. temperature and nature of solvent nature

21. $2C(s) + O_2(g) \rightarrow 2CO(g)$, $\Delta_r G_m^{\ominus}/(\mathrm{J} \cdot \mathrm{mol}^{-1}) = -232600 - 167.7T/\mathrm{K}$, if the temperature rises, then

A. $\Delta_r G_m^{\ominus}$ becomes more negative, the reaction will be more complete

B. $K_p^{\ominus}$ becomes greater, the reaction will be more complete

C. $K_p^{\ominus}$ becomes smaller, the reaction will be more incomplete

D. the direction of the reaction cannot be judged

22. For reaction at 298K, $N_2O_4(g) = 2NO_2(g)$, $K_p^{\ominus} = 0.1132$, when $p(N_2O_4) = p(NO_2) = 1\mathrm{kPa}$, the reaction will

A. goes in the direction of the producing NO_2

B. goes in the direction of the producing N_2O_4

C. be in equilibrium

D. stop

23. At 732K, $NH_4Cl(s) = NH_3(g) + HCl(g)$, $\Delta_r G_m^{\ominus}$ is $-20.8\mathrm{kJ} \cdot \mathrm{mol}^{-1}$, $\Delta_r H_m^{\ominus}$ is $154\mathrm{kJ} \cdot \mathrm{mol}^{-1}$, the $\Delta_r S_m^{\ominus}$ is

A. $239\mathrm{J} \cdot \mathrm{K}^{-1} \cdot \mathrm{mol}^{-1}$ B. $0.239\mathrm{J} \cdot \mathrm{K}^{-1} \cdot \mathrm{mol}^{-1}$

C. $182\mathrm{J} \cdot \mathrm{K}^{-1} \cdot \mathrm{mol}^{-1}$ D. $0.182\mathrm{J} \cdot \mathrm{K}^{-1} \cdot \mathrm{mol}^{-1}$

II. Select the correct options for the following problem (at least two options for each problem).

1. Which of the following is right?

A. for any cycle, $\Delta S_{sys} = 0$, $\Delta S_{cir} = 0$

B. for reversible process, $\Delta S_{sys} = 0$, $\Delta S_{cir} = 0$

C. for irreversible process, $\Delta S_{sys} > 0$, $\Delta S_{cir} > 0$

D. for irreversible cycle process, $\Delta S_{sys} = 0$, $\Delta S_{cir} > 0$

E. for irreversible cycle process, $\Delta S_{sys} = 0$, $\Delta S_{cir} = 0$

2. After adiabatic reversible expansion for non-perfect gas, which of the following are not zero?

A. ΔU B. ΔH C. ΔS D. ΔF E. ΔG

3. Which of the following physical quantities are zero Standard hydrogen electrode?

    A. $\Delta_f H_m^{\ominus}$ (298.15K) of H_2 B. $\Delta_r G_m^{\ominus}$ (298.15K) of H_2

    C. $S_m^{\ominus}$ (298.15K) of H_2 D. $\varphi^{\ominus}$ (298.15K) of standard hydrogen electrode

    E. $\Delta_c H_m^{\ominus}$ (298.15K) of H_2

4. Which of the following variables are zero in the process of the perfect gas's Carnot cycle?

    A. ΔU B. ΔS C. ΔH

    D. ΔF E. ΔG

5. Which of the following properties belong to the colligative property of the solution?

    A. the increase of the freezing point   B. the decrease of the freezing point

    C. the increase of boiling point   D. the decrease of boiling point

    E. the increase of vapour pressure

III. Try to answer the following problem.

In the reversible expansion of ideal gas at constant temperature, $\Delta U = 0$, $Q = -W$, as a result, the entire heat that ideal gas absorbs from a single heat source changes to work. Does it contradict Kelvin's expression of the second law of thermodynamics? Why?

Reference answers

I. 1.B; 2.D; 3.B; 4.C; 5.B; 6.A; 7.D; 8.B; 9.B; 10.B; 11.B; 12.B; 13.B; 14.D; 15.C; 16.D; 17.A; 18.B; 19.A; 20.A; 21.C; 22.B; 23.A.

II. 1.BD; 2. ABCE; 3.ABD; 4.ABCDE; 5.BC.

III. This is not contradictory, the second law of thermodynamics does not say that heat can not be completely converted to work, but that under the condition that there is no additional change, heat can not be completely converted to work. In the above process, the volume and pressure of gas have changed.

Chapter 3   Phase Equilibrium

知识要求

1. 掌握

（1）相律。

（2）相图的一般规律和相图的分析方法。

2. 熟悉

（1）克拉贝龙-克劳修斯方程、蒸馏与精馏的原理以及杠杆规则及相关的计算。

（2）一些常见的相图，如水的相图，完全互溶的二组分气-液平衡系统的 $p-x$ 图、$T-x$ 图，具有最高临界溶解温度的二组分液-液平衡系统的 $T-x$ 图、生成简单低共熔混合物的二组分液-固平衡系统的 $T-x$ 图以及一对部分互溶的三组分系统的相图。

3. 了解

（1）水蒸气蒸馏的基本原理。

（2）相平衡在医药领域中的应用价值。

能力要求

1. 能够利用相律判断系统的自由度数。

2. 能够分析主要的相图。

3. 能够把所学相图的知识应用到实践中，解决某些相关的实际问题。

The process of material transfer from one phase to another in the system is called phase transition process. For example, the melting, evaporation and condensation of material are phase transition processes. When these processes reach equilibrium, they are called phase equilibrium processes, and all phase equilibrium processes follow the phase rule. The phase rule is one of the most universal laws in physical chemistry, which describes the relationship between the number of phases, the independent component number and the degree of freedoms (such as temperature, pressure, composition, etc.) in a multicomponent equilibrium system. Based on the phase rule and some typical phase diagrams, this chapter analyzes how the state of one-component and multicomponent systems varies with the temperature, pressure, and composition of the system.

Phase equilibrium theory is closely related to the pharmaceutical industry, such as distillation, freeze-drying, crystallization, extraction and other operations to separate and purify the required components, and its theoretical basis is derived from the principle of phase equilibrium. In addition, the solubilization, dosage form and compatibility of pharmacy also need the theoretical guidance of phase balance. Therefore, phase equilibrium theory has important practical significance in pharmacy.

Section 1　Basic Concepts

1.1　Phase

A **phase (相)** is a state of matter that is uniform throughout, not only in chemical composition but also in physical state. It is a portion of a system (or an entire system) inside which intensive properties do not change abruptly as a function of position. There are obvious interfaces between different phases in a multicomponent system, and the physical and chemical properties would change dramatically when the interfaces are crossed. The total number of phases in the system of is known as the "number of phases", with "Φ" to represent the symbols.

1.1.1　Gas

A single phase, that is, a gas or a gaseous mixture is a single phase.

1.1.2　Liquid

A homogeneous full miscible solution is a phase; for full immiscible solutions, the number of phase is equal to the number of substance; while for partially miscible solutions, the number of phase can be determined by the degree of mutual solubility, which can be a phase or multiphase coexistence.

1.1.3　Solid

Each solid represents a phase and is independent of its dispersion (except as a uniform solid solution). If the same substance has different crystal types (such as graphite and diamond, etc.), each crystal type is a phase.

In a multicomponent system there can often be several solid phases or several liquid phases at equilibrium. For example, if one system containing mercury, a mineral oil, a methylsilicone oil, water, benzyl alcohol, and a perfluoro compound such as perfluoro (*N*-ethylpiperidine) equilibrates at room temperature, it can obtain six coexisting liquid phases. Each of these phases consists of a large amount of one substance with small amount of the other substances dissolved in it.

1.2　Number of Independent Components

The number of species in a balanced system is called **the number of species (物种数)**, and is represented by the symbol "S". **Number of independent components (独立组分数)** is the minimum number of species necessary to define the composition of all the phases present in a balanced system. It is represented by the symbol "K".

It should be pointed out that the species number "S" and the components number "K" are two different concepts. Whether the values are the same depends on whether chemical equilibrium and other constraints exist in the system. It is illustrated with the following examples:

There is no chemical reaction in the system, and the number of species is equal to the number of components, that is, $K=S$. For example, aqueous solution of NaCl, and the NaCl and H_2O are both species, so $S=K=2$.

There is a chemical equilibrium in the system, for example, any amount of N_2, H_2 and NH_3 is mixed until the chemical equilibrium is reached

$$N_2 + 3H_2 \rightleftharpoons 2NH_3$$

$S=3$, $K=2$ in the system. To determine the composition of the system, you only need to know the amount of two substances or partial pressure of the two substances at equilibrium, and then the amount or partial pressure of the third substance can be determined by the equilibrium constant, and the composition of the system can be determined. Their relationship can be expressed by the following formula: $K=S-R=3-1=2$, where R is the number of independent chemical equilibrium reactions existing in the system, also known as the number of independent chemical equilibrium, pay attention to the word "independent".

For example, there are $H_2O(g)$, $C(s)$, $CO(g)$, $CO_2(g)$ and $H_2(g)$ in the system. Three chemical equilibrium relations between them are as follow:

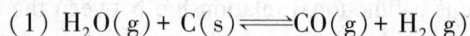

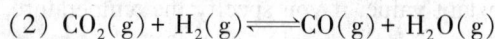

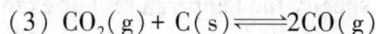

(1) $H_2O(g) + C(s) \rightleftharpoons CO(g) + H_2(g)$

(2) $CO_2(g) + H_2(g) \rightleftharpoons CO(g) + H_2O(g)$

(3) $CO_2(g) + C(s) \rightleftharpoons 2CO(g)$

In the equations above, only two of these reactions are independent, and either one can be obtained by combining the other two reactions. If reaction (3) can be obtained from reaction (1) + (2), its independent chemical equilibrium number $R=2$.

There's a concentration restriction in the system. In the above mixture of N_2, H_2 and NH_3, if we know the input ratio of N_2 and H_2 before the reaction, that is, the concentration of N_2 and H_2 in the mixture before the reaction, then the number of independent components of the described equilibrium system is not $K=2$, but $K=S-R-R'=3-1-1=1$, where R' is the number of concentration restrictions. Because at this point, as long as you know the partial pressure of a substance, such as nitrogen, according to the ratio of inputs, you can know the partial pressure of hydrogen, and based on the equilibrium constant you can determine the partial pressure of ammonium, the composition of the system is determined. Therefore, only one of the three substances is independent.

It should be noted that the concentration restriction can only be applied in the same phase, and the concentration restriction does not apply in different phases. For example, in the decomposition reaction of $CaCO_3$

$$CaCO_3(s) \rightleftharpoons CaO(s) + CO_2(g)$$

Although the amount of CaO (s) produced by decomposition is the same as that of CO_2 (g), since one is in the solid phase and the other is in the gas phase, there is no concentration restriction relationship between them, so the number of independent components $K=2$.

Therefore, the number of independent components of the system can be expressed by the following relation.

$$K = S - R - R'$$

[Example 3–1] A certain amount of NH_4HCO_3 (s) is added to a vacuum container, and the following reactions can occur when being heated. Find the number of independent components of the system at equilibrium:

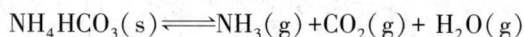

$$NH_4HCO_3(s) \rightleftharpoons NH_3(g) + CO_2(g) + H_2O(g)$$

Solution: The species number $S=4$, there is an equilibrium decomposition reaction in the system,

3.1 例题

医药大学堂
WWW.YIYAODXT.COM

so $R=1$. There are also concentration restrictions in the system, and they are in the same phase, so $R'=2$. According to the formula $K=S-R-R'$, $K=4-1-2=1$, that is, as long as the partial pressure of a substance at equilibrium is known, the composition (or concentration) of the gas phase can be determined.

1.3   Degree of Freedom

The number of variables in an equilibrium system that can be changed within a limited range, without causing the disappearance of the old phase or the creation of the new phase, is called **degree of freedom (自由度数)**, and is represented by the symbol "f". The value of degrees of freedom is the number of variables of the system, such as temperature, pressure, and composition. For example, water in the liquid phase can change temperature and pressure arbitrarily within a certain range and still remain in the liquid phase, that is, $f=2$. When water and water vapor are in a two-phase equilibrium, the variables of the system are still temperature and pressure, but there is a functional relationship between the two. The vapor pressure at a constant temperature has a constant value, if you specify the temperature, you can't specify the pressure. Or if you specify the pressure you can't specify the temperature. For example, under standard pressure, water boils at $100\,^\circ\!C$. If water is kept at $110\,^\circ\!C$, liquid water will disappear and only water in the gas phase will exist. In this time, there's only one independent variable of temperature and pressure, which is $f=1$. As we shall see, these variables are not all independent. The degrees of freedom vary with phase number and the number of independent components, and the relationship between them can be described by phase rule.

1.4   Phase Rule

Phase rule (相律) is a law that describes the relationship between Phase number (Φ), the number of independent components (K) and the degree of freedom (f) in a multiphase equilibrium system. The mathematical expression of the phase law was deduced by Gibbs by means of the theory of thermodynamics. There is an equilibrium system in which there are phases of Φ and species number of S, and they are distributed in each phase. S stands for all kinds of substances. α, β, γ, ...Φ... stand for each phase. When the system reaches equilibrium, it must satisfy

  1. The temperature of all phases is the same. $T^\alpha = T^\beta = T^\gamma = \cdots\cdots = T$
  2. The pressure among all the phases is equal. $p^\alpha = p^\beta = p^\gamma = \cdots\cdots = p$
  3. The chemical potentials of the substances in each phase are the same. $\mu_1^\alpha = \mu_1^\beta = \mu_1^\gamma = \mu_1^\varphi$

All phases of the system should have the same temperature (T) and pressure (p), and each phase should have S concentrations, of which $(S-1)$ is independent, because $\sum x_i = 1$. In all phases of Φ, there are $\Phi(S-1)$ concentration variables, plus two variables of T and p, the total number of variables is $[\Phi(S-1)+2]$. Since the condition for the system to reach phase equilibrium is that the chemical potential of each substance in each phase is equal, that is

$$\mu_1^\alpha = \mu_1^\beta = \mu_1^\gamma = \cdots\cdots = \mu_1^\phi$$

$$\mu_2^\alpha = \mu_2^\beta = \mu_2^\gamma = \cdots\cdots = \mu_2^\phi$$

$$\mu_s^\alpha = \mu_s^\beta = \mu_s^\gamma = \cdots\cdots = \mu_s^\phi$$

These chemical potential equations are associated with the relation between the variables (concentration or composition), because each substance in Φ phase, there are $S(\Phi-1)$ equal equations between the chemical potential. In addition, if there are independent chemical equilibrium equations of R in the system, and there are concentration restrictions of R', the relation between the variables should be $[S(\Phi-1)+R+R']$.

To describe the state of a multiphase equilibrium system, you need to specify the total number of independent variables, the degree of freedom. Therefore, firstly, to find the total number of variables that describe the system state, and secondly, to deduct the non-independent factors, that is, the degree of freedom:

$$f= [\Phi(S-1)+2] - [S(\Phi-1)+R+R'] = [S-R-R']-\Phi+2$$

Since

$$S-R-R' = K$$

So

$$f=K-\Phi+2 \qquad (3-1)$$

Formula (3–1) is the famous mathematical expression, where f is the degree of freedom, K is the number of components, Φ is the number of phase. There are two variables in the equation, one is the temperature and the other is the pressure. The phase rule is applicable to all equilibrium systems, but it only describes the number of phases or the degrees of freedom contained in the system, not the amount of substances contained in each phase. In practice, if temperature or pressure is specified, the above equation can be written as:

$$f = K-\Phi+1$$

In the above equation, we have assumed that each phase contains the substances of S, and if there is no substance in a phase, it does not affect the form of the phase rule. If the "i"th substance is not in the phase, then the concentration variable of the phase will decrease by one, that is, the total number of variables will decrease by one, but it will also decrease by one in the equation of the chemical potential, so the degree of freedom will not change and the phase rule equation will not change either.

[Example 3–2] Try to figure out the degree of freedom in the following equilibrium system:

(1) At 25℃ and standard pressure, KCl (s) coexisted in equilibrium with its aqueous solution;

(2) I_2 (s) and I_2 (g) are in equilibrium;

(3) In a system where you start with any amount of HCl (g) and NH_3 (g), the reaction HCl (g) + NH_3 (g) = NH_4Cl (s) is at equilibrium.

Solution: (1) $K = 2$, $\Phi = 2$, $f = K - \Phi + 2 = 2 - 2 + 2 = 2$.

Due to the specified temperature and pressure, the concentration of saturated salt water is fixed, and the system has no degree of freedom.

(2) $K = 1$, $\Phi = 2$, $f = K - \Phi + 2 = 1 - 2 + 2 = 1$.

That is, there is a functional relationship between p and T in the system, and only one of them is independently variable.

(3) $S = 3$, $R = 1$, $R' = 0$, $K = 3 - 1 = 2$, $\Phi = 2$, $f = K - \Phi + 2 = 2 - 2 + 2 = 2$.

Temperature, total pressure, and concentration of any gas have two independent variables.

Section 2　One-Component System

For a one-component system, the phase rule can be expressed as:

$$f = K - \Phi + 2 = 1 - \Phi + 2 = 3 - \Phi$$

When the $\Phi = 1$, $f = 2$, it is the double variable system. When $\Phi = 2$, $f = 1$, it is a single variable system. When $\Phi = 3$, $f = 0$, it is zero variable system. For a one-component system, the maximum number of phase is 3, the maximum number of degrees of freedom is 2. There are independent intensive variables, that is, both temperature and pressure are variable. The phase diagram of one-component system can be denoted by p–T graph.

2.1   The p–T phase diagram for water

A p–T phase diagram for pure water is shown in Fig. 3–1.

The one-phase regions are the open areas of AOB, AOC and BOC (AOB is the solid phase region, AOC is the liquid phase region and BOC is the gas phase region). In these one-phase regions, $p=1$ and there are 2 degrees of freedom, in that both p and T must be specified to describe the intensive state.

Along the lines (except at point O), two phases are present in equilibrium. Hence, $\Phi = 2$, $f = 1$ along a line. OC line is the liquid-vapor line of water. OB line is the solid-vapor line of ice. OA line is the solid-liquid line of ice. Once T is fixed, then p, the (equilibrium) vapor pressure of liquid water at temperature T, is fixed. On the other hand, if the p is fixed,

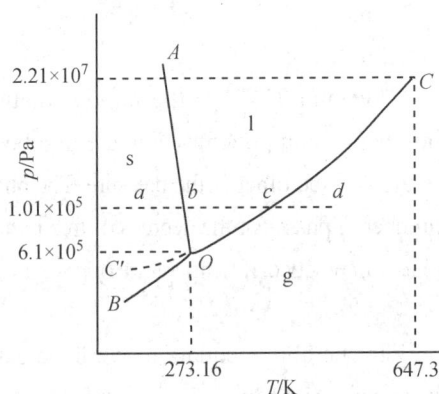

Fig. 3–1   The p–T phase diagram for H_2O

then the T is fixed, it can only be the corresponding temperature on the curve. For example, the vapor pressure of water at 100℃ must be 101.325kPa, the vapor pressure of water at 506.6kPa, the temperature must be 151.1℃, and the vapor pressure of water at 25℃ is 3168Pa.

Fig. 3–1 shows that the boiling point at a given pressure is the maximum temperature at which a stable liquid can exist at that pressure. Line OC gives the boiling point of water as a function of pressure. The H_2O normal boiling point is not precisely 100℃, if T is considered to be the independent variable, line OC gives the vapor pressure of liquid water as a function of temperature. The OC line cannot be extended arbitrarily. It ends at the critical point C, where the temperature is 647.3K and the corresponding pressure is 2.21×10^7Pa. At the critical point, the density of water is equal to that of water vapor, and the gas-liquid interface disappears. If a vertical line is drawn from point C, gas in the area to the left of the vertical line can be liquefied by pressure, while gas in the area to the right of the vertical line cannot be liquefied.

The OB line is a two-phase equilibrium between ice and water vapor (The sublimation line of ice). Any point on the line represents the vapor pressure and temperature (boiling point) at which ice and water vapor balance, and the OB line can theoretically be extended to near absolute zero.

The OA line is the equilibrium between ice and water, and any point on the line represents the relationship between vapor pressure and temperature (melting point) at the equilibrium between water and ice. The OA line also cannot extend upward indefinitely, because when the pressure is 2.0265×10^8Pa, the state diagram becomes more complicated, with six different crystal structures of ice.

The OC' line is an extension of OC line, which represents the metastable equilibrium line between super-cooled water and water vapor. OC' line is above the OB line, and its vapor pressure is higher than that of ice in a stable state at the same temperature, so the super-cooled water is in an unstable state. If a little ice is added to the metastable system, or a little stirring is done, the super-cooled water immediately solidifies.

Point "O" is the intersection of three curves, called triple point. At this point, three phases coexist, $\Phi = 3$, $f = 0$, that is, the temperature and pressure at the triple point are determined by the system and cannot be changed arbitrarily. The triple point of water has a temperature of 273.16K and a pressure of 610.6Pa. It is important to note that the triple point of water is different from the usual freezing point of water. The triple point is strictly for a pure substance, while the freezing point is measured in water with air and external pressure of 101.325kPa. Because of the presence of air in the water, a dilute solution was formed, and the freezing point decreased 0.00242℃ from the triple point. Besides, the vapor pressure of the system at the triple point is 0.6106kPa, while the external pressure of the system at the freezing point is 101.325kPa. Due to the difference in pressure, the freezing point decreases by 0.00747℃, so the freezing point of water decreases by 0.00242+0.00747≈0.01℃ compared with the triple point. It is shown in Fig. 3–2.

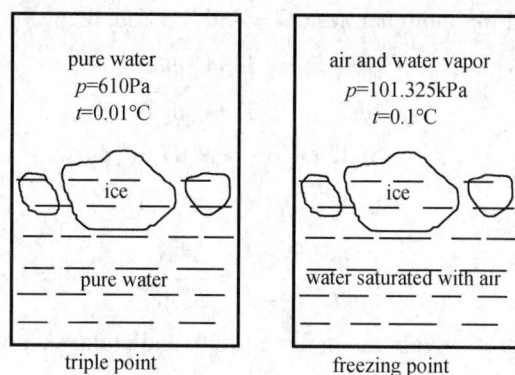

Fig. 3–2 **Triple point and freezing point of water**

The phase diagram can be used to analyze any change process. For example, the isobaric heating process at point "a" is represented by the "$abcd$" horizontal line. Point "a" is ice. When the temperature rises to point "b", the melting point is reached, and liquid water begins to appear. When the ice melts into water and enters the liquid phase, and the temperature rises to point "c", water vapor begins to appear. At this point, the gas and liquid phases coexist, and the water is heated until it is completely vaporized into water vapor, and then enters the gas phase. In addition, the **freeze-drying (冷冻干燥)** process of pharmaceutical preparation can be illustrated by Fig. 3–1: It can be seen from the figure that under pressure and temperature above the triple point "O", a substance can change from solid phase to liquid phase and finally to gas phase. At pressures and temperatures below triple point "O", the solid phase can be changed directly from the liquid phase to the gas phase without passing through the liquid phase. For example, the vapor pressure of ice is 13.3Pa at –40℃ and 1.33Pa at –60℃. If the pressure on the ice at –40℃ is reduced to 1.33Pa, the solid ice will directly turn into water vapor and then turn into ice again on the cooling surface at –60℃. Similarly, sublimation can also occur if ice at –40℃ is heated to –20℃ at 13.3Pa.

Sublimation has important applications in the pharmaceutical technology, such as freeze drying. The drug solution is rapidly and deeply frozen into ice in a short time and the pressure is lowered below the saturated vapor pressure of the ice to sublimate the ice and remove the solvent. After sealing, the loose spongy powder injection can be stored for a long time.

2.2 Clapeyron – Clausius equation

For a one-component system, there is a certain functional relationship between temperature and pressure at two-phase equilibrium, which can be derived from the phase equilibrium condition.

At a certain temperature and pressure, the two-phase equilibrium of a one-component system meets the following conditions:

$$G_m^\alpha(T,p) = G_m^\beta(T,p)$$

If the temperature of the system changes from T to $T + dT$, and the pressure correspondingly changes from p to $p + dp$, then the molar Gibbs function of the system changes to $G_m^\alpha + dG_m^\alpha$, $G_m^\beta + dG_m^\beta$ respectively, and the new equilibrium is reached, then

$$G_m^\alpha + dG_m^\alpha = G_m^\beta + dG_m^\beta$$

Since
$$G_m^\alpha = G_m^\beta$$

So
$$dG_m^\alpha = dG_m^\beta$$

From the basic formula of thermodynamics $dG = -SdT + Vdp$, then

$$dG_m^\alpha = -S_m^\alpha dT + V_m^\alpha dp$$

$$dG_m^\beta = -S_m^\beta dT + V_m^\beta dp$$

Then
$$-S_m^\alpha dT + V_m^\alpha dp = -S_m^\beta dT + V_m^\beta dp$$

$$(V_m^\beta + V_m^\alpha)dp = (S_m^\beta - S_m^\alpha)dT$$

So
$$\frac{dp}{dT} = \frac{S_m^\beta - S_m^\alpha}{V_m^\beta - V_m^\alpha} = \frac{\Delta_\alpha^\beta S_m}{\Delta_\alpha^\beta V_m} \tag{3-2}$$

where, G_m^α, G_m^β, V_m^α, V_m^β are respectively the molar entropy and molar volume of the α, β phase.

Since
$$\Delta_\alpha^\beta S_m = \frac{\Delta_\alpha^\beta H_m}{T}$$

Substituting to (3–2), then

$$\frac{dp}{dT} = \frac{\Delta_\alpha^\beta H_m}{T \cdot \Delta_\alpha^\beta V_m} \tag{3-3}$$

Equation (3–3) is **Clapeyron equation (克拉贝龙方程)**.

The Clapeyron equation shows the change rate of pressure with temperature when the two phases of a one-component system are in equilibrium. Since the equation is not specified in its derivation, it can be applied to the two-phase equilibrium of any pure substance.

If the Clapeyron equation is applied to the gas-solid two-phase equilibrium or gas-liquid equilibrium system, and the vapor is assumed to be an ideal gas, and since the molar volume of the liquid or solid phase is much smaller than that of the gas phase, it can be approximated.

$$\frac{dp}{dT} = \frac{\Delta_\alpha^\beta H_m}{T\Delta_\alpha^\beta V_m} \approx \frac{\Delta_\alpha^\beta H_m}{T \cdot V_m} = \frac{\Delta_\alpha^\beta H_m}{T\left(\frac{RT}{p}\right)} = \frac{p\Delta_\alpha^\beta H_m}{RT^2} \tag{3-4}$$

Or
$$\frac{d\ln p}{dT} = \frac{\Delta_\alpha^\beta H_m}{RT^2} \tag{3-5}$$

Equation (3–4) or (3–5) is the **Clapeyron-Clausius equation (克拉贝龙–克劳修斯方程)**. This formula is applicable not only to gas-liquid two-phase equilibrium, but also to gas-solid two-phase equilibrium. Because the Clapeyron-Clausius equation does not require the value of $\Delta_\alpha^\beta H_m$, it is more convenient than the Clapeyron equation, but it is less accurate than the Clapeyron equation.

If formula (3-5) is integrated between T_1 and T_2, then

$$\ln\frac{p_2}{p_1}=\frac{\Delta_\alpha^\beta H_m(T_2-T_1)}{RT_1T_2} \tag{3-6}$$

This equation is the integral form of the Clapeyron-Clausius equation. The formula can be used to calculate the vapor pressure at different temperatures, boiling point or latent heat of phase change at different external pressures.

In the absence of accurate molar enthalpy data for liquid evaporation, **Trouton empirical rule (特鲁顿经验规则)** can be used to obtain an estimated value. For general non-polar liquids

$$\Delta_1^g H_m = T_b\Delta_1^g S_m \approx T_b \cdot 88\,\text{J}\cdot\text{mol}^{-1}\cdot\text{K}^{-1} \tag{3-7}$$

where, T_b is the boiling point when the external pressure of the liquid is 101325Pa, and $\Delta_1^g S_m$, $\Delta_1^g H_m$ respectively represents the change in molar entropy and molar enthalpy of the liquid when it evaporates.

[Example 3-3] On the Tibetan plateau, with an average altitude of 4500m, the atmospheric pressure is 5.73×10^4Pa. Calculate the boiling point of water there. The heat of vaporization of water is 40.64J·mol^{-1}.

Solution:

$$\ln\frac{p_2}{p_1}=\frac{\Delta_\alpha^\beta H_m(T_2-T_1)}{RT_1T_2}$$

$$\ln\frac{100}{57.3}=\frac{40640(373-T_1)}{8.314\times373T_1}$$

Then
$$T_1=358\text{K}=85℃$$

It is shown that the boiling point of the water there is only 85℃.

Section 3　Two-Component Gas-Liquid System

According to mutual dissolubility of two liquid components, gas-liquidphase diagram of two component systems can be divided into three types, including perfectly miscible system, partially miscible system and full immiscible system. For two-component system, $K=2$, the phase rule is: $f = K - \Phi + 2 = 4 - \Phi$, the minimum value of Φ is 1, and the maximum value of f is 3, there are three independent intensive variable, T, p and composition x. To describe the full state of a two-component system, a three-dimensional phase diagram is required. For convenience, we usually keep one variable constant and plot a two-dimensional phase diagram. This amounts to taking a cross section of a three-dimensional plot. Thus, we can get p–x phase diagram with constant T or T–x phase diagram with constant p comparably for common use. Similarly, we also can get T–p phase diagram with constant composition, but which is not frequently used.

PPT

3.1 Two-component gas-liquid phase diagram of perfectly miscible ideal liquid mixture

Instead of plotting complete phase diagram, we shall usually consider only one part of the phase diagram at a time. This section deals with the gas–liquid part of the phase diagram of a two-component ideal liquid mixture system

3.1.1 Two-component vapor pressure-composition (*p-x*) diagram of ideal liquid mixture

For a two-component system, if the vapor phase is treated as an ideal gas, then Dalton's law of partial pressures says that the total pressure p is the sum of the individual partial pressures. This becomes

$$p = p_A + p_B \tag{3-8}$$

From the Raoult's law

$$p_A = p_A^* x_A \qquad p_B = p_B^* x_B \tag{3-9}$$

That is

$$p = p_A + p_B = p_A^* x_A + p_B^* x_B \tag{3-10}$$

where, p_A^* is saturated vapor pressure of pure A and p_B^* is saturated vapor pressure of pure A. x_A and x_B are the mole fractions of component A and B in the liquid phase, respectively. Because the sum of the mole fractions of the liquid phase must equal 1, so we have

$$x_A + x_B = 1, \text{ or } x_A = 1 - x_B$$

After substitution, the formula (3-10) may be expressed as

$$p = p_A^* (1 - x_B) + p_B^* x_B = p_A^* + (p_B^* - p_A^*) x_B \tag{3-11}$$

If we plot total pressure versus mole fraction of component B, we would get a straight line as shown in Fig. 3-3. Fig. 3-3 suggests that there is a smooth, linear variation in total vapor pressure from p_A^* to p_B^* as the composition of the solution varies.

What are the mole fractions of the two components in the vapor phase? They are not equal to the mole fractions of the liquid phase. We use the variables y_A and y_B to represent the mole fractions of A and B in the vapor-phase. According to Dalton's law of partial pressures and Raoult's law, this becomes

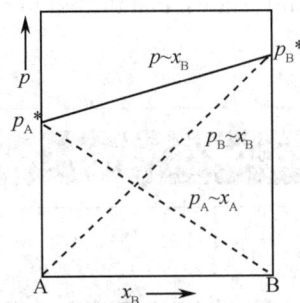

Fig. 3-3　The liquid phase line of p-x_B of ideal liquid mixture

$$y_A = p_A / p = p_A^* x_A / p \tag{3-12}$$

$$y_B = p_B / p = p_B^* x_B / p \tag{3-13}$$

So

$$\frac{y_A}{y_B} = \frac{p_A^* x_A}{p_B^* x_B} \tag{3-14}$$

If $p_B^* > p_A^*$, that is

$$\frac{y_A}{y_B} < \frac{x_A}{x_B}$$

$$x_A + x_B = 1, y_A + y_B = 1 \qquad \frac{1 - y_B}{y_B} < \frac{1 - x_B}{x_B}$$

That is

$$y_B > x_B \quad \text{or} \quad y_A < x_A \tag{3-15}$$

Equation (3–15) shows that the concentration of volatile component with higher vapor pressures in the gas phase is greater than that in the liquid phase, and the concentration of the refractory component with lower vapor pressure is higher in the liquid phase than in the gas phase. This law is known as the **Konowalov's first law(柯诺瓦洛夫第一定律)**. This is why distillation and rectification can separate liquid mixtures.

[Example 3–4] Suppose that ethanol and methanol can form an ideal liquid mixture, the molar fraction of them is 0.5. Given that the vapor pressure of ethanol and methanol at 60℃ is 50kPa and 80kPa respectively. Calculate the composition of the equilibrium vapor of the mixture at 60℃, expressed in mole fraction.

Solution: According to Raoult's law

$$p = p_A + p_B = p_A^* x_A + p_B^* x_B$$
$$= 50 \times 0.5 + 80 \times 0.5 = 65 \, kPa$$

$$p_A = p_A^* x_A = 25 \, kPa \qquad\qquad p_B = p_B^* x_B = 40 \, kPa$$

$$y_A = \frac{p_A}{p} = \frac{25}{65} = 0.385 \qquad\qquad y_B = \frac{p_B}{p} = \frac{40}{65} = 0.615$$

So, y_A is 0.385, y_B is 0.615.

According to the equation (3–11) and (3–13), we can get the formula giving the total pressure as a function of y_B, that is

$$p = \frac{p_A^* p_B^*}{p_B^* + (p_A^* - p_B^*) y_B} \tag{3–16}$$

Thus, we can plot the total pressure of the vapor phase versus the mole fraction of one component y_1. However, it is not an equation for a straight line, instead, it is an equation for a curved line as shown in Fig. 3–4.

According to Fig. 3–4, we can analyze the meanings of points, lines and regions in the phase diagram as follows.

(1) There are three regions in the phase diagram.

Two single phase region: single liquid phase region and single vapor phase region; $\Phi=1$, $f^*=k-\Phi+1=2-1+1=2$ (p and x_B)

One gas-liquid equilibrium phase region: the vapor and liquid phases coexist in equilibrium, $\Phi=2$, $f^*=k-\Phi+1=2-2+1=1$(p or x_B)

(2) There are two lines in the phase diagram.

Line of liquid phase: p–x_B, straight line.

Line of vapor phase: p–y_B, curve line.

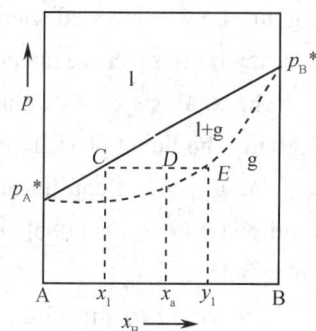

Fig. 3–4   The p-x phase diagram of perfectly miscible ideal liquid mixture

(3) The **system point (物系点)** and the **phase point (相点)**

In the two phase region of p-x diagram, the point "D" stands for the total composition of the system. Draw a line cross point "D" parallel to abscissa, intersect with the liquid phase and vapor phase lines respectively at points "C" and "E". Line CE is called **tie line (联结线)**.

So the point "D" is system point, if system point is fixed, the composition of system x_a will be fixed, the point "C" is liquid phase point and the point "E" is vapor phase point. If the composition of system is x_a, the composition of B in liquid phase is x_1, and the composition of B in vapor phase is y_1.

3.1.2 The level rule

The vapor and liquid phases coexist in equilibrium is shown in Fig. 3–4. According to the material balance principle of component B, we can write $n = n_1 + n_g$ and the overall amount of B is nx_a. The overall amount of B is also the sum of its amounts in the two phases:

$$nx_a = n_1x_1 + n_gy_1$$

So

$$(n_1 + n_g) x_a = n_1x_1 + n_gy_1 \tag{3-17}$$

That is

$$\frac{n_1}{n_g} = \frac{y_1 - x_a}{x_a - x_1} = \frac{\overline{DE}}{\overline{CD}} \tag{3-18}$$

Equation (3–18) is called **the lever rule (杠杆规则)**, which means the relative amount of liquid and vapor phases can be calculated by the rule, that is, the proportions of the two phases are given by the relative lengths of the tie line balanced with the system point as the pivot point. The lever rule can be used in any two-phase equilibrium regions. If the abscissa in the phase diagram is expressed as a mass fraction, then the lever rule

So

$$\frac{m_g}{m_1} = \frac{\overline{DE}}{\overline{CD}} \tag{3-19}$$

By the lever rule, we can calculate the relative amount (the total amount is unknown) or the absolute amount (the total amount is known) of two phases.

3.1.3　Two-component temperature-composition (T-x) diagram of ideal liquid mixture

For ideal liquid mixture, the boiling point-composition diagram is shown in Fig. 3–5. Since the higher the saturated vapor pressure of a liquid, the lower its boiling point, so the T–x diagram and the p–x diagram show an inverted relationship. In addition, the liquidus in the T–x phase diagram is a curve rather than a linear line in the p–x diagram.

The analysis of T–x phase diagram is similar to the p–x phase diagram. The liquid phase region and gas phase region are single phase, $f=2$; The gas-liquid equilibrium region is two phases, $f=1$. The line of liquid phase (T-x_B) is bubble point line and the line of gas phase (T-y_B) is dew point line.

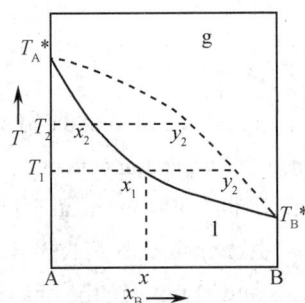

Fig. 3–5　The *T*-*x* diagram of perfectly miscible ideal liquid mixture

According to Fig. 3–5, we can discuss the principle of simple distillation. In the T–x diagram of A–B, the boiling point of pure A is higher than pure B, meaning a higher content of component B in the vapor phase, and also a higher content of component A in the liquid phase When performing a simple distillation, the content of B in the distillate is significantly increased, the content of A is accordingly increased in the residual liquid.

For a two-component solution with a composition of x as shown in Fig. 3–5, it boils at T_1 and the corresponding vapor phase composition is y_1. Obviously, the content of B was significantly increased in the condensing vapor with a composition of y_1, the B content in liquid is decreased. The corresponding liquid composition rises along the line of liquid phase and the boiling point is elevated to T_2, where the gas composition turns out to be y_2. Collecting the fraction between T_1 and T_2, its composition lies between y_1 and y_2. The composition of residual liquid becomes x_2 and the content of A in liquid is increased. A and B are thus roughly separated.

3.2 Two-component gas-liquid phase diagram of perfectly miscible non-ideal liquid mixture

Having examined gas–liquid equilibrium for ideal liquid mixture, we now consider real liquid mixture. Gas–liquid phase diagram for non-ideal liquid mixture systems are obtained by measurement of the pressure and composition of the vapor in equilibrium with liquid of known composition. So there will be deviation, including positive deviation and negative deviation. If the non-ideal liquid mixture is only slightly non ideal, the deviation is general deviation as shown in Fig. 3–6 (a) and (b) in the p–x curve. That is general deviation system, which includes general positive deviation system and general negative deviation system. If the real liquid mixture has a significant deviation from ideality and give a maximum deviation as shown in Fig. 3–6 (c) and (d) in the p–x curve, that is maximum positive deviation system and maximum negative deviation system.

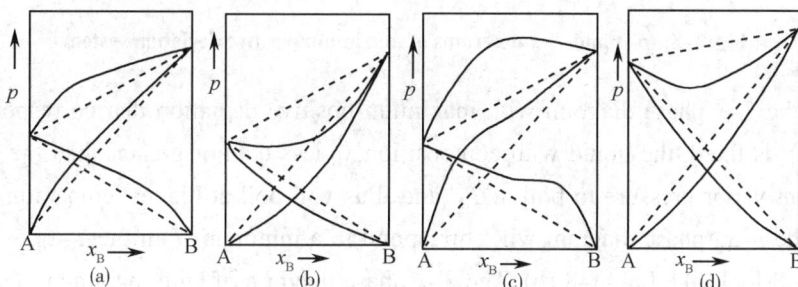

Fig. 3–6 The p–x diagram of perfectly miscible non-ideal solutions

3.2.1 p-x and T-x diagrams of general deviation system

General positive deviation system (一般正偏差) Real vapor pressure is larger than theoretical value calculated by Raoult's law, but in total composition, $p_B^* > p > p_A^*$.

General negative deviation system (一般负偏差) Real vapor pressure is smaller than theoretical value calculated by Raoult's law, but in total composition, $p_B^* > p > p_A^*$.

The phase diagrams of general deviation system are shown in Fig. 3–7 including p–x and T–x diagrams. The analysis of this type of phase diagram is similar to that of ideal liquid mixture, which will not be repeated here.

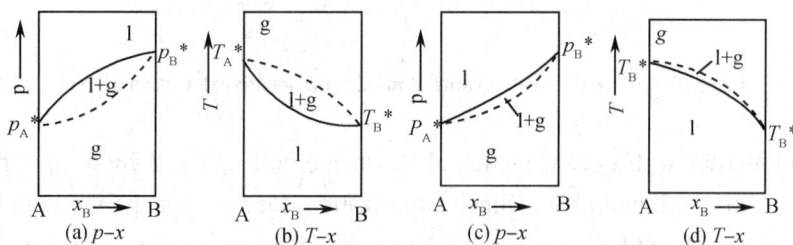

Fig. 3–7 p-x and T-x diagrams of general deviation system

3.2.2 p-x and T-x diagrams of maximum positive deviation and maximum negative deviation system

If the system shows a maximum or minimum p in the p–x curve, the real vapor pressure is larger or smaller than theoretical value calculated by the Raoult's law ($p > p_B^*$, p_A^* or $p < p_A^*$, p_B^*), the phase diagram cannot look like Fig. 3–4 or 3–7. we can draw the phase diagram so that there is a point on the vapor curve with pressure p max or min and the vapor curve overlap with the liquid curve at p max or p min, as shown in Fig. 3–8(a) and 3–8(b).

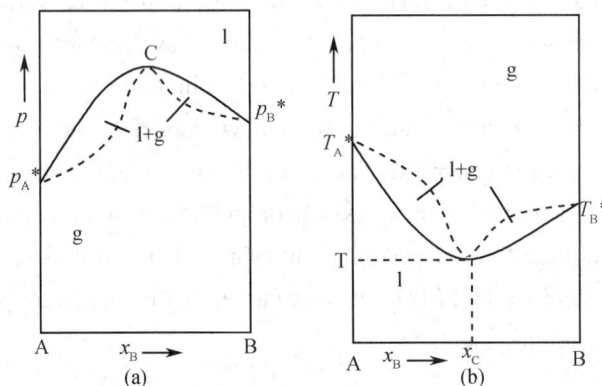

Fig. 3–8 p–x and T–x diagrams of maximum positive deviation system

What does the T–x phase diagram with maximum positive deviation that corresponds to Fig. 3–8 (a) look like? If p is fixed, the liquid with composition x_B less than or greater than the point x_C, it will not have sufficient vapor pressure to boil at T, and thus will boil at higher temperatures. Therefore, a maximum p in the p–x_B phase diagram will correspond to a minimum T in the T–x_B diagram. The T–x phase diagram will look like Fig. 3–8 (b). The T–x phase diagram of with maximum negative deviation that corresponds to Fig. 3–9(a) is shown in Fig. 3–9 (b).

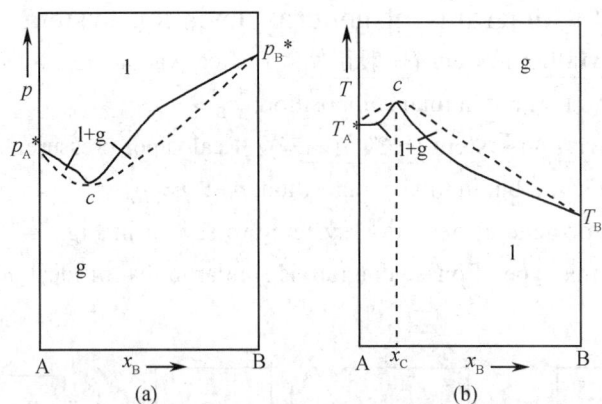

Fig. 3–9 p–x and T–x diagrams of maximum negative deviation system

For the liquid mixture with x_C composition of B, when it boiled, it will yield vapor phase having the same composition with the liquid phase. Since vaporization does not change the liquid's composition, the entire sample of liquid will boil at a constant temperature. Such a constant-boiling solution is called an **azeotrope** (恒沸物) which is a mixture rather than compound and its composition remains constant at constant pressure. If we change the pressure, the temperature of boiling azeotrope and its composition will also change. Thus, an azeotrope can be distinguished from a compound.

The most famous azeotrope is that formed by water and ethanol. When the pressure changes, the azeotropic composition of ethanol-water system changes as shown in Table 3–1. At standard pressure, the azeotropic composition is 95.57% ethanol and the boiling point is 351.31K, which is below the normal boiling points of water and ethanol. Absolute ethanol cannot be prepared by distillation of a dilute aqueous solution of ethanol at standard pressure.

The composition and boiling point of common azeotropic mixture systems are shown in Table 3–2 and 3–3.

Table 3–1 Effect of pressure on composition of ethanol-water azeotrope

Pressure / kPa	101.3	53.3	26.7	21.3	9.33
The azeotropic composition of C_2H_5OH by weight	95.57	96.0	97.5	99.5	100

Table 3–2 The azeotropic mixture having the minimum azeotropic point ($p=p^{\ominus}$)

Component A	Boiling poin /K	Component B	Boiling poin/K	Azeotropic mixture	
				B%(w/w)	Azeotropic point /K
H_2O	373.16	C_2H_5OH	351.5	95.57	351.31
CCl_4	349.91	CH_3OH	337.86	20.56	328.86
CS_2	319.41	CH_3COCH_3	329.31	33	312.36
$CHCl_3$	334.36	CH_3OH	337.86	12.6	326.56
C_2H_5OH	351.46	C_6H_6	352.76	68.24	340.79
C_2H_5OH	351.46	$CHCl_3$	334.36	93	332.56

Table 3–3 The azeotropic mixture having the maximum azeotropic point ($p=p^{\ominus}$)

Component A	Boiling poin /K	Component B	Boiling poin /K	Azeotropic mixture	
				B%(w/w)	Azeotropic point /K
H_2O	373.16	HCl	193.16	20.24	381.74
H_2O	349.91	HNO_3	359.16	68	393.66
H_2O	319.41	HBr	206.16	47.5	399.16
H_2O	334.36	HCOOH	374	77	380.26
$CHCl_3$	351.46	CH_3COCH_3	329.31	20	337.86
C_6H_5OH	351.46	$C_6H_5NH_2$	457.56	58	459.36

3.3 The principle of rectification

There are many types of rectifying towers. Shown in Fig. 3–10 is a schematic diagram of rectifying tower with bubble-cap trays. The bottom of the rectifying tower is the heating region, which has the highest temperature, and the top of the rectifying tower is condenser, which has the lowest temperature. After the rectification, low boiling point component is collected at the top of the tower, high boiling point component left at the bottom.

Illustration the rectification process via the T–x diagram of an ideal fully miscible A-B two-component liquid system is shown in Fig. 3–11. Adding the liquid mixture with composition of "x" to the middle of rectification tower, where the temperature is T_3. The liquid and vapor compositions of state point "O" are x_3 and y_3, respectively.

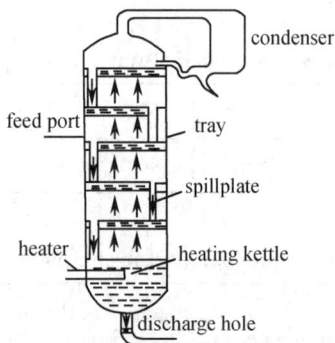

Fig. 3–10 Schematic diagram of the rectifying tower

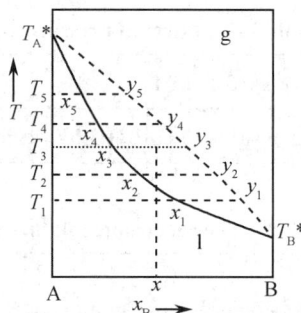

Fig. 3–11 Schematic diagram of rectification process

The vapor phase with composition of y_3 rises in the tower and the temperature decreases to T_2. Part of the liquid with composition of x_2 condenses and the vapor composition becomes y_2, the B content in the vapor is thus increased. The vapor with composition of y_2 continues to rise in the tower and the temperature decreases to T_1, so that until it reaches the top of the tower, where the distillate is almost pure B.

The liquid phase with composition of x_3 drops off the tray after condensation and the temperature rises to T_4. Part of the liquid vaporize and the composition of vapor is y_4, the rest liquid with composition of x_4 further drops off and the temperature continues to increase, the component with high boiling points in the liquid phase increase, so that almost pure A with high boiling point is collected at the bottom of the tower. Every tray experiences a process of heat exchange: the species with high boiling point in vapor condensates on the tray and drops onto the next tray along with the release of condensation heat, while the species with low boiling point in the vapor rises to the above tray after absorbing the heat.

For non-ideal fully miscible two-component liquid mixture systems with large positive and negative deviations, the T–x diagrams is shown in Fig. 3–12. We see that rectification of a solution of two substances that form an azeotrope leads to separation into either pure A and azeotrope or pure B and azeotrope. If the mixture composition lies on the left side of the azeotropic point(if $x_B < x$), only pure A and minimum-boiling azeotrope can be obtained by rectification. If the mixture composition lies on the right side of azeotropic point(if $x_B > x$), only pure B and minimum-boiling azeotrope can be obtained.

Take the water-ethanol system for example, if the ethanol content

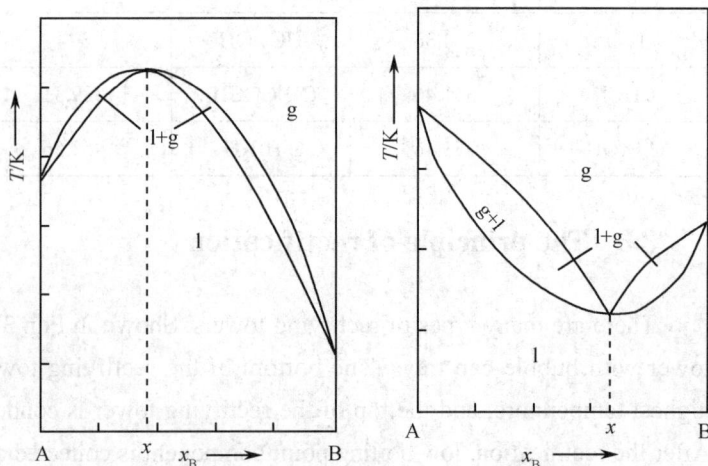

Fig. 3–12 A distillation diagram of a system with azeotropic point

is less than 95.57% (minimum azeotropic point), pure ethanol can never be obtained by rectification. Only by adding water absorbent like $CaCl_2$ or molecular sieves to make the ethanol content exceed over 95.57%, pure ethanol can be obtained from rectification.

3.4   Perfectly immiscible liquid system —— steam distillation

If the solubility of liquids A and B is negligibly small, such as, water-**chlorobenzene (氯苯)**, water- **benzene (苯)**, the vapor pressure is very close to that of the pure component, where the total vapor pressure equals to the sum of the saturated vapor pressure of the two pure components, that is $p = p_A{}^* + p_B{}^*$, so it is actually futile to cover a layer of water on the surface of mercury to reduce mercury vapor. When the two liquids coexist, regardless of their relative amounts, the total pressure is always larger than that of the single component, and the corresponding boiling point being consistently lower than that of the single component.

As shown in Fig. 3–13, OA, OB and OC curves are vapor pressure curves of chlorobenzene, water, and the mixture of water and chlorobenzene. When external pressure is standard pressure, the boiling points of chlorobenzene and water are 403.15K and 373.15K respectively. However, the boiling point is 364K for the mixture of water and chlorobenzene. That is, if chlorobenzene is

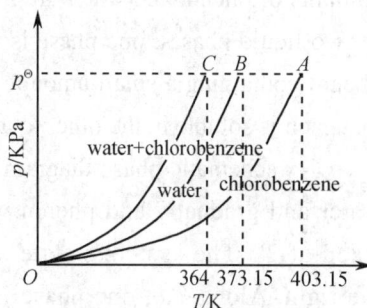

Fig. 3–13   Vapor pressure curve of water, chlorobenzene and the mixture of water and chlorobenzene

distilled together with water, chlorobenzene vaporizes below its boiling point, which is the basic principle of **steam distillation (水蒸气蒸馏)** method.

Steam distillation is especially suitable for extracting volatile active components from plant drugs such as mint, pepper, turmeric, tangerine peel and other herbs. The efficiency of steam distillation can be evaluated by the **water vapor consumption coefficient (水蒸气消耗系数)**. Suppose that the vapor in steam distillation is an ideal gas, according to the partial pressure law, there are the following relations.

$$p_{H_2O}^* = p \cdot y_{H_2O} = p\frac{n_{H_2O}}{n_B + n_{H_2O}} \qquad p_B^* = p \cdot y_B = p\frac{n_B}{n_B + n_{H_2O}}$$

Thus

$$\frac{p_{H_2O}^*}{p_B^*} = \frac{n_{H_2O}}{n_B} = \frac{m_{H_2O}/M_{H_2O}}{m_B/M_B} = \frac{M_B \cdot m_{H_2O}}{M_{H_2O} \cdot m_B}$$

We can write

$$\frac{m_{H_2O}}{m_B} = \frac{p_{H_2O}^* M_{H_2O}}{p_B^* M_B} \tag{3-20}$$

where, p is the total vapor pressure of the system, $p_{H_2O}^*$ and p_B^* false represent the partial pressure of pure water and pure component B respectively; $y_{H_2O}^*$ false and y_B are the mole fraction of H_2O and component B in the gas phase; M_{H_2O} and M_B represent the molar mass of H_2O and component B, respectively; m_{H_2O} and m_B represent the mass of water and component B in the distillate, respectively.

$\dfrac{m_{H_2O}}{m_B}$ is called the water vapor consumption coefficient, and the smaller the vapor consumption factor, the more efficient the vapor distillation.

Section 4　Two-Component Liquid-Liquid System with the Highest Critical Dissolution Temperature

Due to the difference in polarity and other properties, the two liquids cannot be completely soluble, which is called partially miscible two-liquid system, such as water- phenol system. When roughly equal amounts of phenol and water are mixed together at room temperature, we can obtain a system consisting of two liquid phases: one phase is water containing a small amount of dissolved phenol, and the other is phenol containing a small amount of dissolved water. These two liquids are partially miscible, meaning that each is soluble in the other to a limited extent.

T–x schematic phase diagram of water-phenol is shown in Fig. 3–14. Imagining we start with pure water and gradually add phenol while keeping the temperature fixed at T_1. The system's state starts moving horizontally to the right. Along $T_1 a$, one phase is present, a dilute solution of solute phenol in solvent water. At point "a", we have reached the maximum solubility of liquid phenol in liquid water at T_1. Addition of more phenol then produces two phase system for all points between "a" and "b": one phase is a dilute saturated solution of phenol in water and has composition x_1, another phase is a dilute saturated solution of water in phenol and has composition x_2. The overall composition of the two-phase system at a typical point "o" (system point) is x_3. The relative amounts of the two phases present in equilibrium are given by the lever rule.

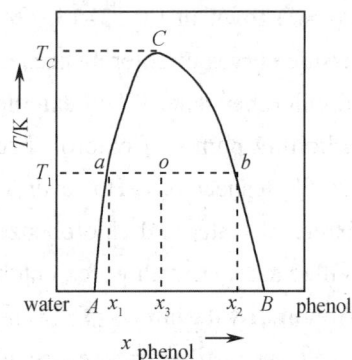

Fig. 3–14　The T–x of water–phenol phase diagram (The pressure is fixed)

[Example 3–5] The water-phenol system is known to be a conjugate solution at 30℃. The mass fraction of phenol in the two liquid phases was 8.75% (W_1) and 69.9% (W_2), respectively. When the system with 100g phenol and 200g water reaches liquid-liquid equilibrium at 30℃, what is the mass of each liquid phase?

Solution:

The mass fraction of phenol in the system is

$$w_{phenol} = \frac{100}{100+200} = 0.3333$$

Let the mass of the water phase be m_1 and the mass of the phenol phase be m_2. According to the lever rule

$$\frac{m_1}{m_2} = \frac{w_2 - w_{phenol}}{w_{phenol} - w_1} = \frac{0.699 - 0.333}{0.333 - 0.0875} = 1.4908$$

$$m_1 + m_2 = 300$$

So:　　　　　　　　$m_1 = 179.6g$　　　$m_2 = 120.4g$

The curve of AC means the change of solubility of phenol dissolved in water. The curve of BC means the change of solubility of water dissolved in phenol. As the temperature increases, the region of liquid-

liquid immiscibility decreases, until at T_C it shrinks to zero. T_C is called the **highest critical dissolution temperature (最高临界溶解温度).** Above T_C, the liquids are completely miscible. As the critical point is approached, the properties of two phases become more and more alike, until at the critical point the two phases become identical, yielding a one-phase system. In the single-phase region, f^* is 2(f^*=2-1+1=2) and in the two-phase region, f^* is 1(f^*=2-2+1=2).

Phase diagrams of this type also include water-**aniline (苯胺)** systems and water-**n-butanol(正丁醇)** system, etc.

Section 5   Two-Component Solid-Liquid System for Forming a Simple Eutectic Mixture

PPT

We now discuss the solid-liquid phase of two-component for forming a **simple eutectic mixture (简单低共熔混合物)**. The effect of pressure on solids and liquids is slight, so we can holds p fixed and examine the T–x_B solid–liquid phase diagram. According to the phase law, f^*=K-Φ+=3-Φ, when f^*=0, Φ_{max}=3, which means that two-component solid-liquid systems coexist at most three phases.

5.1   Drawing the phase diagram by thermal analysis method

One way to determine the solid-liquid phase diagram is by **thermal analysis method (热分析法)** in which a mixture of known composition is heated above its melting point and then allowed to cool slowly. We can record the temperature variation with time during the cooling process, namely **cooling curve (步冷曲线)**, as shown in Fig. 3–15. When the new phase formation, latent heat is released, accompanied with a change in the slope of cooling curve. When Φ =2, then f^*=1, cooling curve will occur a turning point; When Φ =3, then f^*=0, cooling curve will appear a horizontal line (a platform). According to the turning point and horizontal line of cooling curve, we can mark the corresponding points in the T–x phase diagram, then we can get the eutectic T–x diagram.

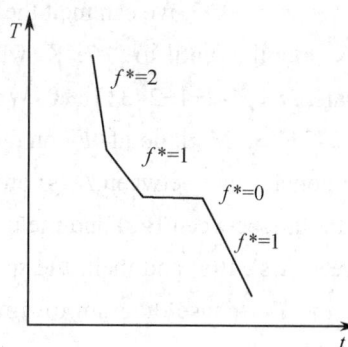

Fig. 3–15   The schematic of cooling curve.

Now, we take a system of o-nitro chlorobenzene (A) and p-nitro chlorobenzene(B) for example, referring to Fig. 3–16, where (a) shows the cooling curves of five samples mole fraction of B from 0 to 1, (b) is the T–x phase diagram obtained.

5.1.1   Curve a and e

When the sample is pure A (x_B= 0), we can get the cooling curve a. Horizontal line appears at 305K, where A (s) appears. The solidification heat offsets the natural cooling. The temperature remains constant, where the degrees of freedom is f^*=K-Φ+1=1-2+1=0. When all liquid melt becomes solid, Φ=1, f^*=1, then the temperature continues to drop. So the melting point of A is 305K. Similarly, on cooling curves e,

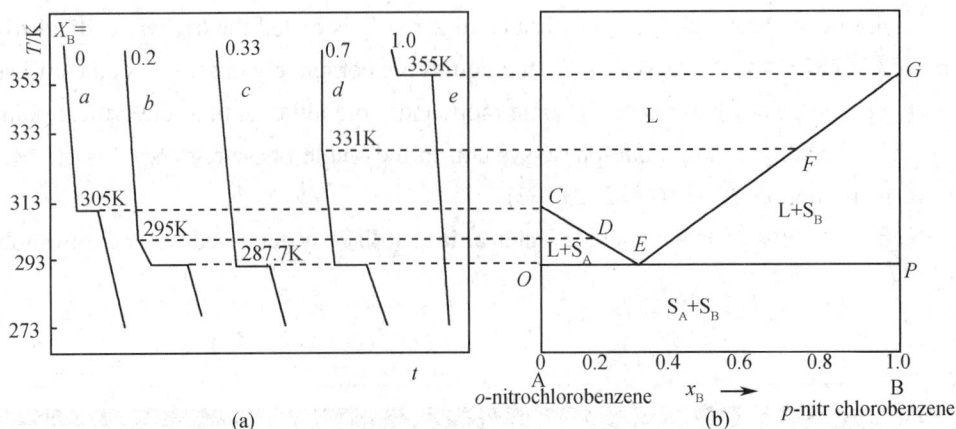

Fig. 3–16　Cooling curve and *T–x* phase diagram of *o*-nitro chlorobenzene and *p*-nitro chlorobenzene system

the melting point of B is 355K. Mark "*C* " and "*G*" points correspondingly on the *T–x* diagram.

5.1.2　Curve *b* and *d*

Melting the mixture of x_B=0.2, recording the cooling curve as show in curve b. At 295K, the curve turns, where A(s) precipitates. The cooling rate slows down, $f^*=K-\Phi+1=2-2+1=1$. Down to 287.7K, B (s) also precipitates, where temperature of the systems remains constant, $f^*=2-3+1=0$; Then the temperature will once again begins to drop, $f^*=2+1-2=1$. A similar cooling curve d can be found for the mixture containing x_B=0.7, but at the turning point(331K), B(s) precipitates first. We can mark the corresponding turning points "*D*" and "*F*" on the *T-x* diagram.

5.1.3　Curve *c*

When x_B=0.33, we can melt the solids and record the corresponding cooling curve *c*. The temperature drops smoothly until to 287.7K, where A(s) and B(s) precipitate simultaneously, and a horizontal line appears, $f^*=K-2+1=2-3+1=0$. When all liquid melt solidifies, the temperature will again drop further, $f^*=2-2+1=1$. Mark point "*E*" on the *T–x* diagram, Connect points "*C*", "*D*" and "*E*", forming the liquid-solid contact line between A (s) and melt; Connect points "*G*", "*F*" and "*E*", forming the liquid-solid contact line between B(s) and melt; Connecting points *D*, *E* and *G*, forming the triple phase contact line between A(s), B(s) and melt; the specific component of the melt is expressed from point "*E*". Then we have the *T–x* phase diagram of *o*-nitrochlorobenzene and *p*-nitrochlorobenzene system shown in Fig. 3–16 (b).

5.2　Analysis of the phase diagram

According to the Fig. 3–17, we can analysis the meanings of points, lines and regions in the phase diagram.

(1) There are four phase regions in the phase diagram:

Above line *CDE*, melt(l) single phase region, $f^*=2$;

Within *CDE*, A(s)+l, two-phase region, $f^*=1$;

Within *EFG*, B(s)+l, two-phase region, $f^*=1$;

Below the line *OEP*, A(s) +B(s), two-phase region, $f^*=1$.

(2) There are three multiphase equilibrium curves:

Line *CDE*, A(s)+melt solid-liquid coexistence line;

Line *EFG*, B(s)+melt solid-liquid coexistence line; The relationship between the quantities of the two phases can also be calculated according to the lever rule. For example, at system point *c*, we can draw the tie line *FM*, thus, $\frac{m_B}{m_1} = \frac{\overline{Fc}}{\overline{cM}}$.

Line *OEP*, A(s)+ melt + B(s) triple phase equilibrium line, the corresponding components of these three phases are reflected in the points of "*O*", "*E*" and "*P*", respectively. Lines *CDE* and *EFG* indicate respectively the decrease of the freezing point of the mixture with the increase of the B and A.

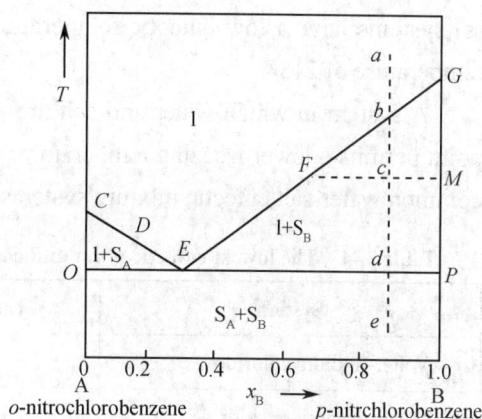

Fig. 3–17 Phase diagram analysis of *o*-nitro chlorobenzene (A) and *p*-nitro chlorobenzene (B) system

(3) There are three special points in the phase diagram:

Point "*C*" and point "*G*" are the freezing points or melting points of the pure A(s) and the pure B (s);

Point "*E*" is three phase coexistence point, A (s) + melt + B (s).

The temperature corresponding to point "*E*" is lower than those of points "*C*" and "*G*", point "*E*" is called **eutectic point (共熔点)**, and the corresponding mixture is called **the lowest eutectic mixture (最低共熔混合物)**, which is not a compound, but comprising two well-mixed phases. The temperature at point E will change with external pressure.

In addition, according to the *T-x* phase diagram, we can also draw the cooling curve. For example, we can plot the cooling curve of the system from point "*a*" to point "*e*" in Fig. 3–17.

5.3 Application of phase diagrams

5.3.1 Determining the purity of the sample by the mixed melting point method

The determination of melting point is a common method to evaluate the purity of samples. It can be seen from the above phase diagram that if there are impurities in the pure sample, the melting point must decrease. The higher the impurity content is, the more the melting point decreases. The mixed melting point method is to measure the melting point of the sample after it is mixed with the standard substance. If the measured melting point is significantly lower than that of the standard substance, it indicates that the two are not the same substance. If the melting point is the same as that of the standard, they are the same substance.

5.3.2 Preparation of powder

If the low eutectic point of two solid drugs is near or below room temperature, the wetting or liquefaction during preparation is called **low eutectic phenomenon (低共熔现象)**, For example, after mixing 45g **camphor (樟脑)** with 55g **phenyl salicylate (水杨酸苯酯)**, whose melting point is 179℃ and 42℃, the melting point is only 6℃. The prescription or process should be adjusted according to the effect of low eutectic on pharmacology.

Prepare a cryogenic solution. In the process of production and scientific research, different cryogenic solutions can be obtained by preparing appropriate water and salt systems. For example, H_2O-NaCl

(s) systems have a low eutectic temperature of 252K and H$_2$O-CaCl$_2$ (s) systems have a low eutectic temperature of 218K.

A system in which water and salt are prepared according to the composition of the lowest eutectic point permits a lower freezing temperature, which will not solidify above the lowest eutectic point. Some common water-salt eutectic mixture systems are shown in Table 3–4.

Table 3–4 The lowest eutectic point and composition of some common water-salt eutectic mixture systems

System	Lowest eutectic point/K	Low eutectic composition / (salt %)
Water-Sodium chloride	252	23.3
Water-Potassium chloride	262.5	19.7
Water - Ammonium chloride	257.8	18.9
Water - Calcium chloride	218.2	29.9
Water - Ammonium sulfate	254.1	39.8

Section 6   Three-Component System

6.1   Composition representation and characteristics of three-component system

For a three-component system, $f = 3 - \Phi + 2 = 5 - \Phi$, $\Phi_{min} = 1$, there are 4 degrees of freedom. To make a two-dimensional plot, we must hold two variables fixed. We shall hold both T and p fixed and use equilateral triangle coordinates to represent the phase diagram of a three-component system.

Take the three-component system composed of A, B and C as an example, and we get the Fig. 3–18(a). The corner of the triangle labeled A, B and C correspond to the pure components A, B and C, respectively. The three edges represent three two-component systems respectively. For example, the edge AB represents a two-component system composed of A and B. The point in the triangle represents a system consisting of three components: A, B and C. The edge *BC* represents the mass fraction of component C from 0 to 1. The edge *CA* represents the mass fraction of component A from 0 to 1, and the edge *AB* represents the mass fraction of component B from 0 to 1.

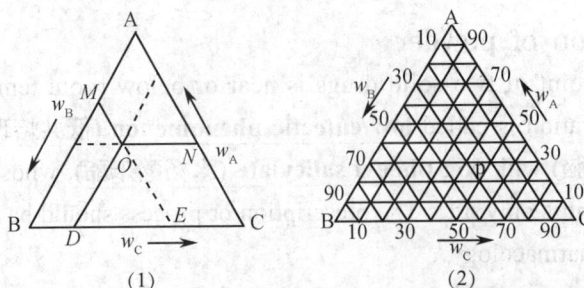

Fig. 3–18   Diagram for plotting the composition of a three- component system

For example, the state point "O", its composition can be determined by the following methods: Making parallel lines parallel to BC, CA and AB at "O" point, they intersect the three edges at points "N", "M" and "D" respectively. So in this three-component system, the mass fraction of A is equal to CN, the mass fraction of B is equal to AM, and the mass fraction of C is equal to BD, Obviously, CN+AM+BD=AC=AB=BC=100%. As shown in Fig. 3-18(b), the composition of this system "P" is that the mass fraction of A is 20 percent, the mass fraction of B is 30 percent, and the mass fraction of C is 50 percent. So any overall composition of the system can be represented by a point in or on the triangle.

An equilateral triangle represents the phase diagram of a three-component system with the following characteristics:

(1) The principle of equal content on a line parallel to side BC which is opposite to vertex A, the overall mass fraction of A is constant. As shown in Fig. 3-19, points "d", "e" and "f" on the line parallel to the bottom edge BC, which have the same percentage of A in the system.

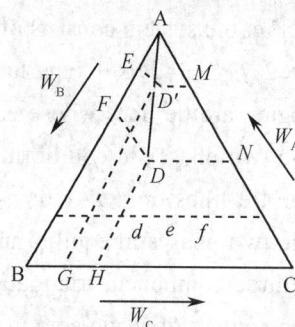

Fig. 3-19 The characteristics (1) and (2) of equilateral triangular coordinates

(2) The principle of equal proportions As shown in Fig. 3-19, we make a line AD through vertex A. All of the systems on the line, the percentage ratio of B to C must be the same. For example, the system points "D" and "D'", the percentage of component B is AE and AF, and the percentage of component C is BG and BH, respectively. That will be:

$$\frac{AE}{AF} = \frac{AD'}{AD} = \frac{BG}{BH} \quad \text{or} \quad \frac{AE}{BG} = \frac{AF}{BH}$$

That is, the ratio of components B and C in D and D' systems is equal.

(3) The lever rule of three-component system. If two three-component systems, "D" and "E", are mixed to form a new three-component system, the new system point "O" must fall on the DE line, as shown in Fig. 3-20. The position of "O" points on the line can be calculated according to the lever rule.

(4) The principle of the center of gravity. If three three-component systems, "F", "M" and "N", are mixed to form a new three-component system, the new system point "Q" must fall on the center of gravity of triangle FMN, as shown in Fig. 3-20. The position of the "O" point on the line can also be calculated based on the lever principle.

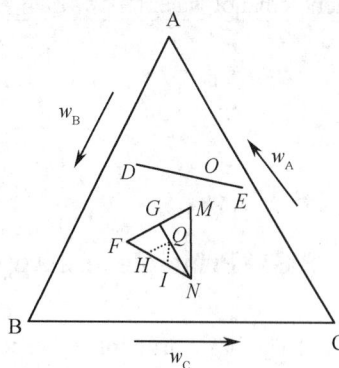

Fig. 3-20 The characteristics (3) and (4) of equilateral triangular coordinates

6.2 The phase diagram of partially miscible three-component system

We shall only consider a pair of partially miscible three-component system such as acetic acid-chloroform-water (醋酸-三氯甲烷-水)system. Consider the system at constant temperature and pressure, water and acetic acid are completely miscible with each other, chloroform and acetic acid are completely miscible with each other, and water and chloroform are partly miscible.

As shown in Fig. 3–21, the curve *DOE* represents the mutual solubility of chloroform and water in the presence of acetic acid. This curve divides the phase diagram into two regions. The region above curve *DOE* is a one-phase area, $\Phi=1$, $f^{**}=3-1+0=2$. For a point in the region below this curve, the system consists of two liquid phases in equilibrium, $\Phi=2$, $f^{**}=3-2+0=1$. The lines a_1b_1, a_2b_2, a_3b_3 and a_4b_4 in this region are tie lines whose endpoints give the compositions of the two phases in equilibrium. For a two-component system, the tie lines on a *T–x* or *p–x* diagram are horizontal, since the two phases in equilibrium have the same *T* and *p*. But on

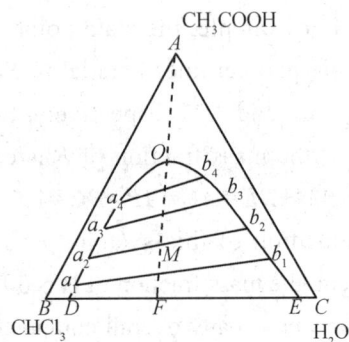

Fig. 3–21 Liquid-liquid phase diagram for acetic acid-chloroform-water

a three-component triangular phase diagram, the tie lines are not parallel to the bottom edge because the content of acetic acid in the two phases is not equal. The locations of the tie lines are determined by chemical analysis of pairs of phases in equilibrium.

If the system point is at point "*F*", addition of certain amount of acetic acid to the two-phase mixture of water-chloroform will produce a one-phase solution. Gradually adding acetic acid to the system, the system point will move along the *FA* line to vertex *A*, when it reaches point "*M*", the phase points of the two phases are a_2 and b_2. Continue adding acetic acid to the system, the solubility of water and chloroform increases, and tie lines are shortened, and the phase points of the two phases gradually get close to each other and finally shrink to one point. The "*O*" point is called the critical point. At this point, the system becomes one phase. Thus, acetic acid can promote the mutual dissolution of water and chloroform.

Phase diagrams of this type also include *n*-butyl alcohol-acetic acid-water (正丁醇–醋酸–水) systems, toluene-ethanol-water (甲苯–乙醇–水) system and benzene -ethanol-water (苯–乙醇–水) system, etc.

Expansion Content

Basic Principle and Application of Supercritical Fluid Extraction

1. The basic principle of **supercritical fluid extraction** (超临界流体萃取)

Early in1879, two British researchers, Hannay and Hogarth, discovered that supercritical fluids have significant solubility to both liquid and solid substances. In their study, they observed that metal halides such as potassium iodide and potassium bromide could be dissolved in supercritical ethanol at increased pressure, and the inorganic salts would recalibrate when the system pressure dropped. The experimental observation shows that the extraction capacity of a solvent to solid and liquid in supercritical state is tens of times or even hundreds of times higher than that in normal temperature and pressure.

As a new extraction and separation technology, supercritical fluid extraction (SFE) has been developed in the past 30 years. Dr. Zosel from Germany successfully applied the supercritical carbon dioxide (SC-CO_2) extraction process to the industrial production of coffee bean decaffeination, and formed the first patent on supercritical carbon dioxide extraction. Dr Zosel is credited with discovering the industrial value of SFE. The principle of supercritical fluid extraction (SFE) technology is to control the extraction of components from the target under conditions above the critical temperature and pressure. When the components are recovered to the normal pressure and room temperature, the dissolved components in the supercritical fluid are immediately separated from the supercritical fluid. As an environmentally friendly extraction and separation technology, supercritical fluid extraction has been widely developed and applied in many fields. At present, this technology has been widely used in chemical industry, medicine, spices and food industry.

2. Characteristics of Supercritical Fluid (SCF or SF)

For some pure substances, there are triple points and critical points C, as shown in the figure below:

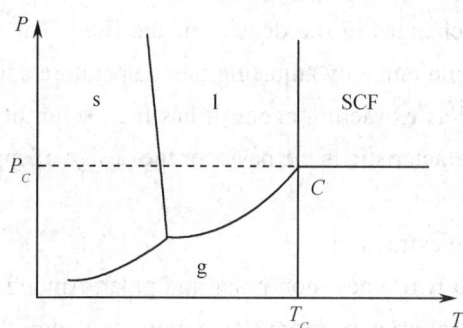

Fig. 3–22　SCF on a p–T diagram　　　　Fig. 3–23　The p–T diagram of CO_2

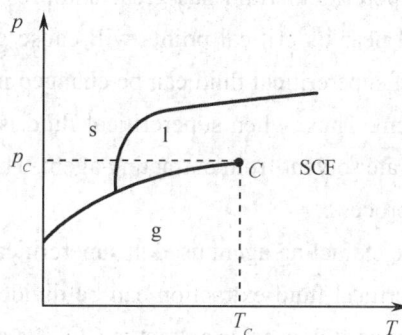

When CO_2 is at the triple point, it is in phase equilibrium of gas, liquid and solid. When it exceeds the critical temperature (T_C) and the critical pressure (p_C), no matter how much pressure is applied, the gas will not liquefy, just increase in density. The properties of the system become uniform rather than gas and liquid, having both the properties of a liquid and the properties of a gas. It is neither a gas nor a liquid, but a special state of matter above the critical pressure and temperature, in the form of a supercritical fluid. In other words, a fluid (gas or liquid) is called supercritical fluid (SCF or SF) when its temperature and pressure exceed its corresponding critical point. Because of its particularity, supercritical fluid has the advantages of both gas and liquid. Its viscosity is small, its diffusion coefficient is large, its density is large, and it has good solubility and mass transfer characteristics. Many substances can be used as SF, such as carbon dioxide, nitric oxide, ammonia, ethylene, propane, propylene, water and so on. Its density is comparable to that of the substance's liquid in its normal state.

According to Fig. 3–23 and Table 3–5, it can be concluded that supercritical fluid has the following four main characteristics.

Table 3–5　Comparison of physical properties of gases, supercritical fluids and liquids

Property ＼ State	Gases	Supercritical fluids	Liquids
Density/(kg · m^{-3})	1.0	7.0×10^2	1.0×10^3
Viscosity/(Pa · s)	$10^{-6} \sim 10^{-5}$	10^{-5}	10^{-4}
Diffusivity/(m^2 · s^{-1})	10^{-5}	10^{-7}	10^{-9}

(1) Because the solubility of solute in the extracting agent is generally proportional to the density, the density of supercritical fluid is close to that of liquid, so that supercritical fluid has the same solubility as liquid.

(2) The diffusion coefficient of supercritical fluid is between that of gas and liquid, its viscosity is close to that of gas, and it has the characteristic of being easy to diffuse and move, so its mass transfer rate is much higher than that of solvent extraction in liquid.

(3) When the fluid state is close to the critical region, the heat of vaporization will drop sharply, and the gas-liquid phase interface disappears at the critical point, when the heat of vaporization is zero. Therefore, the separation near the critical point is more conducive to heat transfer and energy saving than the separation in the gas-liquid equilibrium zone far from the critical point.

(4) Supercritical fluid has great compressibility. Small changes in the pressure and temperature of the fluid near its critical points will cause great changes in the density of the fluid. Therefore, the solubility of supercritical fluid can be changed in a wide range by adjusting the temperature and pressure of the system. Thus, when supercritical fluid is used as extracting agent, it has high solubility and can easily separate solvent from extracting agent. This characteristic is the basis for the design of supercritical extraction process.

(5) The extracting agent used in supercritical fluid extraction.

Supercritical fluid extraction can be divided into two types: non-polar and polar. Among them, the most widely used non-polar extract is CO_2. Its chemical properties are stable, non-toxic, non-flammable, non-corrosive, no pollution, no solvent residue and the ability to dissolve many organic compounds, in the inert environment can avoid the oxidation of products and so on. Up to now, CO_2 has been used as extraction agent in more than 90% of supercritical fluid extraction applications. As far as supercritical fluid extraction is concerned, supercritical CO_2 (SF-CO_2) fluid extraction is the most widely used method for the extraction of Chinese herbal medicine. The main reason is that compared with other conventional extraction methods, this method has the following excellent characteristics.

① Traditional extraction methods often use a large amount of organic solvents, and because of the difficulty of recovery and the loss in the recovery process, organic solvent residues and increased costs. SF-CO_2 extraction is characterized by stable chemical properties, non-toxic, odorless, colorless, non-corrosive, cheap price, easy recovery, easy refining and other advantages, and SF-CO_2 extraction has no solvent residual problems, suitable for the pharmaceutical and food industries.

② Because of the high temperature and longtime of extraction, some heat-sensitive substances in medicinal materials are destroyed by heat. Since the critical temperature of CO_2 is close to room temperature (31.1℃), the extraction temperature of SF-CO_2 selected according to the supercritical fluid extraction conditions can be close to room temperature. It is especially suitable for separating heat-sensitive or easily oxidized components, preventing oxidation and decomposition reactions that may occur in the conventional extraction process, and keeping the original characteristics of each component to the maximum extent.

③ The critical pressure of CO_2 (7.38MPa) is at medium pressure, and the SF-CO_2 extraction pressure selected according to the supercritical fluid extraction conditions is moderate, which is generally easy to achieve at the current industrial level.

④ SF-CO_2 also has the function of anti-oxidation and sterilization, which is beneficial to improve the quality of natural products.

⑤ Due to the good solubility and permeability of SF-CO_2 and the fast diffusion rate, SF-CO_2 extraction is fully extracted and can make full use of traditional Chinese medicine resources.

3. Application of supercritical fluid extraction (SFE)

Traditional natural product separation and refining processes such as pressing, heating, water vapor distillation and solvent extraction often result in the destruction of some of the thermal sensitivity or chemical instability components. It changes the nutrition and unique flavor of food, and the processing process inevitably has solvent residues. Especially with the improvement of people's living standards and the trend of increasingly strict food management around the world, people have been looking for new processing technology of natural products. Since the early 1980s, a lot of research work has been put into the field of supercritical fluid extraction and great progress has been made.

With a long history and a vast territory, China has created and accumulated rich experience in the disease prevention and treatment, forming its unique traditional Chinese medicine theory, which has played a huge role in the prosperity of the Chinese nation. China is rich in resources and varieties of traditional Chinese medicine plants. At the same time, Chinese herbal medicine is very popular because of its characteristics of slow action, long duration, stable curative effect, no side effects and low price. At present, the extraction and preparation of traditional Chinese herbal medicine mostly use water and organic solvents as the solvent, and the extraction takes a long time at a high temperature. This method has problems such as easy loss, decomposition, transformation of active components and residual organic solvents. Supercritical fluid largely avoids the defects of traditional drug extraction process and provides a new method for the modernization of preparation technology and dosage form of traditional Chinese medicine. Although the research and application of supercritical fluid extraction in the extraction of Chinese herbal medicine started late, it has developed rapidly in recent years. This technology has the advantages of being suitable for extracting natural heat-sensitive substances, simple process, convenient operation, high extraction efficiency, low energy consumption, and no solvent residue, which provide a new method of extraction and separation with high efficiency for the modernization of traditional Chinese medicine. Since most Chinese medicinal materials belong to natural plants, the principles and methods of extraction and separation of some natural products can be referred to the extraction of traditional Chinese medicine. Especially with the modernization of traditional Chinese medicine and the improvement of the quality of traditional Chinese medicine, this technology has been very active in domestic research in recent years. At least fifty Chinese herbs have been studied using the SFE method, but most are still in laboratory studies. Only few products have reached industrial production scale. From the Chinese traditional medicine that has been studied, the effective ingredients include alkaloids, quinones, coumarins, lignans, flavonoids, saponins and volatile oils.

Traditional Chinese medicine is the traditional treasure of the Chinese nation. Traditional Chinese herbal compound is multi-component to play the curative effect. Through the combination of traditional Chinese medicine can not only improve and strengthen the curative effect of drugs, but also can reduce the side effects of drugs. SF-CO_2 extraction of Chinese herbal compound must be combined with the efficacy required by traditional Chinese medicine to investigate whether the effective ingredients or effective parts have been extracted and whether their properties are stable. In addition, the synergistic effect and mutual dissolution of traditional Chinese medicine should be considered. This is the reason why SF-CO_2 extraction method has been used to extract traditional Chinese herbal compound, pharmacological research and new drug development literature reports are much less than single traditional Chinese medicine. It is also the most difficult part of traditional Chinese medicine research and the international development. At the same time, it is also a main research direction in the future.

重 点 小 结

相平衡是研究多相平衡系统的状态如何随着温度、压力和组成变化的理论科学，相律是相平衡系统的基本定律。根据实验数据绘制的相图可以直观地表示系统中状态与温度、压力和组成间的相互关系，是研究多相平衡的基本手段。

本章在介绍相、物种数、独立组分数和自由度等基本概念的基础上，重点讨论了单组分系统、完全互溶的理想液态混合物系统、完全互溶的非理想液态混合物系统、部分互溶的双液系统、完全不互溶的双液系统和一对部分互溶的三组分系统的相图的特点和应用。

单组分系统中，以水的相图为例介绍了单组分相图中点、线和各区域的意义。根据水的升华曲线说明了冷冻干燥法的原理；当单组分系统两相平衡时，温度和压力有一定的函数关系，即克拉贝龙 – 克劳修斯方程式，可用于求算液体在不同外压下的沸点和不同温度下的饱和蒸气压。

二组分系统中，分别讨论了完全互溶的理想液态混合物、完全互溶的非理想液态混合物的气液平衡系统的 $p–x$ 相图和 $T–x$ 相图，介绍了系统的类型和对应相图的特点，相图中线的意义、各区域的相数、自由度数。明确了物系点、相点的意义，并推导得到杠杆规则，可用于计算平衡共存两相的量的关系。另外，根据气液平衡系统的 $T–x$ 相图，说明了蒸馏和精馏的原理，可根据系统所属的类型，判断精馏后的产物。根据完全不互溶的双液系统的特点，介绍了水蒸气蒸馏的原理和效率。二组分液 – 液平衡系统中，以水和苯酚的相图为例，讨论了具有最高临界溶解温度系统的 $T–x$ 相图。相图中曲线代表两液体的相互溶解度随温度的变化，在最高临界溶解温度以上，两液体可以任意比例互相溶解。二组分液固平衡系统中，介绍了热分析绘制相图的方法和生成低共熔混合物系统的 $T–x$ 相图的特点。另外，介绍了低共熔相图在药物的配制和检查样品纯度等方面的应用。

三组分系统中，介绍了正三角形坐标的表示方法和特点，以醋酸 – 三氯甲烷 – 水系统为例，详细讨论了一对部分互溶的三组分系统的相图的特点。图中帽形区为两相平衡，帽形区以外为单相。随着醋酸的加入，三氯甲烷和水的相互溶解度逐渐增大，醋酸促进了三氯甲烷和水的相互溶解。

相平衡理论在中药的提取、分离等方面都有着实际的应用。通过本章的学习，对一些基本的相图要熟练掌握，能认识相图并根据相图来分析解决某些实际的问题。

Object detection

I. **Select the correct option for the following problems (one option for each problem).**

1. Which of the following systems is a single-phase system?

    A. Ink

    B. Bleaching powder

    C. Monoclinic sulfur fragments of various sizes

    D. A mixture of dextral and sinistral tartaric acid solid

2. Known, $CaCO_3(s) \rightleftharpoons CaO(s) + CO_2(g)$, in this equilibrium system
　A. $\Phi=3, f=1$ 　　　　　　　　　　B. $\Phi=2, f=2$
　C. $\Phi=2, f=3$ 　　　　　　　　　　D. $\Phi=3, f=2$

3. When the water is in equilibrium at the triple point, and the pressure suddenly increases, what happens to the phase state of the water?
　A. The gas phase and the solid phase disappear, and they all become the liquid phase
　B. The gas phase and the liquid phase disappear and all become the solid phase
　C. The liquid and solid phases disappear and all become the gas phase
　D. The solid phase disappears and the gas and liquid phases coexist

4. In general, the maximum number of phases that can coexist in equilibrium in a two-component system is
　A. 1　　　　　B. 2　　　　　C. 3　　　　　D. 4

5. What systems can the Clapeyron-Clausius equation be used for?
　A. one-component solid - gas and liquid - gas equilibrium system
　B. one-component solid-liquid two phase equilibrium system
　C. one-component solid-solid two phase equilibrium system
　D. any one component two phase equilibrium system

6. At 400K, the vapor pressure of liquid A is 40kPa, and that of liquid B is 60kPa. A and B form an ideal liquid mixture. At equilibrium, the molar fraction of A in the liquid phase is 0.6, and that of B in the gas phase is
　A. 0.31　　　　　B. 0.40　　　　　C. 0.50　　　　　D. 0.60

7. The two-component system composed of A and B has the lowest constant boiling point. The azeotrope is C. If $T_A^* > T_B^*$, the distillate at the top of the rectifying column after rectification is
　A. pure A　　　　B. pure B　　　　C. azeotrope C　　　D. pure A and pure B

8. Equation $\dfrac{d\ln p}{dT} = \dfrac{\Delta H}{RT^2}$ applies to which of the following equilibrium
　A. C (graphite) $\rightleftharpoons$ C(diamond)
　B. $Hg_2Cl_2(s) \rightleftharpoons 2HgCl(g)$
　C. $Hg(s) \rightleftharpoons Hg(g)$
　D. $H_2O(s) \rightleftharpoons H_2O(l)$

9. A two-component system consisting of A and B has the minimum azeotropic point. At the minimum azeotropic point of its T-x phase diagram
　A. $f=0, y_B=x_B$　　B. $f=1, y_B=x_B$　　C. $f=0, y_B>x_B$　　D. $f=1, y_B>x_B$

10. The necessary condition for steam distillation is
　A. the boiling points of the two liquids are similar
　B. both liquids have high vapor pressure
　C. external pressure less than 101kPa
　D. the two liquids do not dissolve in each other or have little solubility

II. Select the correct options for the following problem (at least two options for each problem).

1. Among the points in the following phase diagram, the states of the system that do not belong to a single phase are

A. the minimum azeotropic point   B. the critical point

C. the melting point   D. the eutectic point

2. A and B form an ideal liquid mixture. The mole fractions of A and B in the liquid phase are x_A and x_B, and in the gas phase are y_A and y_B. If $T_A^* > T_B^*$ false, which of the following are incorrect?

     A. $x_A > y_B$ B. $x_A < y_B$ C. $x_A = y_B$ D. $y_B > x_B$

3. In a two-component system T–x or p–x phase diagram, in which of the following regions are system and phase points different?

     A. Single phase region

     B. Two phase equilibrium region

     C. Three phase line

     D. Gas liquid equilibrium line

4. In the description of the azeotrope, the following statements are correct

     A. Has a constant composition as does a compound at a certain external pressure

     B. The boiling point is independent of the external pressure

     C. At equilibrium, the composition of the gas and liquid phases is the same

     D. The constant boiling point varies with external pressure

5. Which of the following statements is true about the scope of the lever rule?

     A. Not suitable for one - component systems

     B. Applicable to any phase region of a two-component system

     C. Suitable for the two equilibrium phases of a two-component system

     D. Suitable for two equilibrium phases of a three-component system

Ⅲ. Try to answer the following problem.

1. What is the difference between the number of component and the number species?

2. When the temperature is the same but the pressure is different, can two phases reach equilibrium? If the pressure in the two phases is the same but the temperature is different, can the two phases reach equilibrium?

3. What are the number of component and the degrees of freedom of the following balanced system?

     A. NH_4Cl (s) is partially decomposed into NH_3(g) and HCl (g)

     B. If a small amount of NH_3(g) is added to the system above

     C. NH_4HS(s) are balanced with any amount of NH_3(g) and H_2S(g)

     D. C(s), O_2(g), CO(g) and CO_2(g) reach equilibrium at 100 ℃

Reference answers

Ⅰ. 1. C;   2. A;   3. A;   4. D;   5. A;   6. C;   7. C;   8. C;   9. A;   10. D.

Ⅱ. 1. ACD;   2. ABC;   3. BCD;   4. ACD;   5. ACD.

Ⅲ. Omitted.

Chapter 4　Electrochemistry

Much of chemistry involves species that have charge. Electrons, cations, and anions are all charged particles that interact chemically. Often electrons move from one chemical species to another to form something new. These movements can be spontaneous, or they can be forced. They can involve systems as simple as hydrogen and oxygen atoms, or as complex as a million-peptide rote in chain. The presence and the value of discrete charges on chemical species introduce a new aspect that we must consider. In considering how charged particles interact, we have to understand the work involved in moving charged particles together and apart, and the energy required to perform that work. Energy, work-these are concepts of thermodynamics. Therefore, our understanding of the chemistry of electrically charged particles, **electrochemistry (电化学)**, is based on thermodynamics.

Electrochemistry is the science of studying the inter-conversion of electrical energy and chemical energy and the related laws in the transformation process. Two aspects are mainly involved. In a **galvanic cell (原电池)**, a chemical reaction produces a flow of electric current, and the chemical energy is converted into the electrical energy. In an **electrolytic cell (电解池)**, a flow of current produces a chemical reaction, and the electrical energy from an external source is converted into chemical energy.

The term electrochemical cell indicates either a galvanic cell or an electrolytic cell. Galvanic cells and electrolytic cells are quite different from each other, and this chapter deals mainly with galvanic cells.

Few people realize the widespread application of electrochemistry in modern life. All batteries and fuel cells can be understood in terms of electrochemistry. Any oxidation-reduction process can be considered in electrochemical terms. The corrosions of metals, nonmetals, and ceramics are electrochemistry. Many vitally important biochemical reactions involve the transfer of charge, which is electrochemistry. The thermodynamics of charged particles are developed in this chapter, and their principles are widely applicable to many systems and reactions.

Section 1　Conductivity of Electrolyte Solution

1.1　Conducting mechanism of electrolyte solution

Materials that conduct electricity are called conductors. Conductors can be divided broadly into two categories. The primary conductors are electronic conductors, which conduct electricity by the directional motion of free electrons in the conductor, such as metal, graphite and some metal compounds. There is no chemical change in the electrical conduction process of the electronic conductor. When the temperature rises, the lattice atoms vibrate more strongly, hindering the motion of electron, thus reducing the conductivity. The second kind of conductors are ionic conductors, they rely on the directional migration of their positive and negative ions, such as electrolytic conductors or molten electrolyte. During conduction, oxidation and reduction reactions occur on the electrode. And when temperature rises, the conductivity is enhanced due to the decrease of the viscosity.

An electrolyte invariably undergoes chemical decomposition as a result of the passage of electric current through its solution.

The phenomenon of decomposition of an electrolyte by passing electric current through its solution is termed **electrolysis**(电解). The apparatus in which the process of electrolysis is carried is called Electrolytic cell. The cell contains water-solution of an electrolyte in which two metallic rods (electrodes) are dipped. These rods are connected to the two terminals of a battery (source of electricity). The two independent, physical systems that contain the reactions are called **half-cells** (半电池). The half-cell that contains the oxidation reaction is called the **anode** (阳极) ,and the half-cell containing the reduction reaction is called the **cathode** (阴极). The two half-cells together make up a system that, for a spontaneous reaction, is called a voltaic cell or galvanic cell.

How the electrolysis actually takes place, is illustrated in Fig. 4-1. The cations migrate to the cathode and form a neutral atom by accepting electrons from it. The anions migrate to the anode and yield a neutral particle by transfer of electrons to it. As a result of the loss of electrons by

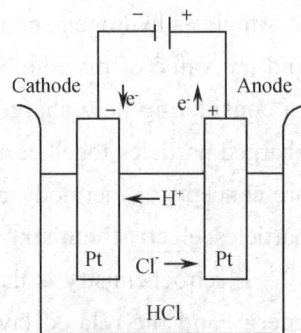

Fig. 4-1　The mechanism of electrolysis

anions and gain of electrons by cations at their respective electrodes chemical reaction takes place.

Let us consider the electrolysis of hydrochloric acid as an example. In solution, HCl is ionised,

$$HCl \rightarrow H^+ + Cl^-$$

In the electrolytic cell Cl^- ions will move toward the anode and H^+ ions will move toward the cathode. At the electrodes, the following reactions will take place.

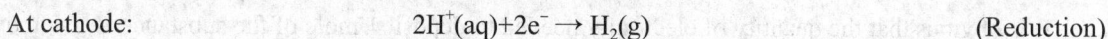

At cathode: $\qquad\qquad 2H^+(aq) + 2e^- \rightarrow H_2(g)$ $\qquad\qquad$ (Reduction)

As you see, each hydrogen ion picks up an electron from the cathode to become a hydrogen atom. Pairs of hydrogen atoms then unite to form molecules of hydrogen gas, H_2.

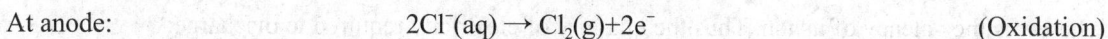

At anode: $\qquad\qquad 2Cl^-(aq) \rightarrow Cl_2(g) + 2e^-$ $\qquad\qquad$ (Oxidation)

After the chloride ion loses its electron to the anode, pair of chlorine atoms unite to form chlorine gas, Cl_2.

The net effect of the process is the decomposition of HCl into hydrogen and chlorine gases. The overall reaction is:

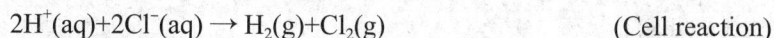

$$2H^+(aq) + 2Cl^-(aq) \rightarrow H_2(g) + Cl_2(g)$$ $\qquad\qquad$ (Cell reaction)

As presented above, when the external circuit is connected, the ions in the solution will move toward the electrodes, and the reaction of electron gain and loss occurs at the interface between electrode and solution, so that the current at the interface can be continuous.

1.2 Faraday's laws

Michael Faraday studied the quantitative aspect of electrolysis. He discovered that there exists a definite relationship between the amounts of products liberated at the electrodes and the quantity of electricity used in the process. In 1834, he formulated two laws which are known as **Faraday's Laws (法拉第定律)**. These are

First Law The amount of a given product liberated at an electrode during electrolysis is directly proportional to the quantity of electricity which passes through the electrolyte solution.

Second Law When the same quantity of electricity passes through solutions of different electrolytes, the amounts of the substances liberated at the electrodes are directly proportional to their chemical equivalents.

If m is the mass of substance (in grams) deposited on electrode by passing Q coulombs of electricity, then

$$m \propto Q$$

We know that $\qquad\qquad Q = It$ $\qquad\qquad\qquad\qquad$ (4−1)

where I is the strength of current in amperes and t is the time in second for which the current has been passed.

Therefore, $m \propto It$ or

$$m = ZIt$$ $\qquad\qquad\qquad\qquad$ (4−2)

where Z is the constant known as the Electrochemical equivalent of the substance (electrolyte).

If $I = 1A$ and $t = 1s$, then $m = Z$.

Thus, the electrochemical equivalent is the amount of a substance deposited by 1A current passing for 1s (i.e., one coulomb).

It has been found experimentally that the quantity of electricity required to liberate one gram-equivalent of a substance is 96,500 coulombs. This quantity of electricity is known as Faraday constant and is denoted by the symbol F.

$$F = Le = (6.022 \times 10^{23} \times 1.6022 \times 10^{-19}) \text{ C} \cdot \text{mol}^{-1}$$
$$= 96,484.6 \text{C} \cdot \text{mol}^{-1} \approx 96,500 \text{C} \cdot \text{mol}^{-1}$$

where L is the Avogadro constant, e is the charge of the elementary charge.

It is obvious that the quantity of electricity needed to deposit 1 mole of the substance is given by the expression.

$$\text{Quantity of electricity} = n \times F \tag{4-3}$$

where n is the valency of its ion. Thus the quantity of electricity required to discharge:

$$1\text{mol of Ag}^+ = 1 \times F = 1F$$
$$1\text{mol of Cu}^{2+} = 2 \times F = 2F$$
$$1\text{mol of Al}^{3+} = 3 \times F = 3F$$

Therefore it means that the quantity of electricity in one Faraday is one mole of electrons. Now we can say that.

$$1 \text{ Faraday} = 96,500 \text{ coulombs} = 1 \text{ Mole electrons}$$

According to this law when the same quantity of electricity is passed through different electrolyte solutions, the masses of the substances deposited on the electrodes are proportional to their chemical equivalents.

Section 2   The Conductance of the Electrolyte Solution

2.1   Conductance of electrolytes

We have seen that electrolyte solutions conduct electric currents through them by movement of the ions to the electrodes. The power of electrolytes to conduct electric currents is termed **conductivity** or **conductance (电导)**. Like metallic conductors, electrolytes obey Ohm's law. According to this law, the current I flowing through a metallic conductor is given by the relation.

$$G = \frac{1}{R} = \frac{I}{E} \tag{4-4}$$

where I is the current intensity (Unit: Amperes, A); E is the External voltage (Unit: Volt, V); R is the resistance measured in ohms (or Ω); and G is the conductance of electrolytes.

2.1.1   Specific conductivity

The resistance R of a conductor is directly proportional to its length, l, and inversely proportional to the area of its cross-section, A. That is,

$$R = \rho \frac{l}{A} \tag{4-5}$$

where ρ (rho) is a constant of proportionality and is called resistivity or specific resistance.

The specific conductivity is denoted by the symbol κ (kappa). Thus,

$$\kappa = \frac{1}{\rho} = \frac{1}{R} \cdot \frac{l}{A} = G \cdot K_{cell} \tag{4-6}$$

Definition of cell constant:
$$K_{cell} = \frac{l}{A} \tag{4-7}$$

Conductance is generally expressed in reciprocal ohms or Ω^{-1}. The specific conductivity's unit can be derived as $\Omega^{-1} \cdot m^{-1}$. The internationally recommended unit for Ω^{-1} is Siemens, S. When S is used, the specific conductivity is expressed as $S \cdot m^{-1}$.

2.1.2 Molar conductivity

Since the number of the charge carriers per unit volume usually increases with increasing electrolyte concentration, the specific conductivity κ usually increases as the electrolyte's concentration increases at low concentration. To get a measure of the current, the molar conductivity of an electrolyte in solution is defined by Λ_m. It is equal to the product of the specific conductivity, κ in $1m^3$ water containing 1mol of the electrolyte.

$$\Lambda_m = \frac{\kappa}{c} \tag{4-8}$$

Where c is the molar concentration. The unit for c is $mol \cdot m^{-3}$, for Λ_m is $S \cdot m^2 \cdot mol^{-1}$.

2.2 Conductivity measurement of electrolyte solution

Conductance is the reciprocal of resistance and the resistance can be determined by a Wheatstone bridge. The basic principle of this method is shown in Fig. 4-2. R_x is the resistance of the solution to be tested, R_1 is the variable resistance, R_3 and R_4 are the slide wire resistor, and G is the galvanometer. When the bridge is balanced (no current passing through the galvanometer), we can get:

$$\frac{R_x}{R_1} = \frac{R_4}{R_3}$$

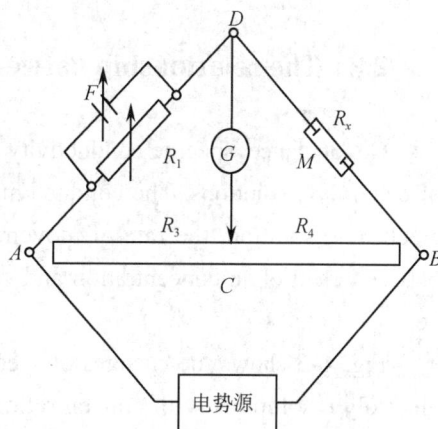

Fig. 4-2   Wheatstone bridge circuit for measurement of conductivity

If we figure out R_x, we then know the conductivity of the electrolyte solution. If the electrode area in the conductance cell, the distance between the electrodes and the concentration of electrolyte solution are known and then the c or Λ_m can be obtained by using equations (4-6) and (4-8).

The exact value of the cell constant (l/A) can be determined by measuring the distance between the electrodes (l) and their area of cross sections (A). Actual measurement of these dimensions is very difficult. Therefore indirect method is employed to determine the value of cell constant.

We know that: $\kappa = \frac{1}{\rho} = \frac{1}{R} \cdot \frac{l}{A} = G \cdot K_{cell}$

$$K_{cell} = \frac{\kappa}{G}$$

To determine the cell constant, a standard solution of KCl whose specific conductivity at a given temperature is known, is used. Then a solution of KCl of the same strength is prepared and its conductance determined experimentally at the same temperature. Substituting the two values in the above expression, the cell constant can be calculated. (Table 4–1)

Table 4–1 Conductivities and molar conductivities of KCl aqueous solutions at 298K, 101.325kPa

$c/(mol \cdot dm^{-3})$	0	0.001	0.01	0.1	1.0
$\kappa/(S \cdot m^{-1})$	0	0.0147	0.1411	1.229	11.2
$\Lambda_m / (S \cdot m^2 \cdot mol^{-1})$	0.0150	0.0147	0.0141	0.0129	0.0112

[Example 4–1] At 298K, $0.0200mol \cdot dm^{-3}$ KCl solution in a conductivity cell, Measured resistance is 82.4Ω. If the same conductivity cell is charged with $0.0050mol \cdot dm^{-3}$ K_2SO_4 solution, the resistance is 376Ω. It is known that the conductivity of a K_2SO_4 solution of $0.0200mol \cdot dm^{-3}$ at this temperature is $0.2786S \cdot m^{-1}$. Try to find: (1) Conductivity cell constant. (2) Electrical conductivity and molar conductivity of K_2SO_4 solution of $0.0050mol \cdot dm^{-3}$.

Solution:

(1) $K_{cell} = \kappa R = 0.2786 \times 82.4 = 23.0 m^{-1}$

(2) $\kappa = \dfrac{1}{R} K_{cell} = \dfrac{1}{376} \times 23.0 = 0.0612 S \cdot m^{-1}$

$$\Lambda_m = \frac{\kappa}{C} = \frac{0.0612}{0.0050 \times 10^3} = 0.0122 S \cdot m^{-2} \cdot mol^{-1}$$

2.3 The relationship between κ and c or Λ_m and c

Conductance, specific conductivity and molar conductivity can be used to describe the conductivity of electrolyte solutions. The conductivity of the electrolyte depends on the concentration of ions in the electrolyte solution, the rate of movement of ions, and the number of valence ions. The relationship between electrolyte concentration and specific conductivity and molar conductivity is mainly discussed here.

Fig. 4–3 shows the changes of specific conductivity of some electrolyte solutions with concentration. For strong electrolyte, the specific conductivity increases sharply with increasing concentration at low concentration, until it reaches the peak value, and then it decreases with concentration increases at high concentration. For weak electrolyte, the specific conductivity is very low in dilute solutions and does not change significantly with the concentration. For neutral salt, its concentration should not be too high, due to the limitation of saturation solubility.

The molar conductivity of a solution does not vary linearly with concentration. The effect of concentration on molar conductivity can be studied by plotting Λ_m values against the square root of the concentration. It has been found that variation of molar conductivity with $\sqrt{c}$ depends upon the nature of electrolyte.

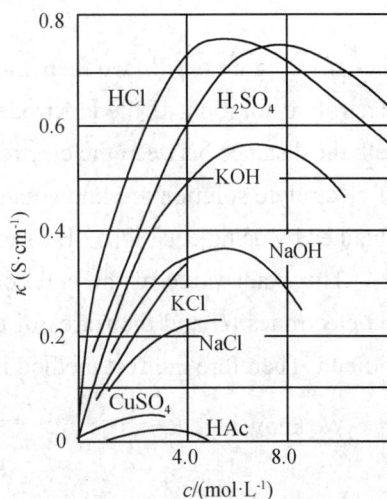

Fig. 4–3 Relationship between κ and c

Fig. 4–4 shows the behavior of strong and weak electrolytes with the change of concentration.

Strong electrolytes are completely ionised at all concentrations (or dilutions). The increase in molar conductivity is not due to the increase in the number of current carrying species. This is, in fact, due to the decrease in forces of attraction between the ions of opposite charges with the decrease in concentration (or increase in dilution). At higher concentration, the forces of attraction between the opposite ions increase. Consequently, it affects the speed of the ions with which they move towards oppositely charged electrodes. This phenomenon is called ionic interference. As the solution becomes more and more dilute, the molar conductivity increases, till it reaches a limitary value. This value is known as molar conductivity at infinite dilution (zero concentration) and is denoted by Λ_m^∞. The relationship of Λ_m and $\sqrt{c}$ of

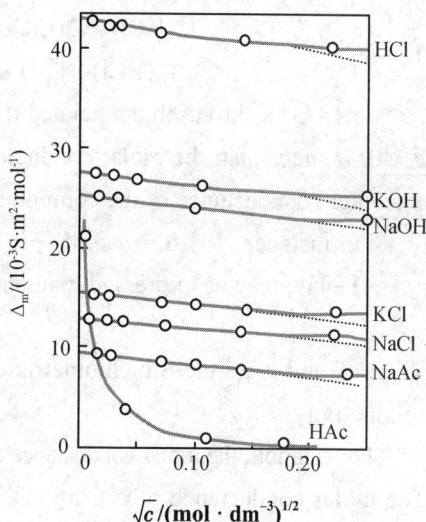

Fig. 4–4   Relationship between Λ_m and $\sqrt{c}$

strong electrolytes at dilute concentration can be expressed by the relation $\Lambda_m = \Lambda_m^\infty - A\sqrt{c}$. Then Λ_m^∞ value of strong electrolyte is obtained by extrapolation.

Weak electrolytes have low ionic concentrations and hence inter ionic forces are negligible. Ionic speeds are not affected with decrease in concentration (or increase in dilution). The increase in molar conductivity with increasing dilution is due to the increase in the number of current carrier species. Thus increase in molar conductivity in case of a weak electrolyte is due to the increase in the number of ions. The rapid increase in Λ_m for weak electrolyte as $c \to 0$ is due to an increase in the degree of dissociation of this weak electrolyte as c decreases. Thus the extrapolation procedure cannot be applied to weakly dissociated electrolytes. Such solutions have lower molar conductivity at higher concentrations, but the values increase greatly with increasing dilution. Because of this steep increase in Λ_m at high dilution, the extrapolation to zero concentration is uncertain and may result in large errors. For this reason, Kohlrausch recommended a different procedure for weak electrolytes.

2.4   Law of the independent migration of ions—Kohlrausch's Law

From a study of the molar conductance of different electrolytes at infinite dilution (Λ_m^∞), Kohlrausch discovered that the difference in Λ_m^∞ for pairs of electrolytes having a common ion is always approximately a constant. Values of Λ_m^∞ for some strong electrolytes at 298.15K are listed in Table 4–2.

Table 4–2 Λ_m^∞ for some strong electrolytes at 298.15K

Electrolyte	$\Lambda_m^\infty/(S \cdot m^2 \cdot mol^{-1})$	$\Delta\Lambda_m^\infty/(S \cdot m^2 \cdot mol^{-1})$	Electrolyte	$\Lambda_m^\infty/(S \cdot m^2 \cdot mol^{-1})$	$\Delta\Lambda_m^\infty/(S \cdot m^2 \cdot mol^{-1})$
KCl	0.014986	34.9×10^{-4}	HCl	0.042616	4.9×10^{-4}
LiCl	0.011503		HNO$_3$	0.04213	
KClO$_4$	0.015004	34.8×10^{-4}	KCl	0.014986	4.9×10^{-4}
LiClO$_4$	0.010598		KNO$_3$	0.014496	
KNO$_3$	0.01450	34.9×10^{-4}	LiCl	0.011503	4.9×10^{-4}
LiNO$_3$	0.01101		LiNO$_3$	0.01101	

From Table 4–2, we can see that

$$\varLambda_m^\infty(KCl) - \varLambda_m^\infty(LiCl) = \varLambda_m^\infty(KClO_4) - \varLambda_m^\infty(LiClO_4) = \varLambda_m^\infty(KNO_3) - \varLambda_m^\infty(LiNO_3)$$

$$\varLambda_m^\infty(HCl) - \varLambda_m^\infty(HNO_3) = \varLambda_m^\infty(KCl) - \varLambda_m^\infty(KNO_3) = \varLambda_m^\infty(LiCl) - \varLambda_m^\infty(LiNO_3)$$

In 1875, Kohlrausch enunciated a generalization which is called the **Kohlrausch's Law (科尔劳施定律)**. It states that: the molar conductance of an electrolyte at infinite dilution is equal to the sum of the equivalent conductance of the component ions.

For instance: $M_{\nu_+}A_{\nu_-} \rightarrow \nu_+ M^{Z+} + \nu_- A^{Z-}$

The law may be expressed mathematically as:

$$\varLambda_m^\infty = \nu_+ \varLambda_{m,+}^\infty + \nu_- \varLambda_{m,-}^\infty \tag{4-9}$$

where ν_+ and ν_- are the Stoichiometric coefficient of cations and anions, $\varLambda_{m,+}^\infty$ and $\varLambda_{m,-}^\infty$ are the ionic molar conductivity.

For example, the molar conductance of NaCl at infinite dilution at 25℃ is found to be 126.45S · m^2 · mol^{-1}. The molar conductance of Na$^+$ and Cl$^-$ ion is 50.11S · m^2 · mol^{-1} and 76.34S · m^2 · mol^{-1} respectively. Thus,

$$\varLambda_m^\infty(NaCl) = \varLambda_m^\infty(Na^+) + \varLambda_m^\infty(Cl^-)$$

Therefore, if the molar conductivity of various ions at infinite dilution can be known, we can calculate the molar conductivity of other strong or weak electrolyte by using the law of the independent motion of ions. For instance: molar conductivity of acetic acid at infinite dilution can be calculated as flowing formula.

$$\varLambda_m^\infty(CH_3COOH) = \varLambda_m^\infty(H^+) + \varLambda_m^\infty(CH_3COO^-)$$
$$= [\varLambda_m^\infty(H^+) + \varLambda_m^\infty(Cl^-)] + [\varLambda_m^\infty(Na^+) + \varLambda_m^\infty(CH_3COO^-)] - [\varLambda_m^\infty(Na^+) + \varLambda_m^\infty(Cl^-)]$$
$$= \varLambda_m^\infty(HCl) + \varLambda_m^\infty(CH_3COONa) - \varLambda_m^\infty(NaCl)$$

Table 4-3 shows the molar conductivity of some ions in limiting dilute solution at 25℃.

Table 4-3　The molar conductivity of some ions in limiting dilute solution at 25℃

Cation	$\varLambda_{m,+}^\infty$/(S · m^2 · mol^{-1})	Anion	$\varLambda_{m,-}^\infty$/(S · m^2 · mol^{-1})
H$^+$	349.82×10^{-4}	OH$^-$	198.0×10^{-4}
Li$^+$	38.69×10^{-4}	Cl$^-$	76.34×10^{-4}
Na$^+$	50.11×10^{-4}	Br$^-$	78.4×10^{-4}
K$^+$	73.52×10^{-4}	I$^-$	76.8×10^{-4}
NH$_4^+$	73.4×10^{-4}	NO$_3^-$	71.44×10^{-4}
Ag$^+$	61.92×10^{-4}	CH$_3$COO$^-$	40.9×10^{-4}
$\frac{1}{2}$Ca$^+$	59.50×10^{-4}	ClO$_4^-$	68.0×10^{-4}
$\frac{1}{2}$Ba^{2+}	63.64×10^{-4}	$\frac{1}{2}$SO$_4^{2-}$	79.8×10^{-4}
$\frac{1}{2}$Mg^{2+}	53.06×10^{-4}		

Section 3　Electromotive Force of Battery

3.1　Galvanic cell

A galvanic cell is the one in which electrical current is generated by a spontaneous redox reaction. A simple primary cell is shown in Fig. 4–5. Here the spontaneous reaction of zinc metal with an aqueous solution of copper sulphate is used.

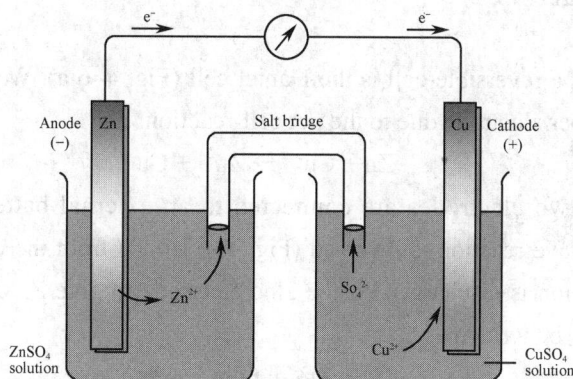

Fig. 4–5　A simple primary cell

$$Zn + Cu^{2+} \rightarrow Zn^{2+} + Cu$$

A bar of zinc metal (anode) is placed in zinc sulphate solution in the left container. A bar of copper (cathode) is immersed in copper sulphate solution in the right container. The zinc and copper electrodes are joined by a copper wire. A salt bridge containing potassium sulphate solution interconnects the solutions in the anode compartment and the cathode compartment.

The oxidation half-reaction occurs in the anode compartment.

$$Zn \rightarrow Zn^{2+} + 2e^-$$

The reduction half-reaction takes place in the cathode compartment.

$$Cu^{2+} + 2e^- \rightarrow Cu$$

When the cell is set up, electrons flow from zinc electrode through the wire to the copper cathode. As a result, zinc dissolves in the anode solution to form Zn^{2+} ions. The Cu^{2+} ions in the cathode half-cell pick up electrons and are converted to Cu atoms on the cathode. At the same time, SO_4^{2-} ions from the cathode half-cell migrate to the anode half-cell through the salt bridge. Likewise, Zn^{2+} ions from the anode half-cell move into the cathode half-cell. This flow of ions from one half-cell to the other completes the electrical circuit which ensures continuous supply of current. The cell will operate till either the zinc metal or copper ion is completely used up.

The flow of electrons from one electrode to the other in an electrochemical cell is caused by the half-reactions taking place in the anode and cathode compartments. The net chemical change obtained by adding the two half-reactions is called the **cell reaction** (电池反应). Thus, for a simple galvanic cell described above, we have

Half-reactions:
$$Zn(s) \rightarrow Zn^{2+}(aq) + 2e^-$$
$$Cu^{2+}(aq) + 2e^- \rightarrow Cu(s)$$

Cell reaction by adding up the half-reactions:
$$Zn(s) + Cu^{2+}(aq) \rightarrow Zn^{2+}(aq) + Cu(s)$$

Electromotive force (电动势): the difference between the reduction reaction's electric potential (φ_+) and the oxidation's electric potential(φ_-), measured between the two terminals with same connecting wires and when there is no flow of current, is called the **emf** of the cell. It is denoted by E.

$$E = \varphi_+ - \varphi_- \qquad (4-10)$$

3.2 Reversible battery

A familiar example of a reversible cell is the Daniel cell (Fig. 4–6 a). We know that electrons flow from zinc electrode to copper electrode due to the net cell-reaction.

$$Zn + Cu^{2+} \rightarrow Zn^{2+} + Cu$$

However, when the two electrodes are connected to an external battery that opposes the cell electromotive force, the above reaction is reversed (Fig. 4–6 b). Cu from the copper electrode dissolves to form Cu^{2+} ion and Zn^{2+} ion is discharged on the zinc electrode to give Zn atom. The overall reaction taking place in the cell may be written as

$$Cu + Zn^{2+} \rightarrow Cu^{2+} + Zn$$

With the help of a potentiometer (Fig. 4–6), the cell electromotive force is exactly balanced by the external electromotive force. At the balance point, no current will flow through the circuit. Now let the external electromotive force increase and then decrease by an infinitesimal amount. A minute current will flow first to the left and then to the right. This reversal of the cell current is accompanied by a corresponding change in the direction of the cell reaction. This type of reversible behavior is a feature of the reversible cells. A reversible cell may be defined as: a cell that operates by reversal of the cell current and direction of cell reaction by infinitesimal change of electromotive force on either side of the balance point.

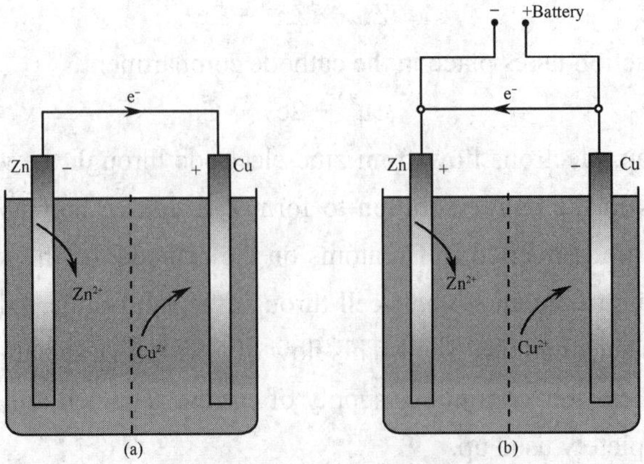

Fig. 4–6 Reversible Daniel cell
(a) Zn-Cu cell in which current flows from left to right;(b) Cu-Zn cell in which current flows from right to left on application of external electromotive force.

3.3   Thermodynamics of reversible battery

3.3.1   Electromotive force

When a cell produces a current, the current can be used to do work. The maximum amount of work obtained from the cell is the product of charge flowing per mole and maximum potential difference, E, through which the charge is transferred.

$$W_{max} = -nFE \qquad (4-11)$$

where n is the number of moles of electrons transferred, F stands for Faraday constant and is equal to 96,500 coulombs and E is the emf to the cell.

According to the thermodynamics, the maximum work that can be derived from a chemical reaction is equal to the Gibbs free energy (ΔG) for the reaction.

$$W_{max} = \Delta G = -nFE$$
$$\Delta_r G_m = W_{max}/\Delta\xi = -nFE \qquad (4-12)$$

According to Gibbs-Helmholtz equation, the decrease in free energy of a system at constant pressure is given by the expression

$$T\left(\frac{\partial \Delta_r G_m}{\partial T}\right)_p = \Delta_r G_m - \Delta_r H_m$$

Substituting the value of ΔG from (4–12)

$$\Delta_r H_m = -nFE + nFT\left(\frac{\partial E}{\partial T}\right)_p \qquad (4-13)$$

$(\partial E/\partial T)_p$ is defined as the temperature coefficient of the emf of the cell.

$$\Delta_r S_m = nF\left(\frac{\partial E}{\partial T}\right)_p \qquad (4-14)$$

[Example 4–2] For cell reaction Zn (s)+CuSO$_4$(aq) = Cu(s) + ZnSO$_4$(aq), given that E=1.103V, $\left(\dfrac{\partial E}{\partial T}\right)_p = -4.6 \times 10^{-4}$ V $\cdot$ K^{-1}, Please calculate $\Delta_r G_m$, $\Delta_r S_m$, $\Delta_r H_m$ of above cell reaction when $T = 298$K.

Solution:

$n=2$

$$\Delta_r G_m = -nFE = -2 \times 1.103 \times 96500 = -2.129 \times 10^5 \text{J} \cdot \text{mol}^{-1}$$

$$\Delta_r S_m = nF\left(\frac{\partial E}{\partial T}\right)_p = 2 \times 96500 \times (-4.6 \times 10^{-4}) = -88.78 \text{J} \cdot \text{K}^{-1} \cdot \text{mol}^{-1}$$

$$\Delta_r H_m = \Delta_r G_m + T\Delta_r S_m = -2.129 \times 10^5 + 298 \times (-88.78)$$
$$= -2.394 \times 10^5 \text{J} \cdot \text{mol}^{-1}$$

3.3.2   Nernst equation

Single electrode potential: The potential of a single electrode in a half-cell is called the Single electrode potential. The amount of the charge produced on individual electrode determines its single electrode potential.

The single electrode potential of a half-cell depends on : (a) concentration of ions in solution; (b) tendency to form ions; and (c) temperature.

When the emf of a cell is determined under standard conditions, it is called the standard emf. The standard conditions are (a) 1M solutions of reactants and products; and (b) temperature of 25℃. Thus standard emf may be defined as: the emf of a cell with 1M solutions of reactants and products in solution measured at 25℃.

A convenient procedure to do so is to combine the given half-cell with another standard half-cell. The emf of the newly constructed cell, E, is determined with a voltmeter. The emf of the unknown half-cell, φ, can then be calculated from the expression

$$E_{measured} = \varphi_R - \varphi_L$$

If the standard half-cell acts as anode, the equation becomes

$$E_{measured} = \varphi_R \qquad (\because \varphi_L = 0)$$

The standard hydrogen half-cell or Standard Hydrogen Electrode (SHE), is selected for coupling with the unknown half-cell. It consists of a platinum electrode immersed in a 1M solution of H^+ ions maintained at 25℃. Hydrogen gas at one atmosphere enters the glass hood and bubbles over the platinum electrode. The emf of the standard hydrogen electrode is arbitrarily assigned the value of zero volts. So, SHE can be used as a standard for other electrodes.

For an oxidation half-cell reaction when the metal electrode M gives M^{n+} ion,

$$M^{n+} + ne^- \rightarrow M$$

The Nernst equation takes the form

$$\varphi = \varphi^\ominus + \frac{RT}{nF} \ln \frac{\alpha_M^{n+}}{\alpha_M} \tag{4-15}$$

The electrode electromotive force of any cell is equal to

$$E = \varphi_+ - \varphi_-$$

Section 4 Application of Conductivity Measurement

4.1 Testing water purity

The pharmaceutical industry often has higher requirements for the purity of water. The purity of water can be measured by measuring the conductivity of water. The conductivity κ of tap water at room temperature is generally about $1.0 \times 10^{-1} s \cdot m^{-1}$, the conductivity κ of ordinary distilled water is about $1.0 \times 10^{-3} s \cdot m^{-1}$, and the κ value of re-distilled water and deionized water is generally less than $1.0 \times 10^{-4} s \cdot m^{-1}$. So the conductivity κ value of water is measured, it can be known whether its purity meets the requirements.

4.2 Determination of ionization and ionization equilibrium constant of weak electrolyte

In the weak electrolyte solution, only the ionized part can assume the task of transferring electricity. In an infinitely dilute solution, the weak electrolyte can be considered to be fully ionized, and its molar conductivity is the sum of the molar conductivity of infinitely diluted ions. The difference between the weak electrolyte Λ_m at a certain concentration and its infinite dilution Λ_m^∞ depends on two factors: one is the degree of dissociation of the electrolyte; the other is the interaction force between the ions. Generally, weak electrolytes have a low degree of ionization and low ion concentration, so the interaction between ions can be ignored. The difference between Λ_m and Λ_m^∞ can be considered to be caused by the difference in the number of ions generated by partial ionization and total ionization.

$$\alpha = \frac{\Lambda_m}{\Lambda_m^\infty} \qquad (4-16)$$

where, α is the degree of ionization of the weak electrolyte at a concentration of c.

Taking weak electrolyte HAc as an example, let its initial concentration be c, then

$$HAc + H_2O \rightarrow H_3O^+ + Ac^-$$

At the beginning: c 0   0
At equilibrium: $c(1-\alpha)$ $c\alpha$ $c\alpha$
dissociation constant

$$K = \frac{\alpha^2}{1-\alpha} \cdot \frac{c}{c^\ominus}$$

Substituting equation (4-16) into

$$K = \frac{\Lambda_m^2}{\Lambda_m^\infty (\Lambda_m^\infty - \Lambda_m)} \cdot \frac{c}{c^\ominus} \qquad (4-17)$$

[Example 4-3] At 25℃, $0.01 mol \cdot dm^{-3}$ aqueous solution of $C_6H_8O_2N_2S$ (磺胺) has a conductivity $\kappa_{(SNH)} = 1.103 \times 10^{-3} S \cdot m^{-1}$, given that $\Lambda_{m(SN-Na)}^\infty = 0.01003 S \cdot m^2 \cdot mol^{-1}$, calculate the degree of dissociation α and the dissociation equilibrium constant K of $C_6H_8O_2N_2S$ solution.

Solution:
According to Table 4-3, $\Lambda_{m(HCl)}^\infty = 0.042616 S \cdot m^2 \cdot mol^{-1}$, $\Lambda_{m(NaCl)}^\infty = 0.012645 S \cdot m^2 \cdot mol^{-1}$.

$$\Lambda_{m(SNH)}^\infty = \Lambda_{m(SN-Na)}^\infty + \Lambda_{m(HCl)}^\infty - \Lambda_{m(NaCl)}^\infty$$
$$= 0.01003 + 0.042616 - 0.012645$$
$$= 0.0400 S \cdot m^2 \cdot mol^{-1}$$

$$\Lambda_m = \frac{\kappa}{c} = \frac{1.103 \times 10^{-3}}{0.01 \times 10^3} = 1.103 \times 10^{-4} S \cdot m^2 \cdot mol^{-1}$$

$$\alpha = \frac{\Lambda_{m(SNH)}}{\Lambda_{m(SNH)}^\infty} = \frac{1.103 \times 10^{-4}}{0.0400} = 0.276\%$$

$$K = \frac{\alpha^2}{1-\alpha} \frac{c}{c^\ominus} = \frac{(2.76 \times 10^{-3})^2}{1-0.00276} \times 0.01 = 7.64 \times 10^{-8}$$

4.3 Determination of solubility of insoluble salts

The solubility of poorly soluble salt in water is very small, and it is generally difficult to measure it directly, but it can be easily calculated by conductivity measurement. The specific method is to first measure the conductivity of pure water κ_w, and then use this water to prepare a saturated solution of the insoluble salt to be measured, and measure the conductivity κ of the saturated solution. The conductivity of the insoluble salt is then obtained (because the solution is extremely dilute, the conductivity contribution of water cannot be ignored). According to equation (4-8), $\Lambda_m = \frac{\kappa}{c}$, where c is the concentration of insoluble salt (unit: mol · m^{-3}). Since the concentration of the insoluble salt in the solution is very small, it can be approximated that $\Lambda_m \approx \Lambda_m^{\infty}$ of the insoluble salt saturated solution. So we can get

$$c_B = \frac{\kappa - \kappa_w}{\Lambda_m} \tag{4-18}$$

Λ_m^{∞} can be obtained by looking up the table. From the above formula, the concentration c of the saturated solution of the insoluble salt can be obtained, that is, the solubility S.

Expansion Content

Conductometric Titration

The method of determining the endpoint of a titration by using the change in the conductance of the solution during the titration is called conductance titration. In volume analysis, conductance titration can often get a very good result when the indicator is not ideally selected or the solution is cloudy and the color is inconvenient.

The principle of conductance titration is to determine the end point of the titration from the change in the conductivity of the solution by changing the ion concentration in the titration process or replacing an ion with another ion with a different rate of its electrical migration. Conductivity titration is commonly used in neutralization and precipitation reactions.

Bioelectrochemistry

Bioelectrochemistry is based on the basic principles of electrochemistry and experimental methods to study the movement of charge and energy in the biological system at the molecular and cellular level, and also study the effects on the activity and function of biological systems. Bioelectrochemistry can understand and study the nature of chemistry in the life process not only at the overall level of individual living organisms and organic tissues, but also at the molecular and cellular level. It has important significance for the development and application of biology.

Bioelectric phenomenon

In 1791 Galvani discovered that a frog leg was inserted between two different wires, and then the other two ends of the two wires were brought into contact. As a result, the muscles of the frog contracted. This shows that there is an interaction between the body tissues of animals and electricity. In fact, all organisms, whether at rest or active, have electrical phenomena, that is, bioelectrical phenomena.

Myoelectricity, electrocardiogram, and electroencephalogram are representative bioelectrical phenomena. The general bioelectricity is very weak, such as the ECG is about 1mV, the brain electricity is about 0.1mV. Therefore, when measuring ECG, EEG, and EMG, electrodes with a relatively large area are usually selected. At the same time, the electrodes have a small resistance and polarization, and can be firmly fixed on the surface of the living body. Generally, silver-silver chloride electrodes are the most commonly used.

Cell membrane potential

Biological cell membranes are a special type of semi-permeable membrane. An electrolyte solution composed of various ions is present on both sides of the membrane. Under normal circumstances, the K^+ ion concentrations inside and outside the nerve cell membrane are $400 mmol \cdot dm^{-3}$ and $20 mmol \cdot dm^{-3}$, respectively. The K^+ ion concentration inside the membrane is about 20 times higher than that outside the membrane; The ion concentrations inside and outside the membrane are $50 mmol \cdot dm^{-3}$ and $440 mmol \cdot dm^{-3}$, respectively. The Na^+ concentration in the membrane is much lower than that outside the membrane. In addition, the cell membrane's permeability to ions can be adjusted. Usually in the resting state, the permeability of nerve cell membranes to K^+ is about 100 times greater than to Na^+. Membrane potential due to different ion concentrations on both sides of the cell membrane, which can be given according to the Goldman equation.

$$\varphi_{membranes} = \frac{RT}{nF} \ln \frac{P(K^+) \cdot a_{extracellular}(K^+) + P(Na^+) \cdot a_{extracellular}(Na^+)}{P(K^+) \cdot a_{intracellular}(K^+) + P(Na^+) \cdot a_{intracellular}(Na^+)}$$

$$= \frac{RT}{nF} \ln \frac{a_{extracellular}(K^+) \cdot P(K^+)/P(Na^+) + a_{extracellular}(Na^+)}{a_{intracellular}(K^+) \cdot P(K^+)/P(Na^+) + a_{intracellular}(Na^+)}$$

In the formula, $a(K^+)$, $a(Na^+)$, $P(K^+)$, and $P(Na^+)$ are K^+ and Na^+ ion activities and permeability, respectively. Footnotes indicate intracellular and extracellular. At 310K, the resting potential is

$$\varphi_{membranes} = \frac{8.314 \times 310}{96500} \ln \frac{20 \times 100 + 440}{400 \times 100 + 50} \approx -0.075V(-75mV)$$

This indicates that the potential of the inner wall in the cell is 75mV lower than that of the outer wall. Therefore, the inside of the cell is negatively charged. The calculated resting potential is close to the experimentally measured value −70mV.

When nerve cells are stimulated electrically, chemically or mechanically, the permeability of the membrane is changed. The permeability of the cell membrane to Na^+ suddenly increases and exceeds the permeability of K^+, $P(Na^+)/(K^+) = 12$. Immediately cause changes in membrane potential. Calculated using the Goldman equation:

$$\varphi_{membranes} = \frac{8.314 \times 310}{96500} \ln \frac{20 \times \dfrac{1}{12} + 440}{400 \times \dfrac{1}{12} + 50} \approx 0.05V(50mV)$$

The sudden change in membrane potential is called potential activation, and it is completed in about 1×10^{-4}s. The stimulated membrane potential is called action potential. Action potentials cause current to propagate along nerve fibers, which is called bioelectricity.

The membrane potential caused by the diffusion caused by the concentration difference is a spontaneous process and does not require energy supply. However, to restore the cells to their original state after stimulation, to maintain the normal uneven distribution of K^+ and Na^+ inside and outside the membrane, this needs to rely on the sodium pump protein on the cell membrane to consume ATP.

The Goldman equation is actually a generalized application of the Nernst equation. However, it should be noted that current is generated when the membrane potential changes suddenly. At this time, the electrode process on both sides of the membrane is actually not a reversible process. The Nernst equation applies only to reversible electrode processes. In addition, different currents are passed through the animal cell membrane and the value of the membrane potential is measured at the same time. Mandle found that the living cell membrane is not a simple resistor. The generation of membrane potential is related to the electrode process. While there is no metabolism on the cell membrane of dead tissue, the cell membrane becomes a simple resistor. Electrochemists believe that the essence of membrane potential generation is a charge transfer process at the membrane-solution interface. On the other side, the reduction reaction of the oxide is carried out. The mechanism of membrane potential generation needs to be further studied. According to the law of membrane potential change, the activity of biological organisms has been studied. That is a very active field in current bioelectrochemical research, and has been widely used. The presence of a membrane potential indicates an electric double layer on each cell. It is equivalent to many electric dipoles distributed on the surface. The measurement of transmembrane potential and the control of membrane potential are of great significance in medicine. Electrocardiogram is the measurement of the change in potential difference over time caused by changes in the dipole moment of the heart between several sets of symmetrical points on the human surface, to check how the heart works. In addition, EEG and electromyograms provide direct and effective detection methods for understanding the activities of brain nerves and muscles.

Biological Sensor

Through sense organs (sensors), people can produce vision, smell, etc. A device that can convert the physical and chemical changes which are caused by the contractions between the biological substance and the substance determined into an electrical signal is called a biosensor. The biological substances are called molecular recognition materials, and they can be divided into two categories: One is a substance with a catalytic function, such as enzymes, complex enzymes (including small organs in cells), microbial cells, etc; the other is a substance capable of forming a stable complex, such as an antibody, a bound protein, and the like. They have strong specificity and sensitivity in molecular recognition. For example, enzymes only recognize their corresponding substrates, antibodies recognize antigens, and so on. Many of these bioidentifiers are water-soluble and unstable, and they are difficult to be used as sensors directly. Usually they are needed to convert into a solid state and fix on the electrode surface.

The main methods are：

(1) By forming a covalent bond, an ionic bond, or a coordination bond, the molecular recognition substance is directly bound to the electrode surface.

(2) The electrode surface is modified with a polymer substance, and the molecular recognition material is embedded or adsorbed in the porous membrane of the polymer carrier.

(3) The polymer is connected to a molecular recognition substance before it is coated on the electrode. In this way, bio-functional electrodes were prepared, which opened up a new way to artificially design and make electrode functions from the molecular level.

The general enzyme sensor is composed of an electrochemical detection device and an enzyme membrane. For example, the glucose enzyme electrode is firstly coated with a polymer film that can be penetrated by oxygen on the surface of the Pt electrode, then put a layer of glucose oxidase (GOD) film on it, an enzyme sensor for measuring glucose was prepared. Insert this sensor into an aqueous glucose solution, and the glucose molecule contacts the enzyme membrane, and an enzymatic reaction occurs:

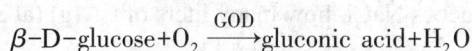

$$\beta-D-glucose+O_2 \xrightarrow{GOD} gluconic\ acid+H_2O$$

The GOD present in the membrane only catalyzes $\beta-D-$glucose and continuously consumes O_2.At the same time, the O_2 dissolved in the solution will also diffuse and reach the surface of the Pt electrode through the enzyme membrane and polymer membrane to be reduced. The rate at which the reduction current of O_2 decreases is related to the concentration of glucose. The glucose content in the blood of diabetic patients can be measured by the glucose oxidase sensor. Only 0.01ml of blood, 20~30s the result is obtained.

A binding protein is a stable protein complex formed by a certain protein and a specific substance. It has excellent molecular recognition function, and can be made into different sensors by using affinity potential determination of binding proteins. For example, vitamin H sensors can be made by antibiotic proteins; In addition, microorganisms can be used as identification materials to make microbial sensors. It can be used for the determination of carcinogens. Because many carcinogens can degenerate microorganisms, damage the DNA in microorganisms, and cause them to lose their respiratory function. Microbial sensors made of certain specific microbial strains can be used to screen for carcinogens. The research and development of biosensors are closely connected with high-tech such as microelectronics, microcomputer technology and ultra-micro electrodes, etc. It will have a very broad prospect in the tracking of physiological processes, living detection, and development of biochips.

重 点 小 结

电化学是研究电能与化学能相互转化及其转化过程中相关规律的科学。 在化学能和电能的转化过程中所用的装置有两类, 原电池是将物质的化学能转化为电能; 而电解池是将电能转化为化学能。 这两种装置中导电物质均为电解质溶液。 本章主要介绍了电解质溶液理论和可逆电池热力学两部分。

电解质溶液是通过正负离子定向迁移而导电, 因此电解质溶液的导电能力除了与温度及溶液浓度有关外, 还与正、 负离子的运动速率有关。 由此提出了电导、 电导率及摩尔电导率的概念。 通过电导的测定可以检测水质的纯度、 计算弱电解质的解离平衡常数以及难溶盐的溶解度。

在可逆电池热力学中, 一方面借助于不同温度下可逆电池电动势的测定, 可以求得相应化学反应的热力学函数的变化, 另一方面也可以利用能斯特方程进行不同温度、 浓度下原电池电动势的计算。

Object detection

I. Select the correct option for the following problems (one option for each problem).

1. One faraday will oxidize _____ mole(s) of Cu to Cu^{2+} ions.

　A. 0　　　　　B. 1/2　　　　　C. 1/4　　　　　D. 1

2. How much time (in hours) is required to plate out 25.0g of gold metal from a solution of

习题题库

Au $(NO_3)_3$ when the current is 2.00 amperes and the electrode efficiency is only 65%?

    A. 9.36h   B. 2.88h   C. 3.11h   D. 7.85h

3. In the electrolysis of aqueous NaCl, how many liters of $Cl_2(g)$ (at STP) are generated by a current of 7.50A for a period of 100min?

    A. 10.4L   B. 45000L   C. 5.22L   D. 0.466L

4. Select the incorrect statement about the chemical activity at electrodes during electrolysis.

    A. anions give up electrons   B. cations take up electrons

    C. oxidation occurs at the anode   D. proton transfer occurs in the reactions

5. Specific conductance is the conductance of

    A. one centimeter cube of solution of an electrolyte

    B. one centimeter cube of a solid electrolyte

    C. one gram of the solution of an electrolyte

    D. one gram of the solid electrolyte

6. The molar conductance of a solution of an electrolyte

    A. increases with dilution   B. decreases with dilution

    C. does not vary with dilution   D. none of these

7. With rise in temperature the conductance of a solution of an electrolyte generally

    A. decreases   B. increases   C. remains constant   D. none of these

8. The cell constant is the ratio of

    A. distance between electrodes to area of electrode

    B. area of electrode to distance between electrodes

    C. specific conductance to area of electrode

    D. specific conductance to distance between the electrodes

9. The units of specific conductance are

    A. $\Omega \cdot cm$ B. $\Omega \cdot cm^{-1}$ C. $\Omega^{-1} \cdot cm$ D. $\Omega^{-1} \cdot cm^{-1}$

10. The units of molar conductance are

    A. $\Omega \cdot cm \cdot mol$ B. $\Omega^{-1} \cdot cm^{-1} \cdot mol^{-1}$

    C. $\Omega^{-1} \cdot cm^2 \cdot mol^{-1}$ D. $\Omega^{-1} \cdot cm^{-2} \cdot mol^{-1}$

11. On passing electrical current through an electrolyte solution

    A. cations move towards anode

    B. anions move towards cathode

    C. cations move towards cathode and anions towards anode

    D. both cations and anions move in same direction

12. Kohlrausch's law can be used to determine

    A. Λ_m^{∞} for weak electrolytes   B. absolute ionic mobilities

    C. solubility of sparingly soluble salts   D. all of these

13. If Λ_m^{∞} is the equivalent conductance at infinite dilution and Λ_m the equivalent conductance of the electrolyte at the dilution, the degree of dissociation is given by

    A. $\alpha = \dfrac{\Lambda_m^{\infty}}{\Lambda_m}$ B. $\alpha = \dfrac{\Lambda_m}{\Lambda_m^{\infty}}$ C. $\alpha = \Lambda_m^{\infty} - \Lambda_m$ D. $\alpha = \Lambda_m - \Lambda_m^{\infty}$

14. The site of oxidation in an electrochemical cell is

    A. the anode   B. the cathode   C. the electrode   D. the salt bridge

15. What is indicated when a chemical cell's voltage ($E^\ominus$) has dropped to zero?

   A. the concentration of the reactants has increased

   B. the concentration of the products has decreased

   C. the cell reaction has reached equilibrium

   D. the cell reaction has completely stopped

16. Standard cell potential is

   A. measured at a temperature of 25℃

   B. measured when ion concentrations of aqueous reactants are 1.00M

   C. measured under the conditions of 1.00atm for gaseous reactants

   D. all of the above

17. The standard reduction potentials in volts for Pb^{2+} and Ag^+ are -0.13 and $+0.80$, respectively. Calculate $E^\ominus_{cell}$ in volts for a cell in which the overall reaction is

$$Pb + 2Ag^+ \rightarrow Pb^{2+} + 2Ag$$

   A. 1.73   B. 0.67   C. 0.93   D. 1.47

18. Given the following information, $Fe^{3+}(aq) + H_2(g) \rightarrow 2H^+ + Fe^{2+}$, $E^\ominus_{cell} = 0.77$. Determine $\varphi^\ominus$ for the reaction:

$$e^- + Fe^{3+}(aq) \rightarrow Fe^{2+}(aq)$$

   A. 1.54   B. 0.77   C. 0.39   D. - 0.77

19. Given $Zn \rightarrow Zn^{2+} + 2e^-$ with $\varphi^\ominus = +0.763$, calculate φ for a Zn electrode in which $Zn^{2+} = 0.025M$.

   A. 1.00V   B. 0.621V   C. 0.810V   D. 0.124V

20. The standard reduction potentials of Cu^{2+} and Ag^+ in volts are $+0.34$ and $+0.80$, respectively. Determine the value of E in volts for the following cell at 25℃ Cu | Cu^{2+} (1.00M) || Ag^+ (0.0010M) | Ag.

   A. 0.37V   B. 0.55V   C. –0.28V   D. 0.28V

II. Try to answer the following problem.

1. Explain Kohlrausch's law of ionic mobility. How does it help in determining the equivalent conductivity of infinite dilution of weak electrolyte?

2. Derive an expression for ΔG, ΔH and ΔS in terms of E of a cell and temperature coefficient.

Reference answers

I. 1.B;　2.D;　3.C;　4.D;　5.A;　6.A;　7.B;　8.D;　9.D;　10.C;　11.C;　12.D;　13.B;　14.A; 15.C;　16.D;　17.C;　18.B;　19.C;　20.D.

II. Omitted.

Chapter 5 Chemical Kinetics

学习目标

知识要求

1. 掌握

（1）简单级数的动力学方程及其特征。

（2）温度对反应速率的影响及阿仑尼乌斯公式的应用。

2. 熟悉

（1）典型复杂反应的动力学方程(可逆反应、平行反应和连续反应)及特点。

（2）溶剂对溶液反应的影响。

（3）催化作用和催化反应的特点。

3. 了解

（1）一级反应与零级反应在药物消除动力学上的应用。

（2）反应级数的确定。

（3）光化学反应的特点。

能力要求

1. 学会根据简单级数反应的动力学特点判断简单反应的级数。

2. 学会利用各类反应的动力学方程计算化学反应速率。

3. 学会利用阿仑尼乌斯方程计算不同温度的化学反应速率常数。

4. 学会利用不同的条件(浓度、温度、溶剂、催化剂、pH、酶)控制反应速率。

There are two basic questions in the reaction. One is the direction, probability, and degree of the reaction, the other is the rate and mechanism of the reaction. The former is the research field of chemical **thermodynamics (热力学)**, which we have discussed in the previous chapters. And the latter is the research field of **chemical kinetics (化学动力学)**, which we will discuss in this chapter.

Chemical kinetics, also called reaction kinetics, is the study of the rates and mechanisms of chemical reactions. How the reaction occurs is the main focus of kinetics. A basic understanding of a process includes foremost, how fast it goes. This is the rate of the reaction. A deeper understanding of a chemical process includes knowing why a particular chemical reaction proceeds as fast or as slow as it does: What are the factors that influence the rate of the reaction? Are the factors controllable, like concentrations or temperatures or available surface area or presence of **catalysts (催化剂)**, or are the factors in herent to the process, like the chemical identity of the reactants and products, or conditions dictated by thermodynamics? These are all factors that must be considered in order to understand the kinetics of a chemical process.

Chemical kinetics is also important in the field of pharmacy, since the production, preparation and storage of the drug are all related to reaction rates. The kinetic method can be always used to study the drug absorption, distribution, metabolism and excretion *in vivo*. The knowledge of chemical kinetics is also very valuable to study on how to improve the drug stability and prevent the drug **degradation (降解)**.

Through the study of chemical kinetics, we can know how to control the reaction conditions and increase the rate of the **main reaction (主反应)** to increase the yield of the product. We also can know how to inhibit or slow down the rate of **side reaction (副反应)** to reduce the consumption of raw materials, reduce the burden of separation operations, and improve product quality.

In the industrial synthesis of compounds, reaction rates are as important as **equilibrium (平衡)** constants. The thermodynamic equilibrium constant tells us the maximum possible yield of NH_3 obtainable at any given T and p from N_2 and H_2, but if the reaction rate between N_2 and H_2 is too low, the reaction will not be economical to carry out. Frequently, in organic preparative reactions, several possible competing reactions can occur, and the relative rates of these reactions usually influence the yield of each product. What happens to pollutants released to the atmosphere can be understood only by a kinetic analysis of atmospheric reactions. An automobile works because the rate of oxidation of hydrocarbons is negligible at room temperature but rapid at the high temperature of the engine. Many of the metals and plastics of modern technology are thermodynamically unstable with respect to oxidation, but the rate of this oxidation is slow at room temperature. Reaction rates are fundamental to the functioning of living organisms. Biological catalysts—**enzymes (酶)** control the functioning of an organism by selectively speeding up certain reactions. In summary, to understand and predict the behavior of a chemical system, one must consider both thermodynamics and kinetics.

Since chemical kinetics is much more complex than thermodynamics, it is relatively immature and many fields remain to be explored. At present, the study of chemical kinetics is very active, and it is one of the subjects with rapid progress. Physical chemist Li Yuanzhe (Chinese American, 1936-) was awarded the Nobel Prize of chemistry in 1986 for his outstanding contributions to the study of cross-molecular beams.

Section 1   Basic Concepts

PPT

1.1   Representation of chemical reaction rate

When we speak of how fast a reaction goes, we are not thinking "fast" as in a **velocity (速度)** in meters per second. Rather, we are thinking about how quickly amounts (that is, moles) of reactants are converted into amounts (moles) of products. The chemical **reaction rate (反应速率)** is defined as the change in concentration of any of reactant or products per unit time. However, since the **stoichiometric coefficients (化学计量系数)** of products and reactants in the reaction equation are not the same, the values may not be same, when the concentration change rate of reactants or products is used to express chemical reaction rate. If chemical reaction rate is defined as the **derivative (导数)** of reaction extent to time, the value is the same no matter which species is chosen.

According to the definition of extent of reaction ξ, consider a generalized chemical reaction in constant-volume,

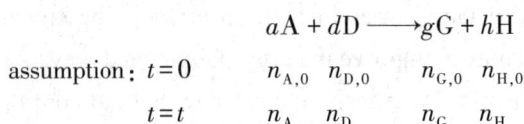

$$aA + dD \longrightarrow gG + hH$$

$$\text{assumption：} \quad t = 0 \quad\quad n_{A,0} \quad n_{D,0} \quad\quad n_{G,0} \quad n_{H,0}$$

$$t = t \quad\quad n_A \quad n_D \quad\quad n_G \quad n_H$$

where the capital letters stand for chemical substances and the lower-case letters stand for stoichiometric coefficients. n_A denotes the molar concentration (in $mol \cdot L^{-1}$ or $mol \cdot m^{-3}$) of substance A, and so on, and t is the time. So extent of reaction ξ can be expressed as

$$\xi = \frac{n_A - n_{A,0}}{-a} = \frac{n_D - n_{D,0}}{-d} = \frac{n_G - n_{G,0}}{g} = \frac{n_H - n_{H,0}}{h} \tag{5-1}$$

where the stoichiometric coefficients are negative for reactants and positive for products. As the rate of change of the extent of reaction

$$J \stackrel{\text{def}}{=} \frac{d\xi}{dt} = -\frac{1}{a}\frac{dn_A(t)}{dt} = -\frac{1}{d}\frac{dn_D(t)}{dt} = \frac{1}{g}\frac{dn_G(t)}{dt} = \frac{1}{h}\frac{dn_H(t)}{dt} \tag{5-2}$$

In view of such relations, the chemical reaction rate (r) can be defined as

$$r = \frac{J}{V} = \frac{1}{V}\frac{d\xi}{dt} \tag{5-3}$$

where V is the volume of the system. For a **homogeneous reaction** (均相反应) in a constant-volume system, the volume V can be taken inside the differential equation and equation (5-3) can be written as

$$r = -\frac{1}{a}\frac{dc_A}{dt} = -\frac{1}{d}\frac{dc_D}{dt} = \frac{1}{g}\frac{dc_G}{dt} = \frac{1}{h}\frac{dc_H}{dt} \tag{5-4}$$

For the gaseous reactions in a constant-volume system

$$2NO + Br_2 \longrightarrow 2NOBr$$

the chemical reaction rate (r) can be expressed as

$$r = -\frac{1}{2}\frac{dc_{NO}}{dt} = -\frac{dc_{Br_2}}{dt} = \frac{1}{2}\frac{dc_{NOBr}}{dt}$$

Obviously, the value of the chemical reaction rate is the same no matter whatever is chosen of the reactants and products.

1.2 Meaning of reaction mechanism

The mechanism of reaction is the microscopic pathway by which reactants are converted into products. It also called reaction process. Most of the chemical equations don't represent the real reaction processes, but just represent the overall stoichiometric formulas. Take the following chemical reaction for example:

$$H_2 + I_2 \longrightarrow 2HI \quad (\text{reaction } I)$$

It is shown in the experiment that the product HI isn't produced directly by the collision of reacting molecules H_2 and I_2. The reaction mechanism of the reaction I is thought to consist of the following steps:

$$(1) \; I_2 \longrightarrow 2I$$

$$(2)\ H_2 + 2I \cdot \longrightarrow 2HI$$

Consider the reaction

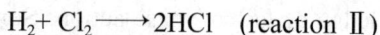

$$H_2 + Cl_2 \longrightarrow 2HCl \quad (\text{reaction } \text{II})$$

The stoichiometric formula is the same as the reaction I, but the reaction processes are different from each other. The reaction mechanism of the reaction II is thought to consist of four steps as follows:

$$(3)\ Cl_2 \longrightarrow 2Cl \cdot$$
$$(4)\ Cl \cdot + H_2 \longrightarrow HCl + H \cdot$$
$$(5)\ H \cdot + Cl_2 \longrightarrow HCl + Cl \cdot$$
$$(6)\ 2Cl \cdot + M \longrightarrow Cl_2 + M$$

where "M" stands for the reactor wall or the other third body molecule. It is an inert substance that only acts as a transfer of energy. If the product in a reaction is produced directly by the collision of reacting molecules, then such reaction is called **elementary reaction (基元反应)**. The elementary reaction is a simple reaction which occurs in a single step. The reaction equation (5) above, for instance, signifies that an H atom attacks a Cl_2 molecule to produce an HCl molecule and a Cl atom. The reaction which consists of only one elementary reaction is called **simple reaction (简单反应)**, it occurs in a single step. And the reaction which consists of two or more than two elementary reactions is called **complex reaction (复杂反应)**, it occurs in two or more steps. Most of the macroscopic reactions are complex reactions. The gaseous phase reactions of hydrogen iodide and hydrogen chloride are representative complex reactions.

1.3   Law of mass action

The rate of reaction depends on concentration of reactants at a given temperature. The exact relation between rate and concentration is determined by study of numerous reactions. It is shown that at a fixed temperature, the rate of a reaction is directly proportional to the reactant concentrations, each concentration being raised to some power.

For a reaction

$$aA + dD \longrightarrow gG + hH$$

The reaction rate with respect to A or D is determined by varying the concentration of one reactant, remaining that of the other constant. Thus the rate of reaction may be expressed as

$$r = k c_A^\alpha c_D^\beta \tag{5-5}$$

The expression which shows how the reaction rate is related to concentration is termed the rate law or rate equation.

Practical experience demonstrated the rate law of elementary reactions is relatively simple at a fixed temperature. The rate of elementary reaction is proportional to the reactant concentrations, each concentration being raised to a power equal to the coefficient that occurs in the chemical equation.

For the elementary reaction equation (2) above

$$H_2 + 2I \cdot \longrightarrow 2HI$$

The rate of reaction is expressed as

$$r = k c_{H_2} c_{I\cdot}^2$$

This law which is proposed by two Norwegian chemists, Guldberg and Waage is called **law of mass action (质量作用定律)**. They studied experimentally a large number of equilibrium reactions and postulated this generalization in 1864.

It's worth noting that not all the rate of reaction can be written by merely looking at the equation with a background of our knowledge of law of mass action. Some of the rates of reactions must be determined by experiment. Therefore, for some elementary reactions or simple reactions, the powers in the rate law may correspond to stoichiometric coefficients. But for the complex reaction, they don't correspond to stoichiometric coefficients. The law of mass action cannot be applied directly to complex reaction.

1.3.1 Reaction order

If the rate law of a reaction can be expressed as $r = kc_A^{\alpha} c_B^{\beta}\cdots$, where the exponents of the concentrations α, $\beta\cdots$are called **reaction orders (反应级数)**. α called the order with respect to A, and β is the order with respect to B, and so on, if other terms exist. The sum $n = \alpha + \beta +\cdots$ is the overall order (or simply the order) of the reaction. Orders are usually small positive whole numbers, but they may be negative whole numbers, zero, or even fractions. For a reaction $H_2+ I_2 \longrightarrow 2HI$, the rate law is $r = kc_{H_2}c_{I_2}$. This reaction is the second order, while the reaction order with respect to H_2 is the first order. For another example $H_2+ Cl_2 \longrightarrow 2HCl$, a reaction having the rate law $r = kc_{H_2}c_{Cl_2}^{1/2}$, is first-order in H_2, half-order in Cl_2, and one-half-order overall. But if the rate law doesn't fit for the form of $r = kc_A^{\alpha} c_B^{\beta}$, the concept of the reaction order can't be used on such reaction. The reaction of hydrogen (H_2) and bromine (Br_2), for example, has a very simple stoichiometry, $H_2+ Br_2 \longrightarrow 2HBr$, but its rate law is complicated $\frac{dc_{HBr}}{dt} = \frac{kc_{H_2}c_{HBr}^{1/2}}{1+k' c_{HBr}/c_{Br_2}}$. The concept of the reaction order can't be used on such reaction.

1.3.2 The reaction rate constant

In the form of the rate law $r = kc_A^{\alpha} c_B^{\beta}\cdots$, the coefficient k is called the **rate constant (速率常数)** for the reaction. The rate constant is equal to the rate of reaction when concentrations of the reactants are unity. The value of the rate constant k should also have units that will give a proper unit for the overall rate (which is usually $mol \cdot s^{-1}$). The rate constant is independent of the concentrations but depends on the temperature, reaction medium (solvent) and catalyst. And it even varies with the shape and nature of the reactor.

The rate constant k is an important physical quantity in chemical dynamics. Its value directly reflects the speed of the reaction.

1.3.3 Molecularity

The **molecularity (反应分子数)** is the number of molecules coming together to react in an elementary reaction. In a **unimolecular reaction (单分子反应)**, a single molecule shakes itself apart or its atoms into a new arrangement, as in the **isomerization (异构)** of **cyclopropane (环丙烷)** to **propene (丙烯)**. In a **bimolecular reaction (双分子反应)**, a pair of molecules collide and exchange energy, atoms, or groups of atoms, or undergo some other kind of change. In a **termolecular reaction (三分子反应)**, the steps involve three particles. Termolecular processes are relatively slow because of the small probability that three molecules will collide or diffuse together at once, and these processes occur less frequently in mechanics than do bimolecular processes. Elementary processes involving four or more reactant particles probably do not occur in chemical reaction mechanisms. Molecularity is defined only for elementary reactions and should not be used to describe **overall reactions (总反应)** that consist of more than one elementary step.

1.3.4 Differences between molecularity and reaction order

The term molecularity is often confused with reaction order. The total number of molecules or atoms which take part in a reaction as represented by the chemical equation is known as the molecularity of the reaction. Molecularity is the number of reacting species undergoing simultaneous collision in the elementary or simple reaction. It is theoretical concept and always a whole number. But it can't have zero value. Molecularity is invariant for a chemical equation. The reaction order is the sum of powers of the concentration terms in the chemical rate equation. It is an experimentally. It can have fractional value and can assume zero value. It also can change with conditions such as pressure, temperature, concentration.

In an elementary reaction, the molecularity is consistent with the reaction order. Thus the unimolecular reaction is the first-order reaction, and the bimolecular reaction is the second-order reaction.

Section 2   Effect of Concentration on Reaction Rate

2.1   Kinetic equation of first-order reaction and its characteristics

2.1.1   Kinetic equation and characteristics for first-order reaction

A first-order reaction is one for which, at a given temperature, the rate of the reaction depends only on the first power of the concentration of a single reacting species. If the concentration of this species is represented by c (for solutions, the units of moles per liter are ordinarily used), and if the volume of the system remains essentially constant in the course of the reaction, the first-order rate equation can be written as

$$r = -\frac{dc}{dt} = kc \tag{5-6}$$

A general first-order reaction is considered as follows

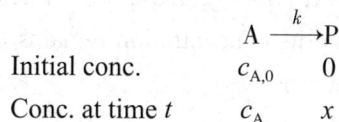

$$A \xrightarrow{\ k\ } P$$

Initial conc.	$c_{A,0}$	0
Conc. at time t	c_A	x

The kinetic data can be treated in terms of the following quantities: $c_{A,0}$ is **initial concentration (初始浓度)** of A, x moles of A have decreased in time t, k is the rate constants of the reaction, thus, $c_A = (c_{A,0} - x)$.

Integrating (积分) equation (5-6) between the limits $t = 0$, $c_A = c_{A,0}$ and $t = t, c = c_A$ gives

$$\int_{c_{A,0}}^{c_A} -\frac{dc_A}{c_A} = \int_0^t k\,dt$$

$$\ln\frac{c_{A,0}}{c_A} = kt \quad \text{or} \quad \ln c_A = \ln c_{A,0} - kt \tag{5-7}$$

$$c_A = c_{A,0}e^{-kt} \tag{5-8}$$

Equation (5-7) can also be written as

PPT

微课

$$k = \frac{1}{t}\ln\frac{c_{A,0}}{c_A} = \frac{1}{t}\ln\frac{c_{A,0}}{c_{A,0}-x} \qquad (5\text{--}9)$$

Characteristics of the first-order reaction are listed below.

(1) The dimension of the rate constant k is $[\text{time}]^{-1}$. Thus its unit is s^{-1}, min^{-1}, and h^{-1}.

(2) As equation (5–7) shows, a plot of $\ln c_A$ versus t gives a straight line. If a straight line is obtained, the **slope (斜率)** of the line is $(-k)$, and the **intercept (截距)** of the line is $\ln c_{A,0}$.

(3) The half-life(半衰期) ($t_{1/2}$) is the time required for the concentration or amount of the reactant to decrease to half its initial value. For a first-order reaction the relation of the half-life to the rate constant can be found from equation (5–9) by inserting the requirement that at $t = t_{1/2}$ the concentration is $c_A = \frac{1}{2}c_{A,0}$. In this way one obtains

$$t_{1/2} = \frac{1}{k}\ln\frac{c_{A,0}}{\frac{1}{2}c_{A,0}} = \frac{\ln 2}{k} = \frac{0.693}{k} \qquad (5\text{--}10)$$

As equation (5–10) shows that for a first-order reaction there is a simple reciprocal relation between k and $t_{1/2}$. The half-life for a first-order reaction is independent of the initial concentration or amount of the reactants.

Examples of first-order reactions are listed below.

(1) **Radioactive decay (放射衰变)**. An example is ${}^{226}_{88}\text{Ra} \longrightarrow {}^{222}_{86}\text{Rn} + {}^{4}_{2}\text{He}$

(2) Most of the **decomposition (分解)**. An example is $N_2O_5 \longrightarrow N_2O_4 + \frac{1}{2}O_2$

(3) The **rearrangement (重排)** and isomerization of some molecules.

(4) The drug absorption and **elimination (消除)** in the body, and the **hydrolysis (水解)** reaction of some drugs.

(5) Inversion of Cane sugar **(sucrose) (蔗糖)**. Sucrose upon hydrolysis in presence of a dilute acid gives glucose and fructose.

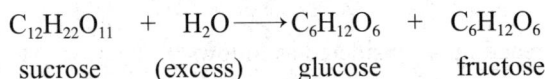

$$\begin{array}{ccccc} C_{12}H_{22}O_{11} & + & H_2O \longrightarrow C_6H_{12}O_6 & + & C_6H_{12}O_6 \\ \text{sucrose} & & \text{(excess)} \quad\quad \text{glucose} & & \text{fructose} \end{array}$$

Here a large excess of water is used, and its concentration remains practically unchanged in the reaction process. Thus the rate law can be written as

$$r = -\frac{dc}{dt} = kc_{H_2O}c_{\text{sucrose}} = k'c_{\text{sucrose}}$$

The reaction is actually second-order but in practice it is found to be first-order. It is called **pseudo-first order (准一级)** reaction.

2.1.2 Application of first-order reaction in medicine field

(1) Application of first-order reaction in predicting the expiration date of drug

The first-order reaction is widely used in predicting the **expiration date (有效期)** of the drug. The drug will lose the potency when 10% of its active ingredient content is degraded. Therefore, the time when the active ingredient content of drug is reduced to 90% is called expiration date. We can get equation (5–11) deduced from the first-order rate equation (5–9) as follows.

$$k = \frac{1}{t}\ln\frac{c_{A,0}}{c_A} = \frac{1}{t}\ln\frac{c_{A,0}}{0.9c_{A,0}} = \frac{0.1055}{t} \qquad \text{or} \qquad t_{0.9} = \frac{0.1055}{k} \qquad (5\text{--}11)$$

Then the expiration date can be calculated through equation (5–11), if the rate constant k is known.

(2) Application of first-order reaction in drug elimination kinetics

The first-order reaction can also be used in the formulation of a reasonable dosing regimen. It is now known that the law of blood concentration changes with time after injection of drugs conforms to the first-order reaction. So the first-order reaction equation can be used to calculate the highest and lowest levels of blood concentration in the body after n times of injections.

It can be known from equation (5–8) that when t is a constant, the value of e^{-kt} is also a constant (γ). So in the same time interval, the same dose ($c_{A,0}$) is injected, $c_A/c_{A,0} = e^{-kt} = \gamma$. After the first injection, the blood concentration is $c_{A,01} = c_{A,0}$, t hours later, after the first injection, the blood concentration is $c_{A,1} = c_{A,0}\gamma$. After the second injection, the blood concentration has increased by $c_{A,0}$ over the previous concentration c_{A1}.

$$c_{A,02} = c_{A,0} + c_{A,1} = c_{A,0} + c_{A,0}\gamma$$

t hours later, after the second injection, the blood concentration is

$$c_{A,2} = c_{A,02}\gamma = (c_{A,0} + c_{A,0}\gamma)\gamma$$

After the third injection, the blood concentration is

$$c_{A,03} = c_{A,0} + c_{A,2} = c_{A,0} + (c_{A,0} + c_{A,0}\gamma)\gamma = c_{A,0} + c_{A,0}\gamma + c_{A,0}\gamma^2$$

t hours later, after the third injection, the blood concentration is

$$c_{A,3} = c_{A,03}\gamma = (c_{A,0} + c_{A,0}\gamma + c_{A,0}\gamma^2)\gamma$$

After the nth injection (the same dose), the blood concentration is

$$c_{A,0_n} = c_{A,0} + c_{A,0}\gamma + c_{A,0}\gamma^2 + \cdots + c_{A,0}\gamma^{n-1} = c_{A,0}(1 + \gamma + \gamma^2 + \cdots + \gamma^{n-1}) \tag{5–12}$$

t hours later, after the nth injection, the blood concentration is

$$c_{A,n} = c_{A,0n}\gamma = c_{A,0}(\gamma + \gamma^2 + \cdots + \gamma^n) \tag{5–13}$$

Equation (5–12) minus equation (5–13)

$$c_{A,0n} - c_{A,n} = c_{A,0} - c_{A,0}\gamma^n$$

$$\text{or} \quad c_{A,0n} = \frac{c_{A,0} - c_{A,0}\gamma^n}{1 - \gamma}$$

When $\gamma < 1$, $n \to \infty$, $\gamma^n \to 0$, the highest blood concentration $c_{A,0max}$ after the nth injection can be obtained as

$$c_{A,0\,max} = \frac{c_{A,0}}{1 - \gamma} \tag{5–14}$$

The lowest blood concentration $c_{A,n\,min}$ after the nth injection can be obtained as

$$c_{A,n\,min} = c_{A,0\,max}\gamma = \frac{c_{A,0}\gamma}{1 - \gamma} \tag{5–15}$$

[**Example 5–1**] The isotope of Plutonium makes a β-radiation. The activity of the isotope decreases by 6.85% after 14 days. Try to calculate the rate constant and half-life for the isotopic decay. And how long does it take to decompose 90.0% of the isotope?

Solution:

If the initial content $c_{A,0}$ of the isotope is 100%, its undecomposed content $(c_{A,0} - x) = (100\% - 6.85\%)$. Substituting the data above in equation (5–9), we get

$$k = \frac{1}{t}\ln\frac{c_{A,0}}{c_{A,0}-x} = \frac{1}{14}\times\ln\frac{100}{100-6.85} = 0.00507\text{d}^{-1}$$

Then substituting the value of k in equation (5–10), gives

$$t_{1/2} = \frac{0.693}{k} = \frac{0.693}{0.00507} = 136.7\text{d}$$

The time for decomposing 90% of the isotope also can be calculated by equation (5–9).

$$t = \frac{1}{k}\ln\frac{c_{A,0}}{c_{A,0}-x} = \frac{1}{0.00507}\times\ln\frac{100}{100-90} = 454.2\text{d}$$

[**Example 5–2**] After the drug is applied to the human body, it establishes a balance with body fluids in the blood on the one hand, and can be eliminated through the kidneys on the other hand. When the equilibrium is reached, the rate of the drug elimination from the blood can be expressed by the first-order rate equation. After 0.5g of the drug was injected into the human body, the blood concentrations were tested at different time intervals. Then the data attained were listed in the following Table 5–1. Try to answer the following questions: (1) The half-life of the drug in the blood. (2) If the blood concentration can't reduce to $0.40 \times 10^{-6}\text{kg} \cdot 0.1\text{dm}^{-3}$, how long does it take to do the second injection?

Table 5–1   The thermodynamic data of the related substances

t / h	4	8	12	16
$c / (\text{kg} \cdot 0.1\text{dm}^{-3})$	0.48×10^{-6}	0.34×10^{-6}	0.24×10^{-6}	0.17×10^{-6}
$\ln c$	−14.55	−14.89	−15.24	−15.59

Solution:

(1) A plot of $\ln c$ versus t gives a straight line as follows (Fig. 5–1)

The slope of the line is −0.0864, thus the rate constant $k = 0.0864\text{h}^{-1}$.

(2) Substituting the value of k in equation (5–10), gives

$$t_{1/2} = \frac{\ln 2}{k} = \frac{0.693}{0.0864} = 8.02\text{h} \approx 8\text{h}$$

Since the concentration of half-life is $0.34 \times 10^{-6}\text{kg} \times 0.1\text{dm}^{-3}$ shown in the Table 5–1, the initial concentration can be attained as $0.68 \times 10^{-6}\text{kg} \cdot 0.1\text{dm}^{-3}$. Then the time to take the second injection is

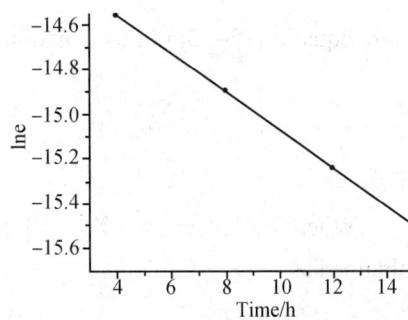

Fig. 5-1   A plot of $\ln c$ versus t

$$t = \frac{1}{k}\ln\frac{c_{A,0}}{c_A} = \frac{1}{0.0864}\times\ln\frac{0.68\times10^{-6}}{0.40\times10^{-6}} = 6.14\text{h} \approx 6\text{h}$$

[**Example 5–3**] According to the data from the above example, if the drug is injected into the body every 6h, what are the highest and lowest concentration of tetracycline in the blood after the nth injections?

Solution:

Substituting the data above in equation (5–7), we get

$$\ln\frac{c_{A,0}}{c_A} = \ln\frac{0.68\times10^{-6}}{c_A} = 0.0864\times6$$

$$c_A = 0.405 \times 10^{-6} \mathrm{kg} \times 0.1 \mathrm{dm}^{-3}$$

$$c_{A,0\,\max} = \frac{c_{A,0}}{1-\gamma} = \frac{0.68 \times 10^{-6}}{1-0.60} = 1.7 \times 10^{-6} \ \mathrm{kg} \times 0.1 \mathrm{dm}^{-3}$$

$$c_{A,n\,\min} = c_{A,0\,\max}\gamma = 1.7 \times 10^{-6} \times 0.60 = 1.0 \times 10^{-6} \mathrm{kg} \times 0.1 \mathrm{dm}^{-3}$$

2.2　Kinetic equation of second-order reaction（二级反应）and its characteristics

A reaction is classified as second-order if the rate of the reaction is proportional to the square of the concentration of one of the reactants or to the product of the concentrations of two species of the reactants.

There are two kinds of second-order reactions are listed below.

$$2A \longrightarrow P$$
$$A + B \longrightarrow P$$

For the second kind of the second-order reaction, if $c_{A,0}$ and $c_{B,0}$ are the initial concentrations of A and B,

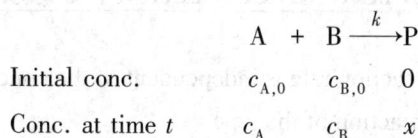

$$
\begin{array}{cccc}
 & A & + \quad B & \xrightarrow{\ k\ } P \\
\text{Initial conc.} & c_{A,0} & c_{B,0} & 0 \\
\text{Conc. at time } t & c_A & c_B & x
\end{array}
$$

After time t, x moles of each reactant is reacted, the concentration of A, B and P will be $c_A = (c_{A,0}-x)$, $c_B = (c_{B,0}-x)$ and $c_p = x$, respectively. k is the rate constants of the reaction, the reaction rate equation gives

$$r = -\frac{dc}{dt} = \frac{dx}{dt} = kc_A c_B = k(c_{A,0}-x)(c_{B,0}-x) \qquad (5\text{-}16)$$

If the two reactants are used up at the same rate and if their initial concentrations are equal ($c_{A,0} = c_{B,0}$), equation (5-16) can be expressed as follows

$$\frac{dx}{dt} = kc_A^2 = k(c_{A,0}-x)^2 \qquad (5\text{-}17)$$

For the first kind of the second-order reaction, the reaction rate equation is the same as equation (5-17). On integration, we get

$$\frac{1}{c_A} - \frac{1}{c_{A,0}} = kt \quad \text{or} \quad k = \frac{1}{t} \cdot \frac{x}{c_{A,0}c_A} = \frac{1}{t} \cdot \frac{x}{c_{A,0}(c_{A,0}-x)} \qquad (5\text{-}18)$$

If it is inconvenient to arrange to have the initial concentrations of A and B equal, the analysis that led to equation (5-18) cannot be used. Integrating equation (5-16), gives

$$\frac{1}{(c_{A,0}-c_{B,0})} \ln \frac{c_{B,0}c_A}{c_{A,0}c_B} = kt$$

$$\text{or} \quad k = \frac{1}{t(c_{A,0}-c_{B,0})} \ln \frac{c_{B,0}c_A}{c_{A,0}c_B} = \frac{1}{t(c_{A,0}-c_{B,0})} \ln \frac{c_{B,0}(c_{A,0}-x)}{c_{A,0}(c_{B,0}-x)} \qquad (5\text{-}19)$$

Characteristics of the second-order reaction are listed below:

(1) The dimension of the rate constant k is $[\text{concentration}]^{-1} \cdot [\text{time}]^{-1}$. If the units of concentration

and time are $mol \cdot dm^{-3}$ and s respectively, k will be given in $dm^3 \cdot mol^{-1} \cdot s^{-1}$. It shows that the unit of k has relations with concentration and time.

(2) As equation (5–18) shows, a plot of $\dfrac{1}{c_A}$ versus t gives a straight line, and the slope of the line can be used to give the values of the rate constant k.

(3) The half-life for the second-order reaction deduced from equation (5–18) is

$$t_{1/2} = \frac{c_{A,0}/2}{kc_{A,0}(c_{A,0}-c_{A,0}/2)} = \frac{1}{kc_{A,0}}$$

This result shows that the half-life is inversely proportional to initial concentration. It is a criterion to classify a reaction as second-order. But if the initial concentrations of reactants are not equal, the reactants have their own half-lives, and they are different with each other. Then the half-life of the reaction is difficult to determine.

The second-order reaction is very common. **Dimerizations (二聚作用)** of **ethylene (乙烯)**, propene or **isobutylene (异丁烯)**, decomposition of $NaClO_3$, **saponification (皂化)** of ethyl acetate, thermal decomposition of **hydrogen iodide (HI)** or **methanal** (甲醛) are all the second-order reactions.

2.3 Kinetic equation of zero-order reaction (零级反应) and its characteristics

In a zero-order reaction, the reaction rate is independent of the concentration of the reaction.

Let us consider a zero-order reaction of the type

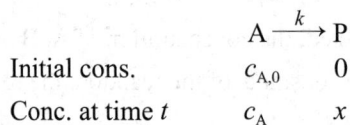

$$A \xrightarrow{\;k\;} P$$

Initial cons.	$c_{A,0}$	0
Conc. at time t	c_A	x

$c_{A,0}$ is initial concentration of A, if after time t, x moles of A decreased, k is the rate constants of the reaction, thus, $c_A = (c_{A,0}-x)$ and $c_P = x$.

The reaction rate equation can be expressed as

$$r = -\frac{dc}{dt} = \frac{dx}{dt} = k$$

On integrating，we get

$$x = kt \quad or \quad k = \frac{x}{t} \tag{5-20}$$

Characteristics of the zero-order reaction are listed below:

(1) The dimension of the rate constant k is $[concentration] \cdot [time]^{-1}$. If the units of concentration and time are $mol \cdot dm^{-3}$ and s respectively, k will be given in $mol \cdot dm^{-3} \cdot s^{-1}$. It shows that the unit of k has relations with concentration and time.

(2) As equation (5–20) shows, a plot of x versus t gives a straight line, and the slope of the line can be used to give the values of the rate constant k.

(3) The half-life for the zero-order reaction is $t_{1/2} = \dfrac{c_{A,0}/2}{k} = \dfrac{c_{A,0}}{2k}$. This result shows that the half-life is proportional to initial concentration.

The zero-order reaction is not common. The surface catalyzed reactions are the most in the zero-order reactions which have been known. Consider the decomposition of **ammonia (NH_3)** on **tungsten**

(钨) as

$$2\,NH_3 \xrightarrow{\;W\;} N_2 + 3H_2$$

Since the reaction takes place only on the surface of the catalyst, the reaction rate is only related to the surface state. If the surface of tungsten is saturated by NH_3, the reaction rate will be not affected by the increase of NH_3. At this situation, the reaction is zero-order reaction.

In order to classify the reaction order conveniently with the characteristics of the reaction, the rate equations and characteristics of the above reactions are listed in Table 5–2.

Table 5–2   The rate equations and characteristics for the simple order reactions

Reaction order	Differential formula	Integral formula	Half life	Linear relation	Dimension of k
1	$\dfrac{dx}{dt} = kc_A$	$\ln \dfrac{c_{A,0}}{c_A} = kt$	$t_{1/2} = \dfrac{0.693}{k}$	$\ln c_A \sim t$	$[\text{time}]^{-1}$
2	$\dfrac{dx}{dt} = kc_A^2$	$\dfrac{1}{c_A} - \dfrac{1}{c_{A,0}} = kt$	$t_{1/2} = \dfrac{1}{kc_{A,0}}$	$\dfrac{1}{c_A} \sim t$	$[\text{concentration}]^{-1} \cdot [\text{time}]^{-1}$
2	$\dfrac{dx}{dt} = kc_A c_B$	$\dfrac{1}{(c_{A,0} - c_{B,0})} \ln \dfrac{c_{B,0}c_A}{c_{A,0}c_B} = kt$	insignificance	$\ln \dfrac{c_{B,0}c_A}{c_{A,0}c_B} \sim t$	$[\text{concentration}]^{-1} \cdot [\text{time}]^{-1}$
0	$\dfrac{dx}{dt} = k$	$x = kt$	$t_{1/2} = \dfrac{c_{A,0}}{2k}$	$c \sim t$ or $x \sim t$	$[\text{concentration}] \cdot [\text{time}]^{-1}$

Section 3   Determination of Reaction Order

PPT

In order to meet the needs of design and applications in industrial production, the regression of dynamic data is usually approximated by equation (5–5) within a certain range, and the empirical rate equation can be established. In such kind of rate equation, only the rate constant k and the reaction order n are kinetic parameters. So the rate equation is found by the determinations of the rate constant k and reaction order n. Since the integral formula of rate equation only dependents on n, independent of k, the determination of reaction order n is the key to determine the rate equation. Experimental data give species concentrations at various times during the reaction. This section discusses how the reaction order n is determined from experimental concentration-versus-time data. The discussion is restricted to cases where the rate equation has the form $r = kc_A^{\alpha} c_B^{\beta} \cdots$

There are at least two different methods to determine the order of a reaction. One is **integration method,** and the other is **differential (微分) method.**

3.1   Integral method

In integral method, the different rate equations in their integrated forms (shown in Table 5–2) are used.

3.1.1　Hit-and-trial method（尝试法）

The reaction under study is performed by taking different initial concentrations of the reactant ($c_{A,0}$) and noting the concentration $c_A = (c_{A,0} - x)$ after regular time intervals (t). The experimental values of $c_{A,0}$, c_A and t are then substituted into the integrated rate equations for the first, second and zero order reactions. The rate equation which yields a constant value of k corresponds to the correct order of the reaction. This method of ascertaining the order of a reaction is essentially a method of **hit-and-trial** but was the first to be employed. It is still used extensively to find the order of simple reactions.

The disadvantage of this method is that it is not sensitive enough and can only be used for simple order reactions. If the experimental data is not enough, it is difficult to determine the reaction order.

3.1.2　Graphical method（图解法）

The integrated rate equations can be rearranged in the form of a linear equation. The reaction order can be determined by seeing whether a graph of the data fits one of the linear rate equations.

If a plot of $\ln c_A$ versus t gives a straight line, the corresponding reaction is of the first order. However, if a curve is obtained, the reaction is not first order.

If a plot of $1/c_A$ versus t gives a straight line, the corresponding reaction is of the second order. However, if a curve is obtained, the reaction is not second order.

If a plot of x versus t gives a straight line, the corresponding reaction is of the zero order. However, if a curve is obtained, the reaction is not zero order.

As the reaction order is determined by seeing whether a graph of the data fits one of the integrated rate equations, the graphical method is also a method of hit-and-trial.

3.1.3　Half-life method（半衰期法）

Two separate experiments are performed by taking different initial concentrations of a reactant. The progress of the reaction in each case is recorded by analysis. When the initial concentration is reduced to one-half, the time is noted. Let the initial concentrations in the two experiments be $c_{A,0}$ and $c'_{A,0}$, while times for completion of half change are $t_{1/2}$ and $t'_{1/2}$, respectively.

We know that half-life period for a first order reaction is independent of the initial concentration. To test for other orders, we can obtain by calculation. When the initial concentrations of the reactants are equal, the half-life of reaction is

$$t_{1/2} = A \times \frac{1}{c_{A,0}^{n-1}} \tag{5-21}$$

where n is the reaction order, while A is a constant. Substituting values of initial concentrations and half-life from the two experiments, we have

$$\frac{t_{1/2}}{t'_{1/2}} = \left(\frac{c'_{A,0}}{c_{A,0}} \right)^{n-1}$$

Taking the logarithm of both sides, it becomes $\log\left(\dfrac{t_{1/2}}{t'_{1/2}} \right) = (n-1) \log\left(\dfrac{c'_{A,0}}{c_{A,0}} \right)$

Solving for n, the reaction order $n = 1 + \dfrac{\log\left(\dfrac{t_{1/2}}{t'_{1/2}} \right)}{\log\left(\dfrac{c'_{A,0}}{c_{A,0}} \right)}$

If the experimental data is enough, n can also be determined by graphical method. Taking the logarithm of equation (5-21), we get

$$\log t_{1/2} = (1-n)\log c_{A,0} + \log A$$

If a plot of $\log t_{1/2}$ versus $\log c_{A,0}$ gives a straight line, the value of n can be calculated from the slope of the line.

The half-life method is more reliable than the first two methods. It is not limited to the half-life $t_{1/2}$, for the half-life $t_{1/2}$ can also be substituted for the reaction time t which is equal to 1/3, 2/3 and so on. The half-life method has the disadvantage that, if data from a single run are used, the reaction must be followed to a high percentage of completion.

3.2　Differential method

The differential method is the method to determine the reaction order by the differential form of the rate equation. If there is only one kind of reactant in the reaction or all concentrations of reactants are the same, the rate equation of the reaction can be expressed as

$$r = -\frac{dc}{dt} = kc^n \tag{5-22}$$

We take the logarithm of both sides of this equation

$$\log r = \log\left(-\frac{dc}{dt}\right) = \log k + n\log c \tag{5-23}$$

Plotting concentration (c) against time (t) with the experimental data, the slope r, at a given time interval is measured by drawing tangents. If a plot of $\log r$ versus $\log c$ gives a straight line, the slope of the line can be used to give the values of n.

It's worth noting that when the differential method is used to calculate the reaction order, it's best to use the initial rate. Plot concentration (c) against time (t) with the experimental data under the different initial concentrations, then the corresponding slops ($-\frac{dc}{dt}$) can be calculated at different initial concentrations. The next step of the method is the same as above. The advantage of the initial concentration method is to avoid the interference of the products in the reaction.

If there are more than two kinds of reactants in the reaction, and the initial concentrations of the reactants are not equal, the reaction rate equation can be expressed as $r = kc_A^{\alpha}c_B^{\beta}\cdots$

It is very difficult to calculate the order α, β…… in such reactions with all of the methods described earlier. In order to solve this problem, the isolation method can be used. This method is employed in determining the order of complicated reactions by "isolating" one of the reactants so far as its influence on the rate of reaction is concerned. For the determination of the order of reaction with respect to A, B is taken in a large excess so that it concentration is not affected during the reaction. Then the rate equation is transformed into

$$r = k'c_A^{\alpha} \tag{5-24}$$

The order of the reaction is then determined by using any of the methods described earlier. Likewise, the order of the reaction with respect to B is determined. Then the order of the reaction n is given by the expression

$$n = \alpha + \beta + \cdots \tag{5-25}$$

Section 4　Complex Reactions

Some reactions proceed in a series of steps instead of a single step and the rate of overall reaction is in accordance with the **stoichiometric equation (计量方程)** of that reaction. These reactions are called complex reactions. For example, **dissociation (解离)** of **hydrogen iodides (HI)**, **bromination (溴化)** of **bromobenzene (溴苯)**, **hydrolyzation (水解)** of **gentianose (龙胆三糖)**, etc. The common typical complex reactions involve **reversible reaction (可逆反应)**, **parallel reaction (平行反应)** and **consecutive reaction (连续反应)**, etc. These are discussed as follows.

4.1　Reversible reaction

There are certain chemical reactions proceed to incompletion. In these reactions the substances react to form products which themselves react to give back the original substances. Thus A and B may react to form C and D which react together to reform A and B.

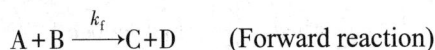

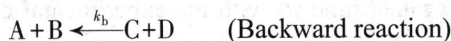

$$A + B \xrightarrow{\ k_f\ } C + D \qquad \text{(Forward reaction)}$$

$$A + B \xleftarrow{\ k_b\ } C + D \qquad \text{(Backward reaction)}$$

A reaction which can go in the forward and backward direction simultaneously is termed a reversible reaction or **opposing reaction (对峙反应)**. Such a reaction is represented by writing a pair of arrows between the reactants and products. The arrow pointing right indicates the forward reaction, while that pointing left shows the reverse reaction.

$$A + B \underset{k_b}{\overset{k_f}{\rightleftharpoons}} C + D$$

In a reversible reaction, when the forward reaction rate is much more comparing to the backward reaction rate, the equilibrium will be far away from the starting end and the reaction may be found to follow a simple and straightforward path as discussed earlier. However, if the reverse reaction cannot be neglected, the kinetics must be taken into consideration for both the direction.

Let us consider the simplest case, a reaction that is first order in both directions

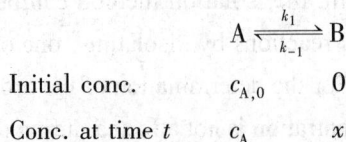

$$A \underset{k_{-1}}{\overset{k_1}{\rightleftharpoons}} B$$

Initial conc.　　　　　$c_{A,0}$　　　0

Conc. at time t　　　c_A　　　x

We denote the rate constant for the forward reaction by k_1 and the rate constant for the backward reaction by k_{-1}. If $c_{A,0}$ is the initial concentration of A and x moles of it have reacted in time t, then $c_A = (c_{A,0}-x)$ and $c_B = x$.

Rate of forward reaction

$$r_{forward} = k_1 c_A = k_1 (c_{A,0}-x) \qquad (5-26)$$

Rate of backward reaction

$$r_{backward} = k_{-1} c_B = k_{-1} x \qquad (5-27)$$

The observable rate of the reaction is a **net rate(净速率)** given by the difference between the forward rate and the reverse rate.

Net rate of reaction

$$r_{net} = \frac{dx}{dt} = r_{forward} - r_{backward} = k_1 c_A - k_{-1} c_B = k_1 (c_{A,0} - x) - k_{-1} x \tag{5-28}$$

or

$$\frac{dx}{k_1 (c_{A,0} - x) - k_{-1} x} = dt \tag{5-29}$$

Integrating equation (5-29), we get

$$\ln \frac{c_{A,0}}{c_{A,0} - \left(\frac{k_1 + k_{-1}}{k_1} \right) x} = (k_1 + k_{-1}) t \tag{5-30}$$

This is the rate equation of reversible reaction that is first order in both directions.

At equilibrium, the forward and back reaction rates are equal (but not zero), therefore, the net rate of reaction will be zero ($r_{net,eq} = dx / dt = 0$). When $x = x_{eq}$,

$$r_{net,eq} = k_1 c_{A,eq} - k_{-1} c_{B,eq} = k_1 (c_{A,0} - x_{eq}) - k_{-1} x_{eq} = 0 \tag{5-31}$$

where x_{eq} is the concentration of A that has reacted into B at equilibrium. From equation (5-31) we get

$$k_{-1} = k_1 \frac{(c_{A,0} - x_{eq})}{x_{eq}} \tag{5-32}$$

Substituting the value of k_{-1} in equation (5-28), gives

$$\frac{dx}{dt} = k_1 (c_{A,0} - x) - k_1 \left(\frac{c_{A,0} - x_{eq}}{x_{eq}} \right) x \tag{5-33}$$

On integration, we get

$$\ln \frac{x_{eq}}{x_{eq} - x} = k_1 \frac{c_{A,0}}{x_{eq}} t \tag{5-34}$$

From equation (5-34) we can find the value of k_1 from the quantities $c_{A,0}$, x_{eq} and x at time t. All these quantities can be measured easily. From the value of k_1 the value of k_{-1} can be calculated by using equation (5-32).

Variation of the amounts of species over time is illustrated in Fig. 5-2. It is clear that, the amounts of reactant c_A and product c_B approach their equilibrium values as a reaction approaches equilibrium. The equilibrium constant K for this reaction is

$$K = \frac{c_{B,eq}}{c_{A,eq}} = \frac{k_1}{k_{-1}} \tag{5-35}$$

K is related to the ratio of forward and backward rate constants for the reaction. A large value for K means that the rate constant for the forward reaction is large compared with that for the reverse reaction. A small value means that the rate constant for the forward reaction is small compared with that for the reverse reaction. The greater the forward rate constant relative to that for the back reaction, the more equilibrium will favor products over reactants. Equation (5-35) can apply to a more

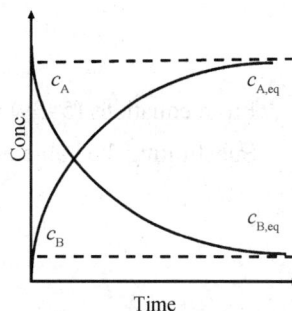

Fig. 5-2 Plots of the amounts of various species versus time for reversible reaction

general case if orders are equal to stoichiometric coefficients.

4.2 Parallel reaction

In these reactions the reacting undergoes in more than one pathway giving rise to different products. The preferential rate of such may be changed by varying the conditions like pressure, temperature or catalyst. The reaction in which the maximum yield of the products is obtained is called the main or major reaction while the other reactions are called parallel or side reactions. It's show in Fig. 5–3.

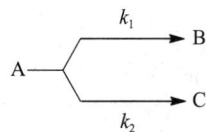

Fig. 5–3 Schematic diagram of parallel reaction

In the above reaction the reactant A gives two products B and C separately in two different reactions with the rate constants k_1 and k_2, respectively. If $k_1 > k_2$, B will be the major product and C will be the side product. Let us assume that both these reactions are first order, the concentration of A, B and C are c_A, c_B and c_C, respectively at time t. The differential rate expressions are

$$r_1 = -\frac{dc_A}{dt} = \frac{dc_B}{dt} = k_1 c_A \tag{5-36}$$

$$\text{and} \quad r_2 = -\frac{dc_A}{dt} = \frac{dc_C}{dt} = k_2 c_A \tag{5-37}$$

The total rate of elimination of A is given by

$$r = -\frac{dc_A}{dt} = r_1 + r_2 = k_1 c_A + k_2 c_A = (k_1 + k_2) c_A = k' c_A \tag{5-38}$$

where k' is the first order rate constant. It is equal to the sum of the two constants k_1 and k_2 of two parallel reactions.

Integrating equation (5–38) as any other first order rate law, we get

$$\ln \frac{c_{A,0}}{c_A} = k't = (k_1 + k_2) t \tag{5-39}$$

$$\text{or} \quad c_A = c_{A,0} e^{-(k_1+k_2)t} \tag{5-40}$$

where $c_{A,0}$ is the initial concentration of the reactant A.

The ratio of the rates for two side reactions is obtained by dividing equations (5–36) by (5–37), we have

$$\frac{r_1}{r_2} = \frac{k_1 c_A}{k_2 c_A} = \frac{k_1}{k_2} \tag{5-41}$$

From equations (5–39) and (5–41) we can calculate the individual rate constant k_1 and k_2.

Substituting the value of c_A to equation (5–36) and (5–37), we get

$$\frac{dc_B}{dt} = k_1 c_{A,0} e^{-(k_1+k_2)t} \tag{5-42}$$

$$\frac{dc_C}{dt} = k_2 c_{A,0} e^{-(k_1+k_2)t} \tag{5-43}$$

These two equations can be integrated in order to determine the concentrations of B and C over time.

$$c_B = \frac{k_1 c_{A,0}}{k_1 + k_2}[1 - e^{-(k_1+k_2)t}] \tag{5-44}$$

$$c_C = \frac{k_2 c_{A,0}}{k_1 + k_2}[1 - e^{-(k_1+k_2)t}] \tag{5-45}$$

The concentrations of B and C all depend on negative **exponentials (指数)**, but in these cases the negative exponential is subtracted from 1. Therefore, as time increases and the negative exponential gets smaller and smaller, the difference gets larger and larger, c_B and c_C increase as the elapsed time increases. Fig. 5–4 illustrates the behavior of c_A, c_B and c_C for a given set of rate constants.

4.3   Consecutive reaction

Frequently a product formed in one of the elementary reactions acts as the reactant for a subsequent elementary reaction. This reaction is termed consecutive reaction or **sequential reaction (顺序反应)**. The overall reaction is a result of several consecutive steps. Every stage has its own reactant and rate constant.

Fig. 5–4   Plots of the amounts of various species versus time for two parallel reactions

Let us consider a simple reaction

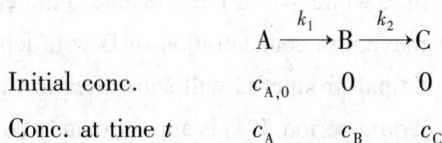

$$A \xrightarrow{k_1} B \xrightarrow{k_2} C$$

Initial conc. $c_{A,0}$ 0 0

Conc. at time t c_A c_B c_C

In the above reaction the product C is formed from the reactant A through intermediate B. k_1 and k_2 are rate constants for the first step and the second step, respectively. The net or overall rate of reaction depends upon the magnitude of the two rate constants.

Let $c_{A,0}$ represents the initial concentration and c_A, c_B and c_C represents the concentrations of A, B and C respectively, at any time t, then

$$c_{A,0} = c_A - c_B + c_C \tag{5-46}$$

The rate of elimination of A is given as
$$r_A = -\frac{dc_A}{dt} = k_1 c_A \tag{5-47}$$

Integrating, we get
$$c_A = c_{A,0}e^{-k_1 t} \tag{5-48}$$

Equation (5–48) gives the concentration of reactant A at any time t.

Rate of formation of B
$$\frac{dc_B}{dt} = k_1 c_A \tag{5-49}$$

Rate of elimination of B
$$-\frac{dc_B}{dt} = k_2 c_B \tag{5-50}$$

Therefore, rate of accumulation of B in the system is
$$r_B = \frac{dc_B}{dt} = k_1 c_A - k_2 c_B \tag{5-51}$$

or
$$\frac{dc_B}{dt} + k_2 c_B = k_1 c_A = k_1 c_{A,0}e^{-k_1 t} \tag{5-52}$$

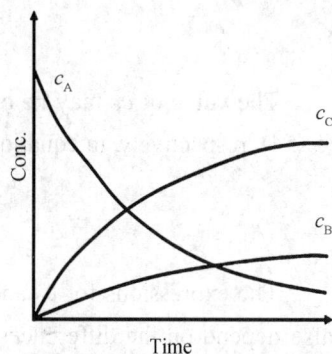

159

and rate of formation of C is

$$r_C = \frac{dc_C}{dt} = k_2 c_B \tag{5-53}$$

The result of linear differential equation (5–52) with constant coefficients of the second order is

$$c_B = \frac{k_1}{k_2 - k_1} c_{A,0} (e^{-k_1 t} - e^{-k_2 t}) \tag{5-54}$$

The value of c_C may be obtained by substituting the values of c_A and c_B from equations (5–48) and (5–54), respectively, in equation (5–46). Thus, we get

$$c_C = c_{A,0} \left(1 - \frac{k_2}{k_2 - k_1} e^{-k_1 t} - \frac{k_1}{k_1 - k_2} e^{-k_2 t} \right) \tag{5-55}$$

The expressions for c_B and c_C are more complicated. Both of them not only depend on k_1 and k_2 but also depend on the differences in the rate constants. When $k_1 \gg k_2$, the second reaction is much slower than the first reaction, equation (5–55) reduces to

$$c_C = c_{A,0} (1 - e^{-k_2 t}) \tag{5-56}$$

However, when $k_2 \gg k_1$, the second reaction is much faster than the first one, equation (5–55) reduces to

$$c_C = c_{A,0} (1 - e^{-k_1 t}) \tag{5-57}$$

The amounts of various species over time are illustrated by Fig. 5–4. It is clear that the concentration of A decreases exponentially with time while that of intermediate B increases, passes through a maximum and then decreases. The value of maximum concentration of B will depend on the rate of its formation and elimination. The formation of final product C will start after formation of a certain amount of B. Consequently, C is formed with a certain period. If k_1 is approximately equal to k_2, the rate of intermediate B formation and elimination are also approximately equal (Fig. 5–5a). The concentration of B is relatively large and tails off to zero towards the end of reaction. If k_1 is much greater than k_2, there is a short-term buildup of the intermediate product B. But over long periods of time, the final product C is formed (Fig. 5–5b). If k_1 is much lower than k_2, there is very little initial buildup of the intermediate product B. The final product C is formed almost immediately (Fig. 5–5c).

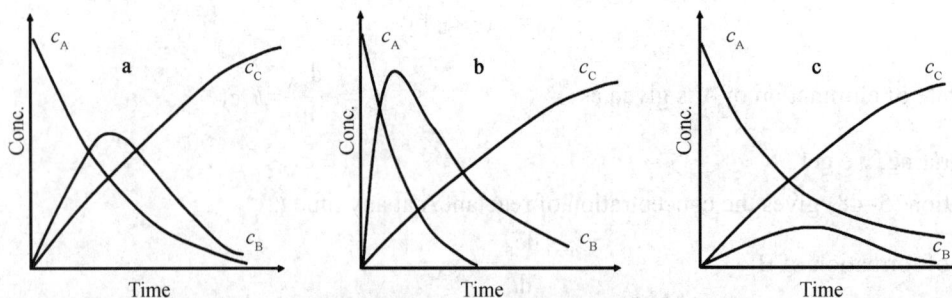

Fig. 5–5 Variation of concentration of reactants and products in a consecutive reaction.

The time at which the concentration of intermediate B is maximum can be calculated as follows.

$$\frac{dc_B}{dt} = \frac{k_1}{k_2 - k_1} c_{A,0} (-k_1 e^{-k_1 t} + k_2 e^{-k_2 t}) = 0 \tag{5-58}$$

Hence
$$k_1 e^{-k_1 t} = k_2 e^{-k_2 t} \quad \text{or} \quad \frac{k_1}{k_2} = e^{(k_1 - k_2) t} \tag{5-59}$$

$$t_{\mathrm{m}} = \frac{\ln\dfrac{k_1}{k_2}}{k_1 - k_2} \tag{5-60}$$

Thus, the value of t_{m} depends on the rate constants k_1 and k_2. And the maximum concentration of intermediate B is

$$c_{\mathrm{B,m}} = c_{\mathrm{A,0}}\left(\frac{k_1}{k_2}\right)^{\frac{k_2}{k_2 - k_1}} \tag{5-61}$$

Section 5　Effect of Temperature on Reaction Rate

Reaction rates depend strongly on temperature, typically increasing rapidly with raising temperature. This is one reason why most declarations of rate constants involve a temperature at which that constant is valid. The first mathematical relation of the rate constant k dependence of absolute temperature T was given by Hood (1878), and various empirical formulas were proposed subsequently.

5.1　Van't Hoff's rule of thumb

A rough rule, valid for many reactions in solution, is that, near room temperature, the rate constant doubles or triples for each 10℃ increase in temperature. Thus the ratio of rate constants of reaction at two different temperatures differing by 10℃ is termed **temperature coefficient (温度系数)**. Mathematically,

$$\text{Temperature coefficient} = \frac{k_{T}+10}{k_{T}} \approx 2 \text{ to } 3 \tag{5-62}$$

5.2　The Arrhenius formula

5.2.1　The Arrhenius equation

In 1889, Arrhenius proposed as simple relation between rate constant for a reaction and the temperature of the system.

$$k = A\mathrm{e}^{-\frac{E_{\mathrm{a}}}{RT}} \tag{5-63}$$

The relation was successfully applied by him to the effect of temperature data for many reactions. This is known as **Arrhenius equation (阿仑尼乌斯方程)** in which the constant A is referred to as the **frequency factor (频率因子)** or Arrhenius **preexponential factor (指前因子)**, E_{a} is the **activation energy (活化能)** for the reaction, R is the gas constant, and T is temperature.

Taking **natural logs (自然对数)** of each side of the Arrhenius equation, it becomes

$$\ln k = -\frac{E_{\mathrm{a}}}{RT} + \ln A \tag{5-64}$$

If k_1 and k_2 are the values of rate constants at temperatures T_1 and T_2, respectively, we can derive

$$\ln\frac{k_2}{k_1}=\frac{E_a}{R}\left(\frac{T_2-T_1}{T_1T_2}\right) \tag{5-65}$$

Arrhenius equation is very valuable because it can be used to calculate the activation energy E_a when the experimental value of the rate constant k is known.

5.2.2 Calculation of E_a using Arrhenius equation

In slightly **rearranged (重排)** form Arrhenius equation (5-64) can be written as

$$\ln k=\left(-\frac{E_a}{R}\right)\frac{1}{T}+\ln A \tag{5-66}$$

Equation (5-66) is a **linear equation (线性方程)**. $\ln k$ and $1/T$ are two **variables (变量)** in this equation. Thus, if we plot $\ln k$ against $1/T$, we will get a straight line (Fig. 5-6). From the slope of the line, E_a can be obtained by calculation. Preexponential factor A can be got from the intercept of the line.

$$\text{Slope}=-\frac{E_a}{R} \quad \text{and} \quad \text{Intercept}=\ln A$$

As shown Fig. 5-7, it is obvious that the activation energy of reaction Ⅰ is less than that of reaction Ⅱ, and the rate constants of reaction Ⅰ is greater than that of reaction Ⅱ. For the reaction with different activation energy, the rate constant varies differently with temperature. The effect of temperature on reaction Ⅱ is greater than reaction Ⅰ. It means the greater the amount of activation energy required, the effect of temperature on rate of reaction will be greater. This rule can be used to control the selectivity of the reaction.

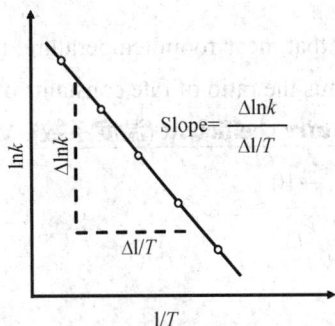

Fig. 5-6 The plot of ln$k$ versus 1/T gives a straight line

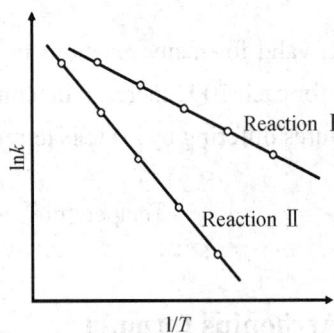

Fig. 5-7 The plot of ln k versus 1/T of two reactions

5.2.3 Calculation of E_a from the values of k at two temperatures

The rate constant k can be measured at two temperatures. Then E_a is calculated using the formula that can be derived as follows from equation (5-64).

At temperature T_1, where the rate constant is k_1

$$\ln k_1=-\frac{E_a}{RT_1}+\ln A$$

At temperature T_2, where the rate constant is k_2

$$\ln k_2=-\frac{E_a}{RT_2}+\ln A$$

The difference between two equations above is

$$\ln k_2 - \ln k_1 = \left(-\frac{E_a}{RT_2} + \ln A\right) - \left(-\frac{E_a}{RT_1} + \ln A\right) = -\frac{E_a}{RT_2} + \frac{E_a}{RT_1}$$

$$\text{or} \quad \ln \frac{k_2}{k_1} = -\frac{E_a}{R}\left(\frac{1}{T_2} - \frac{1}{T_1}\right) \tag{5-67}$$

Thus, the values of k_1 and k_2 measured at T_1 and T_2 can be used to calculate E_a.

[Example 5–4]   For the gas-phase reaction $H_2 + I_2 \longrightarrow 2HI$

At 373.15K, the rate constant is equal to $8.74 \times 10^{-15} L \cdot mol^{-1} \cdot s^{-1}$. At 473.15K it is equal to $9.53 \times 10^{-10} L \cdot mol^{-1} \cdot s^{-1}$. Calculate E_a and A for this reaction.

Solution:

$$\text{Here} \quad \begin{aligned} k_1 &= 8.74 \times 10^{-15} L \cdot mol^{-1} \cdot s^{-1} & T_1 &= 373.15K \\ k_2 &= 9.53 \times 10^{-10} L \cdot mol^{-1} \cdot s^{-1} & T_2 &= 473.15K \end{aligned}$$

Substituting the values in equation (5–67)

$$\ln \frac{k_2}{k_1} = -\frac{E_a}{R}\left(\frac{1}{T_2} - \frac{1}{T_1}\right)$$

$$\ln \frac{9.53 \times 10^{-10}}{8.74 \times 10^{-15}} = -\frac{E_a}{8.314}\left(\frac{1}{473.15} - \frac{1}{373.15}\right)$$

Solving for E_a, gives $E_a = \dfrac{-8.314 \times \ln \dfrac{9.53 \times 10^{-10}}{8.74 \times 10^{-15}}}{\left(\dfrac{1}{473.15} - \dfrac{1}{373.15}\right)} = 1.70 \times 10^5 \ J \cdot mol^{-1}$

$$A = k e^{-\frac{E_a}{RT}} = 8.74 \times 10^{-15} \times \exp\left(\frac{1.70 \times 10^{-5}}{8.314 \times 373.15}\right) = 5.47 \times 10^9 \ L \cdot mol^{-1} \cdot s^{-1}$$

[Example 5–5]   Hydrolyzation of **Aspirin (阿司匹林)** is a first-order reaction. At 373.15K, the rate constant of this hydrolyzation reaction is $7.92d^{-1}$ and the activation energy is about $56.484kJ \cdot mol^{-1}$. Calculate the half-life of reaction at 298.15K.

Solution:

$$\text{Here} \quad \begin{aligned} k_1 &= 7.92d^{-1} & T_1 &= 373.15K \\ E_a &= 56.484kJ \cdot mol^{-1} & T_2 &= 298.15K \end{aligned}$$

Substituting the values in equation (5–67)

$$\ln \frac{k_2}{k_1} = -\frac{E_a}{R}\left(\frac{1}{T_2} - \frac{1}{T_1}\right)$$

$$\ln \frac{k_2}{7.92} = -\frac{56.484 \times 10^3}{8.314}\left(\frac{1}{298.15} - \frac{1}{373.15}\right)$$

Solving for k_2, gives

$$k_2 = 7.92 \times \exp\left[-\frac{56.484 \times 10^3}{8.314}\left(\frac{1}{298.15} - \frac{1}{373.15}\right)\right] = 8.12 \times 10^{-2} d^{-1}$$

Substituting the values of k_2 in equation (5–7)

$$\ln \frac{c_{A,0}}{c_A} = kt$$

$$\ln 2 = k_2 t_{1/2}$$

Solving for $t_{1/2}$ gives

$$t_{1/2} = \frac{\ln 2}{k_2} = \frac{\ln 2}{8.12 \times 10^{-2}} = 8.54d$$

5.3 Concept of activation energy

5.3.1 The Arrhenius activation energy

Arrhenius postulated that only molecules with high energy can react. These molecules possessing high energy is termed **activated molecules (活化分子)**. The minimum amount of energy required to cause a chemical reaction is known as the activation energy. If the potential energy of reactants is greater than the activation energy, the reaction can proceed. Experimental molar activation energy values are usually in the range from 50 to 200kJ · mol^{-1}, somewhat smaller than energies required to break chemical bonds. These magnitudes seem reasonable if we picture the activation process as partially breaking one bond while partially forming another.

Torman used **statistical mechanics (统计力学)** to prove that the activation energy is the difference between the average energy of the activated molecule and the average energy of the reactant molecule for the elementary reaction.

$$E = \overline{E}^* - \overline{E}$$

where $\overline{E}^*$ and $\overline{E}$ represent the average energy of the activated molecule and the average energy of the reactant molecule, respectively.

As evident from the energy diagram of the elementary reaction, if the potential energy of the products is less than that of the reactants (Fig. 5–8a) the energy obtained in going from the activated molecule to products will be more than the activation energy (E_a). Thus, such a reaction will be **exothermic (放热)**. On the other hand, if the potential energy of the products is greater than that of the reactants (Fig. 5–8b), the energy released in going from the activated complex to products will be less than the activation energy and the reaction will be **endothermic (吸热)**.

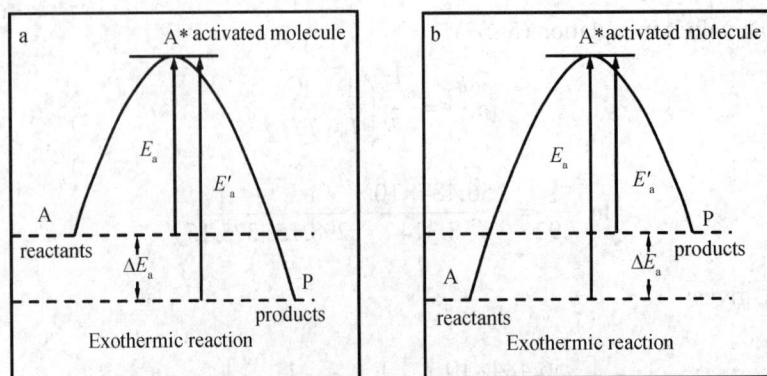

Fig. 5–8　The energy diagram of the elementary reaction

5.3.2　The relation between activation energy and heat of reaction

As shown in Fig. 5-9, for a reversible reaction, when the energy content of the reactants is greater than the activation energy (E_{a1}), the forward reaction can proceed. E_{a1} is called the activation energy of forward reaction. Likewise, when the energy content of the products is greater than the activation energy (E_{a2}), the backward reaction can proceed. E_{a2} is called the activation energy of backward reaction.

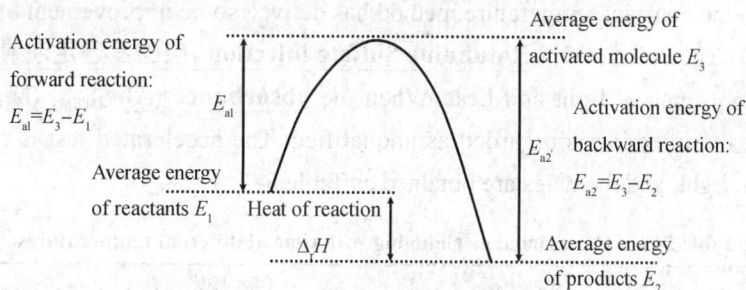

Fig. 5-9　The relation between activation energy and heat of reaction

From Arrhenius equation, we get

$$\frac{\mathrm{d}\ln k_1}{\mathrm{d}T} - \frac{\mathrm{d}\ln k_2}{\mathrm{d}T} = \frac{E_{a1}}{RT^2} - \frac{E_{a2}}{RT^2} \tag{5-68}$$

or

$$\frac{\mathrm{d}\ln(k_1/k_2)}{\mathrm{d}T} = \frac{E_{a1} - E_{a2}}{RT^2} \tag{5-69}$$

At equilibrium, the equilibrium constant K for this reaction is $K = k_1 / k_2$. Substituting the value of K in equation (5-69), we get

$$\frac{\mathrm{d}\ln K}{\mathrm{d}T} = \frac{E_{a1} - E_{a2}}{RT^2} \tag{5-70}$$

The **Van't Hoff equation** (范霍夫方程) is $\dfrac{\mathrm{d}\ln K}{\mathrm{d}T} = \dfrac{\Delta_r H_m}{RT^2}$

Comparing the above two equation, we get

$$E_{a1} - E_{a2} = \Delta_r H_m \tag{5-71}$$

The difference of activation energy in forward and backward reaction is the **reaction heat** (反应热). If E_{a1} is greater than E_{a2}, $\Delta_r H_m$ will be more than zero, such a reaction is an **endothermic reaction** (吸热反应). If E_{a1} is lower than E_{a2}, $\Delta_r H_m$ will be less than zero, such a reaction is an **exothermic reaction** (放热反应).

5.4　Method to predict the storage time of drug

The active ingredients in drugs degrade gradually due to the hydrolyzation and **oxidation**(氧化) during storage. This will result in invalidation of drug. The principle of chemical kinetics can be used in drug storage period prediction. The accelerated degradation experiments are applicable to drug storage period study. The experimental results can be extrapolated to room temperature to obtain the drug storage period at room temperature. The methods of accelerated experiments are classified as **isothermal prediction** (恒温预测) and **nonisothermal prediction** (变温预测).

5.4.1　Isothermal prediction

In the isothermal prediction test, several high temperatures are selected according to the stability of different drugs to determine the change of drug concentration over time. The reaction order of degradation and rate constant k at test temperatures are determined. And then the $\ln k$ against $1/T$ are plotted and a straight line is got based on Arrhenius equation. The straight line can be **extrapolated** (外推) to 298K to obtain the rate constant k_{298K} at room temperature. The drug storage period at room temperature is calculated from k_{298K}. The advantage of isothermal prediction is that the results are accurate. But the experiment workload and drug consumption are large and the experiment period is long. To overcome these shortcomings, the constant temperature method has derived some improvement methods.

[**Example 5–6**] The color of 3% **Rotundine Sulfate injection** (硫酸罗通定注射液) will gradually become darker in presence of light and heat. When the **absorbance (Abs$_{430nm}$)** (吸光度) of injection increases to 0.222, the injection is regarded as unqualified. The accelerated test is carried out at each temperature without light, and the dates are obtained as Table 5–3.

Table 5–3　The asorbance changing with time at different temperatures

333.15K		343.15K		353.15K		361.15K	
t / h	Abs	t / h	Abs	t / h	Abs	t / h	Abs
0	0.088	0	0.088	0	0.088	0	0.088
24	0.131	5	0.110	3.7	0.125	1.2	0.128
48	0.152	10	0.123	7.4	0.151	2.4	0.158
72	0.176	17	0.148	11.1	0.201	3.6	0.173
96	0.206	24	0.177	14.8	0.247	6.0	0.238
120	0.241	34	0.213	25.9	0.371	7.2	0.247
144	0.268	41	0.253	29.6	0.394	8.4	0.299
168	0.298	58	0.306	37	0.489	9.6	0.315
192	0.344	65	0.340			10.8	0.349
216	0.374					12	0.375
240	0.410						
288	0.493						

Calculate the drug storage period in dark at room temperature (298.15K).

Solution:

The absorbance increase indicates that the concentration of degraded products in Rotundine raises. Plotting the absorbance versus time at different temperatures, we get the straight lines as follows (Fig. 5–10).

It is clear that the degradation of Rotundine is a zero-order reaction. The equation of reaction rate is expressed as

$$Abs = Abs_0 + kt$$

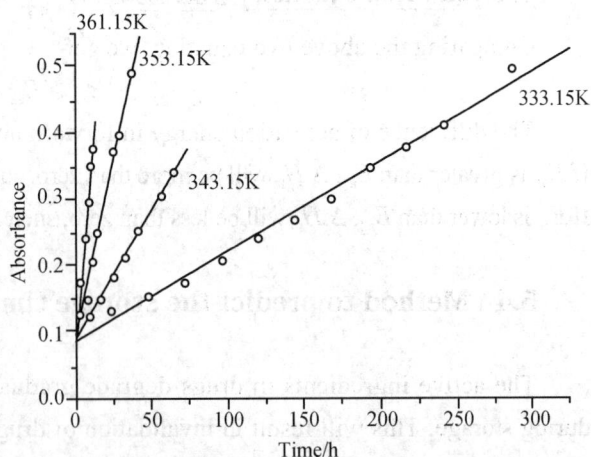

Fig. 5–10　The absorbance versus time at different temperatures

Hence the rate constants at different temperatures are as Table 5–4.

Table 5–4　The asorbance changing with time at different temperatures

T / K	333.15K	343.25K	353.15K	361.15K
$10^3 k$ / (Abs/h)	1.33	3.82	10.05	24.0

Plotting $\ln k$ versus $1/T$ gives a straight line which is illustrated as Fig. 5–11.

The **linear regression equation (线性回归方程)** is

$$\ln k = -\frac{12415}{T} + 30.61$$

where 12415 is equal to E_a / R, and 30.16 is equal to $\ln A$.

Solving for E_a and A, gives

$$E_a = 12415 \times R = 12415 \times 8.314$$
$$= 1.03 \times 10^5 \mathrm{J} \cdot \mathrm{mol}^{-1}$$
$$A = e^{30.61} = 1.97 \times 10^{13} \mathrm{Abs/h}$$

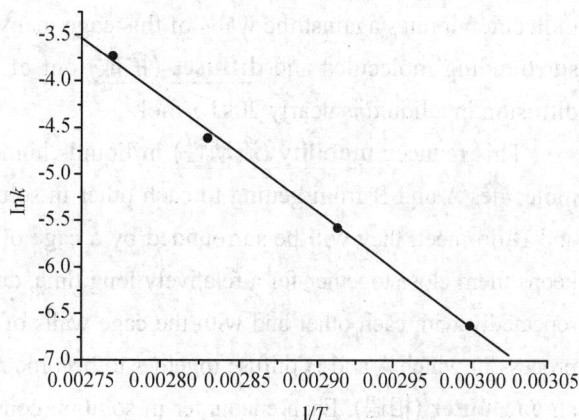

Fig. 5–11 A plot of $\ln k$ versus $1/T$

Substituting the values of temperature (T=298.15K) in equation, we get

$$\ln k_{298K} = -\frac{12415}{T} + 30.61 = -\frac{12415}{298.15} + 30.61 = -11.03$$

Solving for k_{298K}, gives

$$k_{298K} = e^{-11.03} = 1.62 \times 10^{-5} \mathrm{Abs/h}$$

Substituting the values of k_{298K} in equation of degradation reaction rate, we get

$$\mathrm{Abs} = \mathrm{Abs}_0 + kt = 0.088 + 1.62 \times 10^{-5} t_{298K} = 0.222$$

Solving for t_{298K}, gives

$$t_{298K} = \frac{0.222 - 0.088}{1.62 \times 10^{-5}} = 8271.6\mathrm{h} = 344.6\mathrm{d}$$

5.4.2 Nonisothermal prediction

The nonisothermal prediction test change the temperature continuously in a certain temperature range. The required kinetic parameters (activation energy, rate constant and storage period, etc.) can be obtained by one test. This method can reduce the amount of sample and test time comparing with the isothermal prediction. The heating methods of nonisothermal prediction involve programmed heating and flexible heating. The programmed heating changes the temperature continuously with temperature-programming. The heating laws consist of reciprocal heating, linear heating and logarithmic heating. Instead of temperature control in isothermal prediction and the programmed heating, the flexible heating utilizes the computer to record the test temperature automatically without fixed temperature-programming.

Section 6 Effect of Solvent on Reaction Rate

In a gas, the molecules are relatively far apart and can move freely between **collisions (碰撞)**, while they cannot move freely in a liquid due to the little empty space between each other. Instead, a given molecule can be seen as being surrounded by a **cage (笼)** formed by other molecules. A given molecule vibrates against the walls of this cage many times before it squeezes through the closely packed surrounding molecules and **diffuses (扩散)** out of the cage. The activation energy for the process of diffusion in a liquid is nearly $20kJ \cdot mol^{-1}$.

This reduced **mobility (流动性)** in liquids hinders two reacting solute molecules A and B from getting to each other in solution. However, once A and B do meet, they will be surrounded by a cage of solvent molecules that keeps them close together for a relatively long time, during which they collide repeatedly with each other and with the cage walls of solvent molecules. The process in which A and B diffuse together to become neighbors is regarded as an **encounter (相遇)**. Each encounter in solution consists of many collisions between A and B while they remain trapped in the solvent cage (Fig. 5–12). In a gas, there is no distinction between an encounter and a collision.

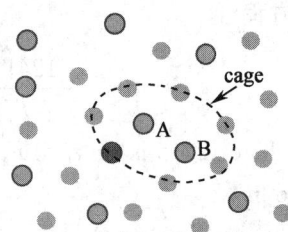

Fig. 5–12 Molecules A and B in a solvent cage

Theoretical estimates indicate that in water at room temperature, two molecules in a solvent cage will collide 20 to 200 times with each other before they diffuse out of the cage. Although the rate of encounters per unit volume between pairs of solute molecules in a liquid solution is much less than the corresponding rate of collisions in a gas, the **compensating effect (补偿作用)** of a large number of collisions per encounter in solution makes the collision rate roughly the same in solution as in a gas at comparable concentrations of reactants.

Direct evidence for this is the near constancy of rate constants for certain reactions on going from the gas phase to a solution (see the data on the N_2O_5 decomposition in Table 5–5). Although the collision rate is about the same in a gas and in solution, the pattern of collisions is quite different, with collisions in solution grouped into sets, with short time intervals between successive collisions of any one set and long intervals between successive sets of collisions.

Table 5–5 Decomposition of N_2O_5 in different mediums at 25℃

Medium	$10^5 k / s^{-1}$	$\ln (A / s^{-1})$	$E_a / (kJ \cdot mol^{-1})$
In gas	3.38	31.3	103.3
CCl_4	4.09	31.3	101.3
$CHCl_3$	3.72	31.3	102.5
$C_2H_2Cl_2$	4.79	31.3	102.1
CH_3NO_2	3.13	31.1	102.5
Br_2	4.27	30.6	100.4

The reasons of solvent affecting the rate constant are rather complicated and still unclear. There are some qualitative introductions as follows:

6.1 Effect of solvent's polarity and solvation

The influence of solvent **polarity (极性)** on the reaction velocity varies enormously according to the reaction. If the polarity of the product is larger than that of the reactant, the rate of reaction increases in the polar solvent. Conversely, if the polarity of the reactant is larger than that of the product, the rate of reaction decreases in the polar solvent. For example, in the reaction of

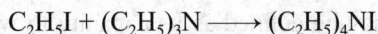

$$C_2H_5I + (C_2H_5)_3N \longrightarrow (C_2H_5)_4NI$$

The polarity of product which is a quaternary **ammonium salt (季铵盐)** is greater than that of the reactant, so the rate of reaction is enhanced with the increase of the polarity of the solvent. While, in the reaction of

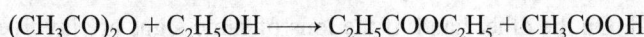

$$(CH_3CO)_2O + C_2H_5OH \longrightarrow C_2H_5COOC_2H_5 + CH_3COOH$$

The polarity of two products is less than that of the reactant, so the reaction rate is retarded with the increase of the polarity of the solvent. The results are summarized in Table 5–6.

Table 5–6　The influence of solvent polarity on the rate constants

Solvent	$C_2H_5I + (C_2H_5)_3N \longrightarrow (C_2H_5)_4NI$ $k / s^{-1}(373K)$	$(CH_3CO)_2O + C_2H_5OH \longrightarrow C_2H_5COOC_2H_5 + CH_3COOH$ $k / s^{-1} (323K)$
Hexane	0.00018	0.0119
Benzene	0.0058	0.00462
Chlorine Benzene	0.023	0.00433
P-methoxybenzene	0.04	0.00293
Nitrobenzene	70.1	0.00245

The **solvation (溶剂化)** of the species of reaction may also affect the rate of reaction. In a solution, the species of reaction are usually solvated that are bound to one or more solvent molecules. And the degree of solvation changes with change in solvent, thus affecting reaction constant k. If the reactant is solvated to a lower extent comparing with the activated complex, the rate of reaction is faster than that in a non-solvating solvent. It is because the activity coefficient of the complex is less than it is in a solvent that does not solvate it. This reduces the potential energy of activated complex or causes a decrease in the activation energy of the reaction (Fig. 5–13a). Conversely, if the reactant is solvated, while the activated complex is not, the activation energy is increased and consequently the rate of reaction is reduced (Fig. 5–13b). Moreover, when the reactant and activated complex are both solvated, the overall effect on both the activation energy and reaction rate may be little.

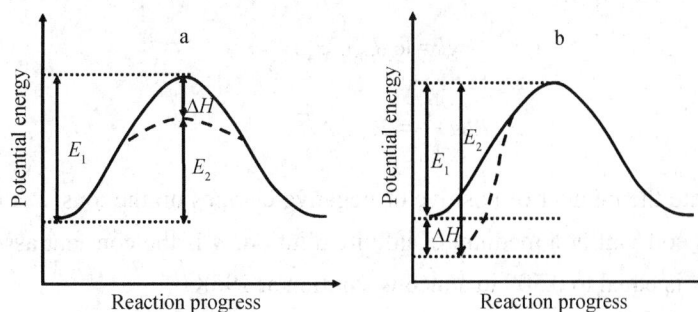

Fig. 5–13　(a) The activation energy is reduced by solvation of the active complex
(b) The activation energy is raised by solvation of the reactant

6.2　Effect of solvent's dielectric constant

Most reactions in solution involve ions or **polar molecules (极性分子)** as reactants or reaction intermediates, and here the electrostatic attraction and repulsion between the reacting species are influenced by the **dielectric constant (介电常数)** of a solvent, thus affecting the reaction rate. The dielectric constant of a solvent may be defined as its capacity to weaken the force of attraction between the electrical charges immersed in that solvent. As evident from the above definition, the force between ions of opposite signs decreases as the dielectric constant of the medium is increased. Therefore, if the ions of opposite signs are involved in the reaction, the rate constant decreases as the dielectric constant of solvent is increased. On the other hand, if the ions of same signs are involved in the reaction, the rate constant increases as the dielectric constant of solvent is increased.

For example, hydrolyzation of **benzyl bromide (溴苄)** catalyzed by OH^- ion is a reaction between ions of opposite charges.

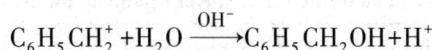

$$C_6H_5CH_2^+ + H_2O \xrightarrow{OH^-} C_6H_5CH_2OH + H^+$$

The ions of opposite charges can attract each other easily in solvent with lower dielectric constant, therefor the rate of reaction is higher in this medium. Addition of substances with smaller dielectric constant than water, such as glycerol, ethanol or propylene glycol etc., will enhance the rate of reaction.

Hydrolyzation of **barbiturates (巴比妥盐)** catalyzed by OH^- ion in aqueous solution is a reaction between ions of same charges. Addition of glycerol or ethanol will retard the rate of reaction.

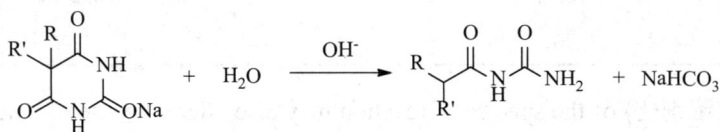

6.3　Effect of ionic strength

The rate of reaction can be effected by the inert ionic or non-reacting species in the solution. This influence is especially great for ion-ion reactions, where rate of reaction is altered even at low concentrations. The effect of a charged species on the rate of reaction is termed as **salt effect(原盐效应)**. This effect is important in the study of ionic reactions in solutions.

In a dilute solution, the relationship between the rate of ionic reaction and the ionic strength of the solution is as follows:

$$\log k = \log k_0 + 2z_A z_B A\sqrt{I} \tag{5-72}$$

$$\text{or} \quad \log \frac{k}{k_0} = 2z_A z_B A\sqrt{I} \tag{5-73}$$

where z_A and z_B indicate the number of positive or negative charges on the ions. I is ionic strength of the medium, k_0 is the rate constant in a medium of infinite dilution, A is the constant associated with solvent and temperature, i.e. A is equal to 0.509 in aqueous solution at 298K.

Equation (5-72) indicates that when reactants possess same charges, the rate of reaction is accelerated as the ionic strength of solvent is increased. Whereas when reactants possess opposite charges, the rate of reaction is slowed as the ionic strength of solvent is increased. When a reactant is not charged, the reaction rate is not affected by the ionic strength.

Section 7   Catalysis

There are certain substances that participate in chemical reactions by altering the reaction rate without changing themselves at the end of the reaction. Such a substance is defined as **catalyst(催化剂)** and the process is called **catalysis(催化作用)**. As evident from the above definition, a catalyst may increase or decrease the rate of a reaction. If a catalyst which enhances the reaction rate is called **positive catalyst(正催化剂)** and the process is known as **positive catalysis(正催化作用)** or simply **catalysis**. If a catalyst which retards the reaction rate is called **negative catalyst(负催化剂)** or **inhibitor(抑制剂)** and the process is known as **negative catalysis (负催化作用)**. When a product itself acts as a catalyst for the reaction, the phenomena is referred to as **autocatalysis(自催化作用)**. When a reaction influences the rate of some other reaction which does not occur under ordinary conditions, the phenomenon is referred to as referred to as **induced catalysis(诱导催化作用)**. Sometimes the activity of the catalyst can be increased by addition of small amounts of another substance. This another substance which, though itself is not a catalyst, promotes the activity of a catalyst, is termed **promoter(促进剂)**. Sometimes the catalyst loses its effectiveness due to the presence of a small quantity of impurities in the reactants. Such a substance, which destroys the activity of catalyst, is termed **poison(毒剂)** and the process is called **catalytic poisoning(催化剂中毒)**.

The catalysis is mainly divided into **homogeneous catalysis (single-phase catalysis) (均相催化)** and **heterogeneous catalysis (multi-phase catalysis) (非均相催化)**. In homogeneous catalysis, the catalyst exists in the same phase as the reactants and is evenly distributed throughout. This type of catalysis can occur in gas phase or the liquid (solution) phase. In heterogeneous catalysis, the catalyst exists in a different physical phase from the reactants. The most important of such reactions are those in which the reactants are in the gas phase while the catalyst is a solid. The process is also called **contact catalysis (接触催化)** since the reaction occurs by contact of reactants with the catalyst surface. This form of catalysis has great industrial importance. Also, there is another type of catalysis known as **enzyme catalysis(酶催化)** which is largely of biological interest. Enzyme catalysis can belong to homogeneous catalysis or heterogeneous catalysis because of the different state of the enzyme.

7.1   Basic characteristics of catalysis

7.1.1   Characteristics of catalytic reactions

Although there are different types of catalytic reactions, the following features or characteristics are common to most of them.

(1) A catalyst undergoes no change in chemical composition and mass after reaction, however, it may undergo physical change.   The catalyst itself remains chemically unchanged at the end of the reaction. However, the physical properties of catalyst may change, e.g. appearance, crystal form, etc. The granular **manganese dioxide (MnO_2)** used as a catalyst in the thermal decomposition of **potassium chlorate ($KClO_3$)** is left as a fine powder at the end of the reaction.

$$KClO_3 \xrightarrow[\text{heat}]{MnO_2} KCl + O_2 \quad \text{(Decomposition)}$$

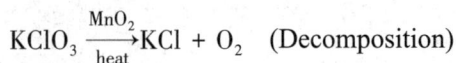

(2) A small amount of catalyst can produce an appreciable effect on the reaction rate. The catalyst is not consumed during the reaction, so a small quantity of catalyst can participate in numerous reactions, e.g. $1/10^7$ of its mass of finely divided platinum is sufficient to catalyse the decomposition of hydrogen peroxide. While, there are some reactions need relatively large amount of catalysts to accelerate the rate. Thus in Friedel-Crafts reaction **anhydrous (无水的)** aluminium chloride (AlCl₃) functions as a catalyst effectively when present to the extent of 30 percent of the mass of benzene in the

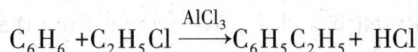

$$C_6H_6 + C_2H_5Cl \xrightarrow{AlCl_3} C_6H_5C_2H_5 + HCl$$

(3) A catalyst alters the reaction rate but does not initiate the reaction. Since the catalyst is reproduced at the end of reaction, it does not contribute any energy to the system. The free energy change thus will be same in presence or in absence of the catalyst. An impossible reaction in thermodynamics will not occur with the catalyst.

(4) The catalyst shortens the time required to establish the equilibrium but does not alter the final state of equilibrium. It implies that the catalyst effects the rate constants of forward and backward reactions equally in a reversible reaction. Therefore, the equilibrium constant (the ratio of rate constant for forward and backward reactions) $K = k_f / k_b$ remains unchanged.

The effect of a catalyst on the time required for equilibrium to be established for the reaction

$$A \underset{k_b}{\overset{k_f}{\rightleftharpoons}} B$$

is illustrated in Fig. 5–14. At the beginning of the reaction, the concentrations of A and the forward rate is maximum, while the initial concentration of B is zero and the backward rate is lowest. As the time passes, the forward rate decreases and backward reaction increases till the equilibrium is established. Similar curves of the rates of reactions with the catalyst show that the rates of the forward reaction and the reverse reaction are altered in same proportion but the equilibrium is established earlier.

Fig. 5–14 The effect of a catalyst on the time required for the equilibrium to be established

(5) A particular catalyst is specific in its action. A particular catalyst can catalyse one reaction, however, it will not necessarily catalyse another reaction. In addition, different catalysts can bring about completely different reactions for the same reactant. For example, ethanol (C₂H₅OH) gives ethanal (CH₃CHO) when passed over hot copper at the temperature of 473 to 520K.

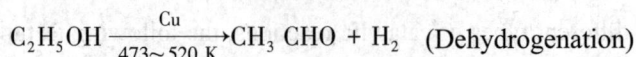

$$C_2H_5OH \xrightarrow[473\sim520\ K]{Cu} CH_3CHO + H_2 \quad \text{(Dehydrogenation)}$$

but with hot aluminium oxide at the temperature of 623 to 633K it gives ethene (C₂H₄).

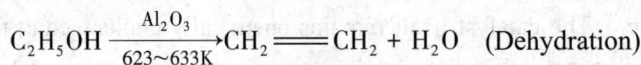

$$C_2H_5OH \xrightarrow[623\sim633K]{Al_2O_3} CH_2 = CH_2 + H_2O \quad \text{(Dehydration)}$$

(6) Temperature change alters the rate of a catalytic reaction as it would do for the same reaction in absence of catalyst. Some catalysts are physically altered by a rise in temperature and hence their

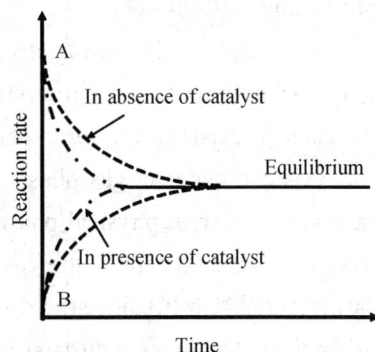

catalytic activity may be decreased. In such a case the reaction rate increases up to a certain value and then gradually decreases. The reaction rate is maximum at a particular temperature called the **optimum temperature** (最适温度).

7.1.2　Mechanism of catalysis and activation energies of catalyzed reactions

The catalyst works as an agent to provide an alternative path for the transformation in which the required activation energy is reduced. To be effective, a catalyst must combine with a reactant or an intermediate forming an intermediate **complex** (复合物). After the reaction has taken place, the catalyst is freed and combines with another reactant or intermediate in a subsequent reaction. The simplest mechanism describing a catalytic process is as follows

$$A+D \xrightarrow{\ K\ } AD$$

$$A+K \underset{k_{-1}}{\overset{k_1}{\rightleftharpoons}} AK$$

$$AK+D \xrightarrow{\ k_2\ } AD+K$$

where A and D is the reactant, K is the catalyst. AK is the intermediate complex which reacts with D to give product AD with elimination of the catalyst. The differential rate expression for product formation is

$$\frac{dc_{AD}}{dt}=k_2 c_{AK} c_D \tag{5-74}$$

Given that AK is an intermediate, we write the differential rate expression for this species and apply the **steady-state approximation** (稳态近似法).

$$\frac{dc_{AK}}{dt}=k_1 c_A c_K - k_{-1} c_{AK} - k_2 c_{AK} = 0 \tag{5-75}$$

$$c_{AK}=\frac{k_1 c_A c_K}{k_{-1}+k_2} \tag{5-76}$$

Substituting the expression for c_{AK} into equation (5–74), the rate of product formation becomes

$$\frac{dc_{AD}}{dt}=\frac{k_1 k_2}{k_{-1}+k_2} c_K c_A c_D = k' c_A c_D \tag{5-77}$$

In equation (5–77), k' is referred to as the apparent rate constant of overall reaction and is equal to

$$k'=\frac{k_1 k_2}{k_{-1}+k_2} c_K \tag{5-78}$$

As shown in the energy diagram of a reaction (Fig. 5–15), where E_1 and E_2 are the activation energy of forward reaction and backward reaction respectively for

$$A+K \underset{k_{-1}}{\overset{k_1}{\rightleftharpoons}} AK$$

E_3 is the activation energy for reaction

$$AK+D \xrightarrow{\ k_2\ } AD+K$$

E_a and E_0 represent the activation energy of reaction with and without the catalyst, respectively.

The peaks of each curve represent the average energy of the activated molecules. Depending upon the system and conditions, the relationship between the overall activation energy of a catalyzed reaction and activation energies of the individual steps may be considered as

$$E_a = E_1 + E_3 - E_2$$

It clearly shows the catalyst lowering the activation energy by providing an alternative pathway.

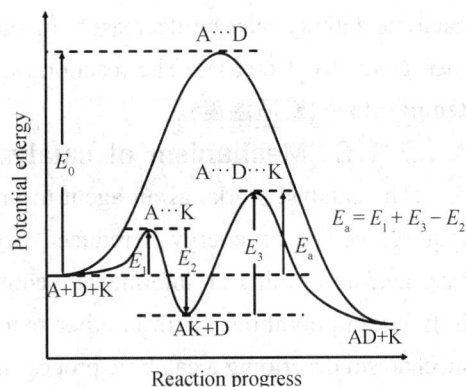

Fig. 5-15   Energy diagram of a reaction with and without the catalyst

7.2   Single-phase catalytic reaction

Single-phase catalyst (homogeneous catalyst) is a catalyst that exists in the same phase as the species involved in the reaction.

7.2.1   Acid base catalysis

Many homogeneous catalytic reactions in solutions are catalysed by acids and bases, e.g. inversions of sucrose by H^+ ions, decomposition of **nitrosotriacetone-amine(亚硝基三丙酮胺)** by OH^- ions, hydrolyzation of ester by both H^+ and OH^- ions etc. These are known as **specific acid base catalysis (专属酸碱催化)**. While, the catalysis brought about by Brönsted proton acid base is termed **general acid base catalysis (广义酸碱催化)**.

(1) General acid base catalysis   Brönsted pointed out that acid are **proton donors (质子供体)** and bases are **proton acceptors (质子受体)**. In general acid base catalysis, not only H^+ ions but all **Brönsted acids (proton donors)) (布朗斯台德酸)** cause acid catalysis. Thus the general acid catalysts include H^+, undissociated acids, cations of weak bases (NH_4^+) and water (H_2O). Moreover, not only OH^- ions but all **Brönsted bases (proton acceptors) (布朗斯台德碱)** act as base catalyst. Thus the general base catalysts include OH^-, undissociated bases, anions of weak acids (CH_3COO^-) and water (H_2O).

(2) Mechanism of general acid base catalysis   In acid catalysis, a proton is transferred from an acid to the **substrate (底物)**:

$$S + HA \longrightarrow SH^+ + A^- \longrightarrow P + HA$$

In acid catalysis, the H^+ (or Brönsted acid) donates a proton to form an intermediate complex with the reactant, which then reacts to give back the proton. For example, the mechanism of **keto-enol tautomerism (酮-烯醇互变异构)** of **acetone (丙酮)** is

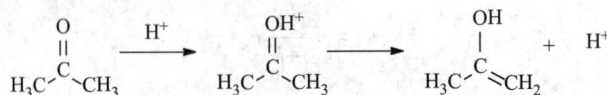

In base catalysis, a proton is transferred from the substrate to a base

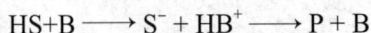

$$HS + B \longrightarrow S^- + HB^+ \longrightarrow P + B$$

In base catalysis, the OH^- ion (or any Brönsted base) accepts a proton from the reactant to form an intermediate complex which then reacts or decomposes to regenerate the OH^- (or Brönsted base). For example, the decomposition of **nitramide (硝胺)** by OH^- ions and CH_3COO^- ions may be explained as follows.

By OH⁻ ions:

$$NH_2NO_2+OH^-\longrightarrow H_2O+NHNO_2^-\ (\text{intermediate complex})$$
$$NHNO_2^-\longrightarrow N_2O+OH^-$$

By CH_3COO^- ions:

$$NH_2NO_2+CH_3COO^-\longrightarrow CH_3COOH+NHNO_2^-\ (\text{intermediate complex})$$
$$NHNO_2^-\longrightarrow N_2O+OH^-$$
$$OH^-+CH_3COOH\longrightarrow H_2O+CH_3COO^-$$

(3) The relation between the value of pH and the catalytic constants for H^+ or OH^- ions　If a reaction is catalysed simultaneously by H^+ and OH^- ions and reaction also can occur without these ions, the rate of reaction is expressed as

$$r=-\frac{dc_S}{dt}=k_0c_S+k_{H^+}c_{H^+}c_S+k_{OH^-}c_{OH^-}c_S=(k_0+k_{H^+}c_{H^+}+k_{OH^-}c_{OH^-})c_S \tag{5-79}$$

where S is the substrate, k_0 is the rate constant without catalyst, k_{H^+} and k_{OH^-} are catalytic constants for H^+ and OH^- ions, respectively.

The first order rate constant is, therefore, given by

$$k=\frac{r}{c_S}=k_0+k_{H^+}c_{H^+}+k_{OH^-}c_{OH^-} \tag{5-80}$$

or

$$k=k_0+k_{H^+}c_{H^+}+k_{OH^-}\frac{K_W}{c_{H^+}} \tag{5-81}$$

or

$$k=k_0+k_{H^+}\frac{K_W}{c_{OH^-}}+k_{OH^-}c_{OH^-} \tag{5-82}$$

In most of the cases, one of these terms containing concentration is small compared with other terms and can be neglected.

For example, if reaction is carried out in acidic solutions $(0.1\text{mol}\cdot\text{dm}^{-3})$, term $k_{H^+}c_{H^+}$ would be $k_{H^+}\times10^{-1}$, while term $k_{OH^-}\dfrac{K_W}{c_{H^+}}$ would be $k_{OH^-}\times10^{-13}$ which is negligible compared to $k_{H^+}\times10^{-1}$ therefore, rate constant may be given as

$$k=k_0+k_{H^+}c_{H^+} \tag{5-83}$$

When the concentration of acidic solution is high enough, the first term can also be neglected, rate constant may be simplified as

$$k=k_{H^+}c_{H^+} \tag{5-84}$$

Taking logarithm of each side of equation (5-84), it can be put in a more useful form

$$\log k=\log k_{H^+}+\log c_{H^+}=\log k_{H^+}-\text{pH} \tag{5-85}$$

The $\log k$ reduces linearly with increasing pH. Similarly, if the concentration of basic solution is high enough, k_0 and $k_{H^+}c_{H^+}$ term can be neglected, rate constant may be simplified as

$$k=k_{OH^-}\frac{K_W}{c_{H^+}} \tag{5-86}$$

Or

$$\log k=\log k_{OH^-}+\log K_W-\log c_{H^+}=\log k_{OH^-}+\log K_W+\text{pH} \tag{5-87}$$

As shown in Fig. 5–16, a variety of possibilities that may arise in the reactions are illustrated in a plot of $\log k$ against the pH of the solution. Curve a represents a most general type of behavior for catalysis by H^+ and OH^- ions. The rate in the intermediate region is equal to $k_0 c_S$ so that k_0 can be determined directly from the rate in this region. A curve of the type a is given by the **mutarotation (变旋)** of glucose, if k_0 is sufficiently small, the horizontal part of the curve is found to be missing. Two limbs of the curve intersect sharply in case of hydrolysis of carboxylic esters (curve b). If either k_{H^+} or k_{OH^-} is negligibly small, the corresponding sloping limb of the curve is not found. If k_{H^+} is negligible, we obtain curve c and if k_{OH^-} is

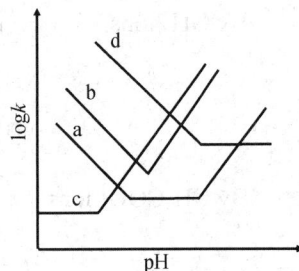

Fig. 5–16 Variation of rate constant with pH for acid base catalyzed reaction

negligible, we get curve d. If a reaction without the catalyst is very slow and reaction rate is negligible, these curves will be simple straight lines with either a positive slope (curve c) or a negative slope (curve d). In addition, there are level region in curve a, c and d in which H^+ and OH^- ions have little effect on catalysis, k_0 is relatively large and k is independent of pH.

When pH of the system is varied, the rate of reaction passes through a minimum at certain pH called the most stable pH, expressed as pH_m. The rate is higher at other values of pH. There are two methods for determination of the most stable pH. One is plotted by experiment, the other is calculation. This is very useful for the preparation of drug solutions. We may obtain the value of pH_m for drug solution by a plot of $\log k$ against the pH or direct calculation. The calculation is as follows.

Taking **derivation (求导)** for c_{H^+} of each side of equation (5–81), gives

$$\frac{dk}{dc_{H^+}} = k_{H^+} - k_{OH^-} \frac{K_W}{c_{H^+}^2} \tag{5-88}$$

At pH_m, $\frac{dk}{dc_{H^+}} = 0$, the equation becomes

$$k_{H^+} = k_{OH^-} \frac{K_W}{c_{H^+}^2} \quad \text{or} \quad c_{H^+} = \left(\frac{k_{OH^-} K_W}{k_{H^+}}\right)^{\frac{1}{2}} \tag{5-89}$$

The negative logarithm of equation (5–89) is expressed as

$$pH_m = \frac{\log k_{H^+} - \log k_{OH^-} - \log K_W}{2} \tag{5-90}$$

If k_{H^+} and k_{OH^-} of a drug solution are known, the pH_m of the drug can be calculated.

7.2.2 Enzyme catalysis

Enzymes (酶) are complex protein molecules which serve as catalysts to accelerate numerous organic reactions in living cells. There are many examples of the biochemical reactions catalysed by enzymes, such as inversion of sucrose into **glucose (葡萄糖)** and **fructose (果糖)** by **invertase (蔗糖转化酶)** present in yeast, conversion of glucose into **ethanol (乙醇)** by **zymase (酿酶/酒化酶)** present in yeast, hydrolyzation of **starch (淀粉)** into glucose by **amylase (淀粉酶)** present in oral cavity, hydrolysis of **urea (尿素)** into ammonia and **carbon dioxide (CO_2)** by **urease (脲酶)** present in soya bean, etc. These processes are referred to as **enzyme catalysis (酶催化)**.

(1) Characteristics of enzyme catalysis　When enzymes exist in solution and catalyze reactions that

occur in solution, they can serve as homogeneous catalysts. They are unique in their efficiency and high degree of specificity. Some important features of enzyme catalysis are listed below.

① The catalytic efficiency of enzyme is very high at extremely low concentrations.

Compared with inorganic substances catalyzed reaction, the enzyme catalyzed reactions proceed at very high rate, e.g. 1mol of cooper may transform 0.1mol of ethanol per second at 473K. While 1mol of alcohol dehydrogenase can convert 720mol of ethanol into acetaldehyde per second at room temperature.

② Enzyme catalysis shows absolute selectivity.

An enzyme generally catalyses just one reaction with a particular substance. For example, amylase can only catalyse the hydrolysis of starch, while hydrochloric acid can not only catalyse the hydrolysis of starch, but also catalyse the hydrolysis of protein and fat. Urease which is derived from soya bean catalyses the hydrolysis of urea and no other amide, not even **methylurea (甲基脲)**.

③ Rate of enzyme catalysed reactions is maximum at the optimum temperature.

The rate of enzyme catalysed reaction with increase of temperature gives a parabolic curve as shown in Fig. 5–17. The rate is increased with the temperature rise but up to a certain point. Thereafter the rate is gradually decreased because the protein structure of enzyme is destroyed. The temperature at which the reaction rate is maximum is called the Optimum temperature. Most human enzymes have an optimal temperature range from 35℃ to 40℃.

④ Rate of enzyme catalysed reactions is maximum at the **optimum pH (最适pH)**.

When pH of the system is varied, the rate of enzyme reaction passes through a maximum at certain pH called the Optimum pH. The enzyme activity is lower at other values of pH (Fig. 5–18). Thus, most mammalian enzymes function are best at pH of about 7 to 8, which is similar to the cellular environment where they are found in.

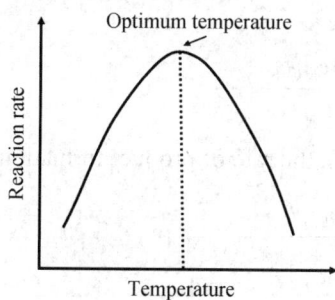

Fig. 5–17　The variation of rate of an enzyme catalysed reaction with rise of temperature

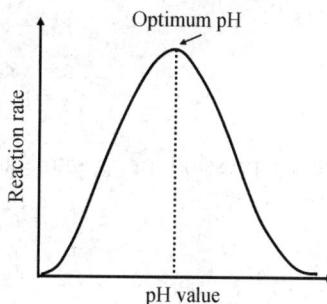

Fig. 5–18　The variation of rate of an enzyme catalysed reaction with increase of pH

⑤ **Activators (辅因子)** or **coenzymes (辅酶)** can greatly enhance the catalytic activity of enzyme.

Metal ions are served as activators which bind to enzyme weakly and promote their catalytic action. For example, addition of sodium chloride (Na^+) makes amylase catalytically very active. A small nonprotein (vitamin) is termed a coenzyme when present along with an enzyme, promotes the catalytic activity.

⑥ Enzymes are often inhibited or poisoned.

The catalytic activity of an enzyme is often inhibited or destroyed completely by addition of other substances. These inhibitors or poisons could interact with the active site on the surface of enzyme.

(2) Michaelis-Menten enzyme kinetics　The simplest mechanism of an enzymatic process may be

described as follows.

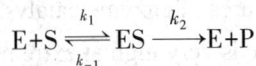

$$E + S \underset{k_{-1}}{\overset{k_1}{\rightleftharpoons}} ES \xrightarrow{k_2} E + P$$

In this mechanism, S represents substrate, E is enzyme, ES is the intermediate complex, and P is product. The enzyme catalysis mechanism is identical to the general catalysis mechanism described earlier in equation except that the catalyst K is now the enzyme E, the intermediate AK is now the ES.

In the enzyme catalyzed reactions, the molar concentration of enzyme is usually much less than that of substrate. Thus, very few of substrate is bound to the enzyme. The total concentration of enzyme $c_{E,0}$ should be regarded as the sum of the concentration of the enzyme c_E and concentration of complex c_{ES}, i.e. $c_{E,0} = c_E + c_{ES}$.

The rate of reaction is defined as

$$r = \frac{dc_P}{dt} = k_2 c_{ES} \tag{5-91}$$

Applying the steady-state approximation to the intermediate ES, we get

$$\frac{dc_{ES}}{dt} = k_1 c_E c_S - k_{-1} c_{ES} - k_2 c_{ES} = 0 \tag{5-92}$$

$$c_{ES} = \frac{k_1}{k_{-1} + k_2} c_E c_S = \frac{c_E c_S}{K_M} \tag{5-93}$$

where $K_M = \dfrac{k_{-1} + k_2}{k_1}$ is known as **Michaelis Menten constant (米氏常数)**.

c_E can be determined in terms of $c_{E,0}$ as $c_E = c_{E,0} - c_{ES}$. Substituting the value of c_E into equation (5-93), hence, c_{ES} is given as

$$c_{ES} = \frac{(c_{E,0} - c_{ES}) c_S}{K_M} = \frac{c_{E,0} c_S}{K_M + c_S} \tag{5-94}$$

Substituting the expression for c_{ES} into equation (5-91), the rate of product formation becomes

$$r = \frac{dc_P}{dt} = k_2 c_{ES} = \frac{k_2 c_{E,0} c_S}{K_M + c_S} \tag{5-95}$$

When c_S is sufficiently small, where $c_S = K_M$ and $K_M + c_S \approx K_M$, the rate law becomes

$$r = \frac{k_2}{K_M} c_{E,0} c_S \tag{5-96}$$

The reaction will be first order with respect to the substrate and the plot of rate versus c_S will be linear at lower substrate concentrations.

At higher substrate concentrations, where $c_S \gg K_M$ and $K_M + c_S \approx c_S$, the rate law becomes

$$r = k_2 c_{E,0} \tag{5-97}$$

The reaction will be zero order with respect to the substrate and the plot of rate versus c_S will be horizontal to concentration axis as shown in Fig. 5-19. When c_S is quite high, the rate will be maximum, i.e. $r_{max} = k_2 c_{E,0}$. Again at this stage, the rate law may be written as

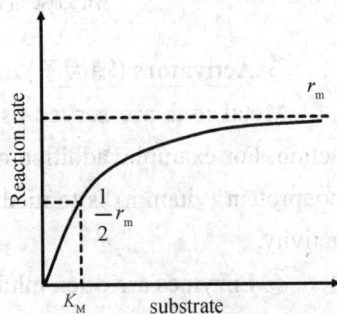

Fig. 5-19 Plot of rate versus concentration of substrate for enzyme catalyzed reaction

$$r = \frac{r_{\max} c_S}{K_M + c_S} \quad \text{or} \quad \frac{r}{r_{\max}} = \frac{c_S}{K_M + c_S} \tag{5-98}$$

Similarly, when $K_M = c_S$, the rate is half the maximum $r = \frac{1}{2} r_{\max}$.

Therefore, K_M is equal to the concentration of the substrate at which the rate is half of its maximum value. The value of K_M for an enzyme depends on the substrate and experimental conditions like temperature, pH, ionic strength, solvent, etc. K_M gives an idea of strength of binding and saturation of enzyme and substrate.

When equation (5-95) is written in its reciprocal form, it becomes

$$\frac{1}{r} = \frac{K_M + c_S}{k_2 c_S c_{E,0}} = \frac{K_M}{k_2 c_S c_{E,0}} + \frac{1}{k_2 c_{E,0}} \tag{5-99}$$

Thus, a plot of $1/r$ versus $1/c_S$ would give a straight line. The values of k_2 and K_M can be determined from the intercept $1/k_2 c_{E,0}$ and slope $K_M/k_2 c_{E,0}$ of the plot.

Section 8　Photochemical Reaction

The phenomenon of **photochemical reaction (光化学反应)** has been well known. The primary event in vision involves the absorption of a **photon (光子)** by the visual pigment **rhodopsin (视紫红质)**. **Photosynthesis (光合作用)** refers to the conversion of light energy into chemical energy by plants and bacteria. **Ozone (臭氧)** production and decomposition occurs in the atmosphere that is critical to life on Earth. The active ingredients in drugs gradually degrade under light, causing drugs to lose their potency. As illustrated by these examples, photochemical reactions are an extremely important in a wide variety of areas and they are explored in this section.

8.1　Mechanism of photochemical reaction

Ordinary reactions occur by absorption of heat from outside. The reactants are activated, and then the reaction is brought about. These reactions which are caused by heat and without light are termed **thermal reactions (热反应)** or **dark reactions (暗反应)**.

There are some reactions in which the activation is implemented by electromagnetic radiations in **ultraviolet and visible region (紫外和可见光区)** having wavelength about between 100 to 1000nm. These reactions are named Photochemical reactions. If a photon from high energy **electromagnetic radiations (电磁辐射)** such as X- ray and γ-ray is used, the chemical processes are called **Radiolytic reactions (放射反应)**.

There are many differences between photochemical reactions and thermal reactions. These differences are summarized in the following Table 5-7. According to **the second law of thermodynamics (热力学第二定律)**, chemical reactions are **spontaneous (自发的)** in the direction of decreasing **Gibbs free energy (吉布斯自由能)**, at constant temperature and pressure. However, the direction of photochemical reaction is irrelevant to the change of Gibbs free energy. Because **non-expansion work**

(非体积功) may be done on a system by the surroundings in form of light. Some spontaneous process of photochemical reactions is usually consistent with the direction of increasing Gibbs free energy. For example, ammonia decomposition under photochemical process and photosynthesis, etc. The activation energy of thermal reaction is obtained through molecular **thermal motion (热运动)**, so the reaction rate is greatly affected by the temperature. While the energy of photochemical reaction is from photon, so the reaction rate depends on the **illumination intensity (照度)** and is less affected by the temperature. The reaction rate of thermal reaction is mostly related to the reactant concentration, while the reaction rate of photochemical reaction depends only on the radiation intensity without relation to the reactant concentration, so it is zero-order reaction. In addition, photochemical reactions are usually more selective than thermal reactions.

Table 5-7　Difference between photochemical reactions and thermochemical reactions

	Photochemical reactions	Thermochemical reactions
Energy	Photochemical reactions involve absorption of light radiations	Thermochemical reactions involve absorption or evolution of heat
Light effect	Light is the primary requirement for reactions to occur	The reactions can occur in dark as well as in light
Temperature effect	The rate is almost independent of temperature	The rate depends on temperature significantly
ΔG	ΔG may be negative or positive	ΔG is always negative
Selectivity	Photochemical activation is highly selective.	Thermochemical activation is not selective

8.2　The law of photochemical equivalent

The processes of photochemical reactions are governed by two basic principles, viz. the **Grotthus-Draper law (first law of photochemistry) (格罗特斯–德拉波定律)** and the **Stark-Einstein law of photochemical equivalence (second law of photochemistry) (斯塔克–爱因斯坦光化学当量定律)**.

8.2.1　Grotthuss-Draper law

Grotthuss-Draper Law states that only those radiations which are absorbed can be effective in producing the chemical change. Although photochemical reaction is caused by absorption of light, it may not always lead to chemical change. When the conditions are not favorable for reaction, the absorption of photon may only increase the internal energy or be reemitted.

8.2.2　Stark-Einstein law of photochemical equivalence

Stark and Einstein studied the quantitative aspect of photochemical reactions by application of Quantum theory of light and propounded the law of photochemical equivalence. This law states that absorption of a single photon causes the reaction of one molecule in the primary step of a photochemical process.

The law of photochemical equivalence is illustrated in Fig. 5-20, where the molecule A absorbs a photon of radiation, the energy contained in the photon is transferred

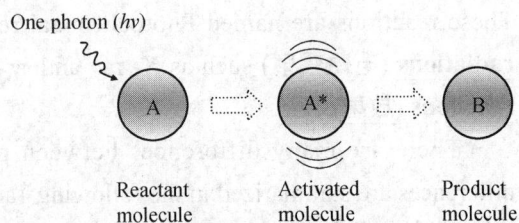

One photon (hv)

Reactant molecule　　Activated molecule　　Product molecule

Fig. 5-20　Illustration of Law of Photochemical equivalence

to the molecule. The molecule A gets activated. The activated molecule A* then decomposes to yield B.

The amount of energy contained by a photon is given by the **Planck equation (普朗克方程)**.

$$E_{photon} = h\nu = \frac{hc}{\lambda} \tag{5-100}$$

$$E = Nh\nu = \frac{Nhc}{\lambda} = \frac{11.96}{\lambda} \text{ J} \cdot \text{mol}^{-1} \tag{5-101}$$

If λ is expressed in Å (1Å = 10^{-8} cm), $E = \frac{1.196 \times 10^9}{\lambda} = \text{J} \cdot \text{mol}^{-1}$.

In equation (5-101), h is Planck's constant 6.626×10^{-34} J, c is the speed of light in a vacuum 2.998×10^8 ms^{-1}, ν is the frequency of light, N is **Avogadro's number (阿佛加德罗常数)** 6.02×10^{23} mol^{-1} and λ is the corresponding **wavelength (波长)** of light, respectively. A mole of photons is referred to as an **Einstein (爱因斯坦)**, and the energy contained by an Einstein of photons is Avogadro's number times E_{photon}. As $E \propto \frac{1}{\lambda}$, so one Einstein corresponding to UV radiations would involve more energy than that in the visible region.

8.2.3　Primary and secondary reactions

Photochemical reactions involve two steps. The primary step consists of raising of the electronic quantum level of molecule or atom by absorption of energy from photon. Photons can be regarded as reactants, and initiation of the reaction occurs when the photon is absorbed. The secondary step includes a succession of process which occurs subsequent to the primary step. These two steps are continuous and difficult to separate.

For example, in the **photolysis (光解)** of HI, absorption of photon leads to destruction of two HI molecule. The primary step is

$$\text{HI} + h\nu \longrightarrow \text{H} \cdot + \text{I} \cdot$$

and the secondary step consists of

$$\text{H} \cdot + \text{HI} \longrightarrow \text{H}_2 + \text{I} \cdot$$
$$2\text{I} \cdot \longrightarrow \text{I}_2$$

The total reaction is

$$2\text{HI} + h\nu \longrightarrow \text{H}_2 + \text{I}_2$$

Evidently, the primary reaction only obeys the law of photochemical equivalence strictly. The secondary reactions have no concern with the law.

8.3　Quantum efficiency

It has been shown that not always a photochemical reaction obeys law of photochemical equivalence. The number of molecules reacted or decomposed is often found to be markedly different from the number of quanta or photons of radiation absorbed in a given time. The number of molecules reacted or formed per photon of light absorbed is expressed in terms of quantum yield, ϕ. ϕ is defined as

$$\phi = \frac{\text{Number of molecules reacted or formed}}{\text{Number of photons absorbed}} \tag{5-102}$$

Quantum yield of some photochemical reactions are listed in Table 5-8. It is clear that the quantum yield is not equal to 1 for most reaction. When the activated molecules transfer part of the energy to the ordinary molecules reducing inactivation or the **free atom (自由原子)** or **radical (自由基)** combined as the original molecules before the reaction, the number of molecules taking part in chemical change would be less than the number of quanta of energy absorbed. When every molecule activated in primary absorption directly decomposes, the number of molecules undergoing chemical change would be equal to the number of quanta of energy absorbed. However, a molecule activated photochemically may initiate a sequence of reactions so that many reactant molecules through a chain mechanism would undergo chemical change. In such cases the number of molecules participating chemical changes will be many times of the quanta of energy absorbed.

Table 5-8　The quantum yield of certain photochemical reactions

Reactions in the gas phase	Wavelength (λ) / Å	Quantum yield (ϕ)
$2NH_3 \longrightarrow N_2 + 3H_2$	~ 2100	0.2
$CH_3COCH_3 \longrightarrow CO + C_2H_6$	~ 3000	0.3
$SO_2 + Cl_2 \longrightarrow SO_2Cl_2$	~ 4200	1
$2HI \longrightarrow H_2 + I_2$	2070 ~ 2820	2
$2Cl_2O \longrightarrow 2Cl_2 + O_2$	3130 ~ 4360	3.5
$H_2 + Cl_2 \longrightarrow 2HCl$	4000 ~ 4360	10^3

重 点 小 结

本章首先介绍了化学动力学的一些基本概念：反应级数、反应分子数、基元反应、反应机制、简单反应、复杂反应等。重点介绍了一级、二级、零级反应动力学方程及其特征，并讨论了温度对反应速率的影响。简单介绍了反应级数的测定方法以及可逆反应、平行反应、连续反应三种复杂反应的动力学特征。简要讨论了溶剂的极性、介电常数、离子强度、pH以及酶催化等因素对反应速率的影响。

Object detection

I. Select the correct option for the following problems (one option for each problem).

1. Which of the following includes all the aims of kinetics?

　A. to be able to predict the rate of a reaction

　B. to be able to establish the mechanism by which a reaction occurs

　C. to be able to control a reaction

　D. all of the above

2. The reaction, $2NO(g) \rightarrow N_2(g) + O_2(g)$, proceeds in a single elementary step. This reaction is thus

　A. the molecularity cannot be determined from the given information

　B. termolecular

　C. bimolecular

　D. unimolecular

3. If the reaction, 2A + 3D → products, is first-order in A and second-order in D, then the rate law will have the form: $r=$

    A. $kc_A c_D^2$ B. $kc_A^2 c_D$ C. $kc_A^2 c_D^2$ D. $kc_A c_D$

4. The rate law relates the rate of a chemical reaction to

    A. the concentrations of reactants   B. the temperature

    C. the activation energy   D. the reaction mechanism

5. For a reaction, A → products, a graph of c_A versus t is found to be a straight line. What is the order of this reaction?

    A. zero order   B. first order   C. second order   D. third order

6. For first-order reactions the rate constant k, has the unit(s)

    A. mol^{-1} B. $time^{-1}$ C. $(mol \cdot L^{-1})^{-1} \cdot time^{-1}$ D. $time \cdot mol^{-1}$

7. For a first-order reaction of the form A → P, $t_{1/2}$ = 9 hours. If the initial concentration of A is $0.042 mol \cdot L^{-1}$, how many moles of A will remain after 24 hours?

    A. 0.0026   B. 0.0066   C. 0.0052   D. 0.022

8. The half-life of radioactive sodium is 15.0 hours. How many hours would it take for a 64g sample to decay to one-eighth of its original concentration?

    A. 3   B. 15   C. 30   D. 45

9. The reaction A → B is a second-order process. When the initial concentration of A is $0.50 mol \cdot L^{-1}$, the half-life is 8.0 minutes. What is the half-life if the initial concentration of A is $0.10 mol \cdot L^{-1}$?

    A. 1.6 minutes   B. 8.0 minutes   C. 40.0 minutes   D. 16.0 minutes

10. Here is a second order reaction A → P. If the initial concentration of A 0.0818mol goes down 30.0% in 3.15 minutes, what is the rate constant for the reaction?

    A. $0.00781 mol^{-1} \cdot min^{-1}$ B. $1.7l mol^{-1} \cdot min^{-1}$

    C. $9.1l mol^{-1} \cdot min^{-1}$ D. $16l mol^{-1} \cdot min^{-1}$

11. Reaction rates can change with

    A. temperature   B. the addition of a catalyst

    C. reactant concentrations   D. all of these

12. At equilibrium

    A. the rate of forward reaction is equal to zero

    B. a change in reaction conditions may shift the equilibrium

    C. the reverse reaction will not continue

    D. the rate constant of forward reaction is equal to that of backward reaction

13. Which of the following will lower the activation energy for a reaction?

    A. increasing the concentrations of reactants

    B. raising the temperature of the reaction

    C. adding a suitable catalyst

    D. there is no way to lower the activation energy of a reaction

14. The minimum amount of energy required to start a chemical reaction is called

    A. entropy   B. enthalpy   C. free energy   D. activation energy

15. A catalyst is a substance which

    A. increases the equilibrium concentration of the products

    B. changes the equilibrium constant of the reaction

    C. supplies energy to the reactions

    D. shortens the time to reach the equilibrium

16. A reaction has an activation energy of 40.0kJ · mol^{-1}. At what temperature will the rate of this reaction be triple that at 300K?

    A. 281K   B. 322K   C. 1.89 × 10^{-4}K   D. 0.638K

17. As temperature increases, the reaction rate will

    A. decrease than increase   B. decreases

    C. increases   D. stays the same

18. Species that are formed in one step of reaction mechanism and used up in another step are called

    A. catalysts   B. intermediates   C. inhibitors   D. activated complexes

19. For any chemical reaction at equilibrium, the rate of the forward reaction is

    A. less than the rate of the reverse reaction

    B. greater than the rate of the reverse reaction

    C. equal to the rate of the reverse reaction

    D. unrelated to the rate of the reverse reaction

20. For the reaction A → B, the activation energy is E_a = 125kJ · mol^{-1} and the heat of reaction, ΔH = 50kJ · mol^{-1}. What is the E_a for the reverse reaction?

    A. −75kJ · mol^{-1} B. 125kJ · mol^{-1} C. 175kJ · mol^{-1} D. 75kJ · mol^{-1}

21. Why do most chemical reaction rates increase rapidly as the temperature rises?

    A. the fraction of the molecules with kinetic energy greater than the activation energy increases rapidly with temperature

    B. the average kinetic energy increases as temperature rises

    C. the activation energy decreases as temperature rises

    D. more collisions take place between particles so that the reaction can occur

22. The rate constant for a reaction depends upon each of the following, except

    A. solvent for solutions   B. temperature

    C. concentration of reactants   D. nature of reactants

23. Which of the following does not affect the rate of a chemical reaction?

    A. enthalpy of the reaction   B. concentration of reactants

    C. temperature   D. surface area

24. Which of the following statements about the photochemical reactions is true?

    A. the presence of light is the primary requirement for reactions to take place

    B. temperature has a very little effect on the rate of photochemical reactions

    C. ΔG for photochemical spontaneous reactions may be negative or positive

    D. all of the above

25. The number of molecules reacted or formed per photon of light absorbed is called

    A. yield of the reaction   B. quantum efficiency

    C. quantum yield   D. quantum productivity

Ⅱ. **Try to answer the following problem.**

Plateau value (坪值) is also called **steady-state plasma concentration** (稳态血药浓度). It is the blood concentration at when the dosing rate and the elimination rate are equal. According to the needs of clinical treatment, most of the drugs require multiple dosing. If the kinetics of drug elimination is first-order reaction and giving the same dose every other half-life, do you know how many half-lives pass when the blood concentration is equal to steady-state concentration?

Reference answers

Ⅰ. 1.D; 　 2.D; 　 *3*.A; 　 4.A; 　 5.B; 　 6.B; 　 7.D; 　 8.C; 　 9.B; 　 10.D; 　 11.B; 　 12.C; 　 13.D; 　 14.D; 15.B; 　 16.C; 　 17.B; 　 18.C; 　 19.D; 　 20.A; 　 21.C; 　 22.A; 　 23.D; 　 24.C.

Ⅱ. Omitted.

Chapter 6　Surface Phenomena

From early chapter, we all knew that a phase of substance is a form of matter that is uniform throughout in chemical composition and physical state. When two phases coexist, the physical boundary between the adjacent phases is named an **interface(界面)**. Conventionally, if one of the phases is gas, the interface is also named **surface(表面)** of the non-gas phase, such as solid surface and liquid surface. It is worth noting that the interface between any two phases is not a sheer geometric plane, but a thin layer with several molecular thicknesses, so it is more accurate to be called the interface layer. Surface phenomena are the special properties of the interface, which are different from either of the coexisting phases. For example, water in the glass capillary will automatically rise up a certain height; solid surfaces tend to automatically absorb adjacent substances; the water drop on the leaves of plants will automatically be of spherical shape; the tiny liquid droplets are easy to evaporate, and so on.

The underlying cause of surface phenomena is that there is an imbalanced force performed on the surface molecules. Take liquid surface as an example. It is well known that there exist short-range forces of attraction between liquid molecules. A molecule in the bulk liquid phase is, on average, subjected to equal forces of attraction in all directions. So there is no net force on a molecule in the bulk liquid. In contrast, an interface molecule experiences unbalanced attractive forces resulting in a net inward pull (Fig.

6–1), for the liquid phase is much denser than the gas phase. As a result, the surface molecules tend to get into the bulk of the liquid as more as possible to minimize the energy of the system. That is why a water droplet will spontaneously assume a spherical shape.

The characteristic of substance interface will also have an influence on other properties of the substance, which becomes more evident with increase in the degrees of dispersion. Surface phenomena and related properties are important for modern scientific and technological research, especially for the field of pharmaceutical preparation.

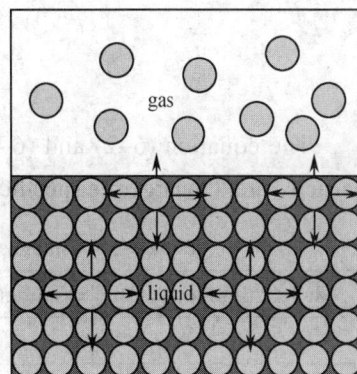

Fig. 6–1   Schematic representation of a liquid molecule at the surface and in the bulk liquid

Section 1   Specific Surface Area and Specific Surface Energy

PPT

1.1   Specific surface area

Surface phenomena become more significant as the degree of dispersion of a substance increases. So it is necessary to define a variable to measure the degree of dispersion. Given a certain amount of substance, it is evident that the higher the degree of dispersion is, the larger its surface area. For example, when a cube with side length of 10^{-2}m is cut into 10^9 smaller cubes with side length of 10^{-5}m, the total surface area will be increased by 10^3 times, as shown in Table 6–1. So usually **specific surface area(比表面积)** is used to measure the degree of dispersion of a system, which is defined as the total surface area of a material per unit of volume(a_S) or per unit of mass(a_W)

$$a_S = \frac{A}{V} \quad \text{or} \quad a_W = \frac{A}{m} \tag{6-1}$$

where A is the surface area, V and m are the volume and mass of the material respectively. For materials having exact geometric shapes, the specific surface can easily be calculated by using well-known geometric formulas. For example, for a cube with edge length of l, the specific surface area can be calculated as follows

$$a_S = \frac{A}{V} = \frac{6l^2}{l^3} = \frac{6}{l} \text{m}^{-1} \tag{6-2a}$$

$$a_W = \frac{A}{m} = \frac{6l^2}{\rho l^3} = \frac{6}{\rho l} \text{m}^2 \cdot \text{kg}^{-1} \tag{6-2b}$$

where ρ is the bulk density of the material with unit of kg $\cdot$ m^{-3}. Similarly, for a spherical particle with diameter of d, its specific surface area is

$$a_S = \frac{A}{V} = \frac{4\pi r^2}{\frac{4}{3}\pi r^3} = \frac{6}{d} \, \text{m}^{-1} \tag{6-3}$$

The equation (6–2) and (6–3) demonstrate that for a certain amount of material, the smaller its particles are, the larger its specific surface area and the higher the degree of dispersion.

Table 6–1   Changes of total and specific surface area of particles with particle size

Side length of a cube/m	Number of cubes after cutting	Total surface area/m^2	Specific surface area/m^{-1}
10^{-2}	1	6×10^{-4}	6×10^2
10^{-3}	10^3	6×10^{-3}	6×10^3
10^{-4}	10^6	6×10^{-2}	6×10^4
10^{-5}	10^9	6×10^{-1}	6×10^5
10^{-6}	10^{12}	6×10^0	6×10^6
10^{-7}	10^{15}	6×10^1	6×10^7
10^{-8}	10^{18}	6×10^2	6×10^8
10^{-9}	10^{21}	6×10^3	6×10^9

1.2   Specific surface Gibbs function

For a given condensed phase, the energy of a surface molecule is different from that in the bulk phase. For example, in a gas-liquid equilibrium system, the molecules in liquid are kept close to each other by the cohesion force. A molecule in the bulk liquid is attracted by others in all directions, thus is in a physical balance state with zero net force. However, because there are very few molecules on the vapor side compared with the liquid side, a surface molecule will experience a net force pulling it back into the bulk liquid. So the surface molecules are in a state of higher energy than those in the bulk liquid. This means that work must be done to pull a molecule from the bulk to the surface, which is called **surface work**(表面功,W'_B). According to the thermaldynamic principle, under the condition of constant pressure and temperature, the surface work $\delta W'_R$ done reversibly to create a surface area dA is equivalent to the increase in Gibbs function of the system(dG), i.e. $dG = \delta W'_R$. There is therefore an energy change associated with the formation of a liquid surface, which is called the **surface Gibbs function** (表面吉布斯函数) or **surface free energy**(表面自由能).

Usually, if the surface of system is constant, the Gibbs function can be expressed as

$$G = f(T, p, n_1, n_2, \cdots)$$

However, if the surface of a system occurs obvious changes, the contribution of the surface area to the Gibbs function must be explicitly considered. In this case, the Gibbs function will be of the following form

$$G = f(T, p, n_1, n_2, \cdots, A) \tag{6-4}$$

Correspondingly, the differential change of Gibbs function(dG) of a system during any process is

$$dG = \left(\frac{\partial G}{\partial T}\right)_{p, n_1, n_2, \ldots, A} dT + \left(\frac{\partial G}{\partial p}\right)_{T, n_1, n_2, \ldots A} dp + \sum_B \mu_B dn_B + \left(\frac{\partial G}{\partial A}\right)_{T, p, n_1, n_2, \ldots} dA \tag{6-5}$$

$$\sigma = \left(\frac{\partial G}{\partial A}\right)_{T,p,n_1,n_2,\cdots} \tag{6-6}$$

The variable σ is called **specific surface Gibbs function**(比表面吉布斯函数) with unit of $J \cdot m^{-2}$, representing the increase in surface Gibbs function when the surface area is increased by one unit, i.e. $1m^2$, under the condition that the temperature, pressure and the composition of the system remain constant. Under the same condition, the equation (6–5) reduces to

$$dG = \sigma dA \tag{6-7}$$

The integration of the above formula gives

$$G = \sigma A \tag{6-8}$$

which indicates that the amount of surface Gibbs free energy is directly proportional to the two variables of σ and A.

1.3   Surface tension

The previous analysis indicates that a molecule on the liquid surface is subject to a net inward attraction perpendicular to the surface. So a liquid surface tends to contract to the smallest possible surface area for a given volume. It is just like there is an elastic membrane covering the surface of a liquid, which cause resistance of the liquid to an increase in its surface area. So work must be done on the liquid to increase or extend its surface area.

Fig. 6–2 shows an idealized system used to analyze the mechanical property of a liquid surface, where a movable metal bar is put on a metal frame and the formed rectangle is covered with a liquid film. To increase the rectangular surface area, we have to exert dragging force on the metal bar and against the inward pulling forces from the liquid film. Assume the magnitude of the exerted force is f and the bar is moved out by an infinitesimal distance dx, then the infinitesimal amount of work done on the system $\delta W' = f dx$, which is the exact analogy of the physical definition

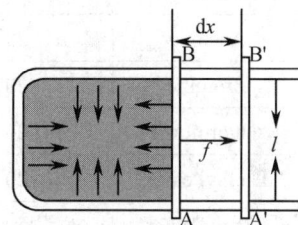

Fig. 6-2   Schematic illustration of surface tension

of work. If the process occurs reversibly, then the work $\delta W'$ is equal to the increase in surface free energy dG, i.e., $f dx = \sigma dA$. It is obvious that the rectangular liquid film has two sides, so the infinitesimal change in its surface area, $dA=2ldx$, where l is the width of the metal track, as demonstrated in Fig. 6-2. The equation $f dx = \sigma dA$ can be rewritten as

$$f dx = \sigma 2l dx \tag{6-9}$$

which can be further reduced to

$$\sigma = \frac{f}{2l} \tag{6-10}$$

The above equation indicates that the variable σ can also be viewed as the force acting on any line of unit length on the liquid surface along the tangent direction of the surface with unit of N/m. So it is called the **surface tension**(表面张力). However, this definition is somewhat misleading, since there is no such force at the surface of a liquid. The observed shrink tendency at the liquid surface results from the same inward pull of the bulk molecule on the surface molecules described above, rather than some new forces on the surface molecules.

Surface tension for a given liquid is affected by several factors including intermolecular forces, second medium, temperature, etc. Table 6–2 lists surface tensions of some common liquids. It is obvious that the strength of surface tension is mainly determined by the intermolecular force of a liquid. The stronger the force is, the larger the surface tension. For example, the water liquid has a larger surface tension than most organic liquid, due to the strong hydrogen bonds between water molecules. In fact, other than mercury, water has the greatest surface tension of any liquid at normal temperature. When the same substance contacts with different medium, the interface molecules will subject to different force field. Since the surface tension origins from the unbalanced force on the surface molecule exerted by the different bulk molecules, the second medium interfacing with the given liquid will also affect the resulting surface tension.

Temperature also plays a role in altering the surface tension of a liquid. As the temperature rises, the distance between the liquid molecules increases. As a result, the attraction of bulk molecules to the surface molecules decreases. In addition, increase in temperature will also raise the density of gas phase, which in turn increases the attraction of gas molecules to the surface molecule. With the increase in temperature, the two effects act synergistically in reducing the surface tension. At the critical temperature, the surface tension becomes zero as the interface between liquid phase and gas phase disappear.

Table 6–2 Surface tensions of various liquids

Liquid	Temperature / ℃	Surface tension / ($\times 10^{-3}$ N $\cdot$ m^{-1})	Liquid	Temperature / ℃	Surface tension / ($\times 10^{-3}$ N $\cdot$ m^{-1})
Acetic acid	−30	27.8	Helium	−270	0.24
Acetone	25	23.7	Mercury	25	485,5
Bromine	20	41.5	Water	0	75.6
Chloroform	20	27.1	Water	10	74.22
Diethyl ether	20	17.0	Water	20	72.75
Diethyl ether	50	13.5	Water	60	66.18
Ehanol	20	22.8	Water	100	58.9
Glyecrine	20	63.4			

It is worth noting that the specific surface energy and the surface tension are closely related to each other. In fact, they are the same phenomenon described from two different perspectives, energetic or mechanic respectively. They share the same physical dimension, but have different physical meaning. Usually, the specific surface energy is used to describe the thermodynamic properties of the system, while the surface tension is used to describe the mechanical properties of the system.

1.4 Thermodynamic criteria for studying surface phenomena

Gibbs function is widely used to discuss the potential of spontaneous procedure. We apply the Gibbs function to discuss the thermodynamic criteria of surface phenomena. According to the expression of surface Gibbs function ($G = \sigma A$), the differential of surface Gibbs function may be expressed as

$$dG_{T, p} = d(\sigma A) = \sigma dA + A d\sigma \qquad (6-11)$$

According to the second thermodynamic principle, under the condition of constant temperature and pressure, a process is spontaneous if dG is negative. At certain temperature and pressure, equation (6–8) indicates that the surface Gibbs function depends on two variables, surface tension σ and surface area A. For a single component system, the σ is constant, i.e. dσ = 0, so dG = σdA. Because σ must be a positive number, this implies that for a spontaneous process the requirement of dG<0 can only be achieved by dA<0. That is, for a system with a single component, the reduction in surface Gibbs function can only be achieved by decreasing surface area. That explains why water droplets spontaneously assume a spherical shape. As indicated by equation (6–6), the σ is a function of the composition of the system. For a system with multiple components, variation in the composition of the surface may reduce the σ, which may also lead to a negative dG. This is reason for adsorption and absorption phenomena, which will be discussed in more details in the later section of this chapter.

Section 2   Wetting and Spreading

2.1   Wetting

Wetting(润湿) refers to the process by which the gas absorbed on a solid surface is replaced by a liquid. The degree of wetting (wettability) is determined by the change in surface tension involved in the process. The more the surface tension is reduced, the higher the wetting degree.

Fig. 6–3 shows the wettability of different liquid on a solid surface, where the point O is the intersection point of solid, liquid and gas phases. The angle between the solid-liquid interfacial tension (denoted by $\sigma_{s,l}$) and the liquid-vapor surface tension (denoted as $\sigma_{s,g}$) is defined as θ. The wettability of a surface can be quantitatively measured by the contact angle. For a stationery droplet, the three surface tensions must be balanced, leading to the following expression

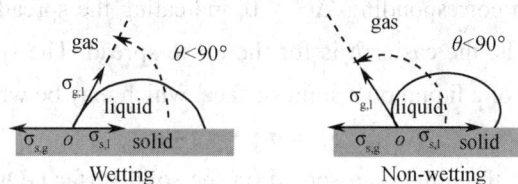

Fig. 6–3   The wettability of liquids on the solid surface

$$\sigma_{s,g} = \sigma_{s,l} + \sigma_{g,l} \cos \theta$$

which can be rewritten as

$$\cos\theta = \frac{\sigma_{s,g} - \sigma_{s,l}}{\sigma_{g,l}} \tag{6–12}$$

Thomas Young derived the formula in 1805, so it was named Young relation, which indicates that the behavior of the liquid on the solid surface is dependent on the relative magnitude of the three interfacial surface tensions. Specifically, in terms of the above formula, the wettability can be divided into the following cases.

(1) If $\sigma_{s,g} = \sigma_{s,l}$, then $\cos\theta = 0, \theta = 90°$, indicating that the droplet lies at the critical point distinguishing wetting or non-wetting.

(2) If $\sigma_{s,g} > \sigma_{s,l}$, then $\cos\theta > 0, \theta < 90°$, indicating that the droplet would spread out on the solid surface, which is called (partial) wetting.

(3) If $\sigma_{s,g} < \sigma_{s,l}$, then $\cos\theta < 0, \theta > 90°$, indicating that the droplet can't spread, instead, forms a spherical cap resting on the solid surface, which is called (partial) non-wetting.

(4) If $\sigma_{s,g} \approx \sigma_{s,l} + \sigma_{g,l}$, then $\cos\theta \to 0, \theta \to 0°$, indicating that the droplet may spread on the solid surface without any limit, which is called total wetting

(5) If $\sigma_{s,g} + \sigma_{g,l} \approx \sigma_{s,l}$, then $\cos\theta \to -1, \theta \to 180°$, indicating that the droplet would take on an almost spherical shape, which is called total non-wetting.

2.2 Spreading

The phenomenon that a drop of liquid spontaneously forms a film on the surface of another immiscible liquid is called **spreading(铺展)**. The essence of spreading can be understood in terms of the change in the surface free energy. Suppose a drop of oil is dripped on a clean water surface. The original water-gas interface disappears, which is replaced with an oil-water and oil-gas interfaces. Ignoring the tiny surface area of the oil droplet, the change in surface Gibbs function during the dripping process is

$$\Delta G = (\sigma_{o,w} + \sigma_{o,g} - \sigma_{w,g})A \qquad (6-13)$$

where $\sigma_{o,w}$, $\sigma_{o,g}$ and $\sigma_{w,g}$ are the interface tensions on oil-water, oil-gas, water-gas respectively, and A is the area of the newly-formed interface. According to second-law of thermodynamics, only if the change in surface Gibbs function $\Delta G < 0$, can the oil droplet spontaneously spread on the water surface under the conditions of constant temperature and constant pressure. The above formula indicates that the sign of ΔG is determined by the relative magnitude of surface tensions after and before the spreading, since A is always positive. So a new variable S, named **spreading coefficient(铺展系数)**, is defined by rearranging equation (6-13) into the following form

$$S_{o,w} = -\Delta G/A = \sigma_{o,w} + \sigma_{o,g} - \sigma_{w,g} \qquad (6-14)$$

Obviously, if $S > 0$, then corresponding $\Delta G < 0$, indicating the spreading can occur. Otherwise, it can't occur. The larger the S is, the easier it is for the oil to spread. The spreading coefficient can also apply to predict the spreading of a liquid on a solid surface, which may be written as

$$S_{l/s} = \sigma_{s,g} + \sigma_{s,l} - \sigma_{s,g}$$

Likewise, if $S_{l/s} > 0$, then the liquid can spread on the solid surface. Otherwise, the spreading can't take place.

Spreading, wetting and dewetting are of great practical significance in pharmaceutical field. For instance, to prepare a stable emulsion, it is necessary to spread a suitable film of surfactant on the surface of the oil drop. In order to make the eye ointment spread evenly on the conjunctiva, the formulation of the ointment matrix should be designed carefully to improve the spreading effect. Since all preparations based on mineral oil can not spread evenly on the skin, adding some lanolin is a must to ameliorate the spreading effect, thus improving drug efficacy.

[Example 6-1] At 20℃, it is know that the surface tensions of oleic acid and water are $\sigma_o = 32 \times 10^{-3}$ N·m^{-1} and $\sigma_w = 73 \times 10^{-3}$ N·m^{-1} respectively. The interface tension between pure oleic acid and pure water is $\sigma_{o,w} = 32 \times 10^{-3}$ N·m^{-1}. At the end, the two liquids form a pair of mutual saturated solution, the corresponding interface tensions are $\sigma'_o = \sigma_o$ and $\sigma'_w = 40 \times 10^{-3}$. Based on the above data, speculate on the beginning and end shapes of oleic acid, when it was dripped on the water surface?

Solution:

We need to calculate the spreading factors based on the surface tension data. When the oleic acid is dripped on the water surface:

At the beginning, $S_{o/w} = \sigma_w - \sigma_o - \sigma_{o,w} = (73 - 32 - 12) \times 10^{-3} = 29 \times 10^{-3} \text{N} \cdot \text{m}^{-1} > 0$

At the end, $S'_{o/w} = \sigma'_w - \sigma'_o - \sigma_{o,w} = (40 - 32 - 12) \times 10^{-3} = -4 \times 10^{-3} \text{N} \cdot \text{m}^{-1} < 0$

According to the calculated results, we can conclude that when the oleic acid is dripped on the water surface, at the beginning it will spontaneously spread on the water surface, forming a thin film. At the end, after forming mutual saturated solution, the oleic acid will contract into an ellipsoid on the water surface due to the change in the surface tension. That is, the oleic acid can't spread on the water surface anymore.

Section 3   Effect of High Dispersion on Physical Properties

3.1   Additional pressure on curved liquid surface——Laplace Equation

The plane surfaces of two connected water pools are always at the same height. This indicates that in addition to the gas pressure, no **additional pressure(附加压力)** is performed on the water surfaces. But this is not for the liquid with curved surface area, such as bubble or droplet. A common apparatus used to demonstrate additional pressure is a capillary tube. For instance, if a glass capillary is placed vertically into a bow of mercury, a convex meniscus forms inside the capillary, as shown in Fig. 6-4. Since surface tensions are always acting along the tangential line of a curved surface, the surface tensions of the convex meniscus produces an additional pressure pointing towards the mercury. Consequently, the mercury inside the capillary experiences a larger pressure than that outside, being lower than that outside. Oppositely, a concave meniscus appears in the glass capillary tube placed in a bow of water, which produces an additional pressure pointing towards the air. As a result, the surface inside the capillary will rise up higher than the liquid surface outside, as shown in Fig. 6-5.

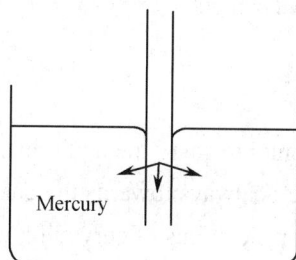

Fig. 6-4   Mercury surface in the capillary tube

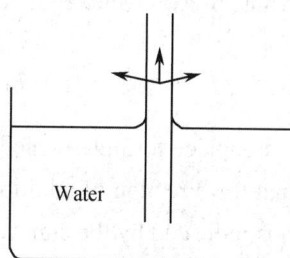

Fig. 6-5   Water surface in the capillary tube

What factors determine the strength of additional pressure? In around 1805, Young and Laplace independently derived the formula relating extra pressure to surface tension and curvature radius, namely, Young-Thomas formula, which can be derived as following. Generally, for an arbitrary curved surface, the curvature at any point may be defined by assigning two radii of curvature as shown in Fig. 6-6.

Take a small rectangle *ABCD* on an arbitrary curved surface with an area *xy*, where the radii of curvature of arc *AB* and *BC* are r_1 and r_2 respectively. Choose two normal planes that cut the rectangle along two principal curvature sections. The intersecting line of the two planes is the normal of the rectangular center *O*. Move the curved surface *ABCD* a distance of d*z* along the normal *OO'*, yielding a new surface *A'B'C'D'* with area of $(x + dx)(y + dy)$.

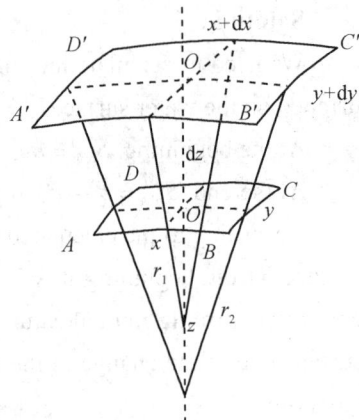

Correspondingly, the change in the curvature surface area during the expansion of *ABCD* into *A'B'C'D'* is

$$dA = (x + dx)(y + dy) - xy$$
$$= xdy + ydx + dxdy$$
$$= xdy + ydx$$

Fig. 6-6　Expansion of arbitrary curved surface

With the increased surface area, the increase in surface Gibbs function is

$$dG = \sigma dA = \sigma(xdy + ydx)$$

Due to the additional pressure on the curved surface, work has to be done on the system to increase the surface area

$$\delta W = p_s dV = p_s \cdot xydz$$

where d*V* is the increase in the volume of the system and p_s is the additional pressure of the curved surface.

If the process is carried out reversibly, then $dG = \delta W$, substitute d*G* and δW with the above equations, yielding

$$\sigma(xdy + ydx) = p_s \cdot xydz \qquad (6\text{-}15)$$

According to the principle of similar triangles,

$$\frac{x+dx}{r_1+dz} = \frac{x}{r_1} \quad \text{or} \quad dx = \frac{x}{r_1}dz$$

$$\frac{y+dx}{r_1+dz} = \frac{y}{r_1} \quad \text{or} \quad dy = \frac{y}{r_1}dz$$

Substituting the value of d*x*, d*y* into equation (6-15), we can get

$$p_s = \sigma\left(\frac{1}{r_1} + \frac{1}{r_2}\right) \qquad (6\text{-}16)$$

This is the famous Laplace formula, which is fundamental to study the additional pressure of curved liquid surface. Note that the direction of additional pressure is always towards the curvature center of the curved surface, which is indicated by the sign convention for the radius of curvature, which is positive for convex surface($r>0$), but negative($r<0$) for a concave surface.

For a spherical surface, such as a tiny bubble in a liquid, the two curvature radii are equal, i.e., $r_1=r_2=r$, the formula reduces to

$$p_s = \frac{2\sigma}{r} \qquad (6\text{-}17)$$

A plane surface may be viewed as a curved surface with a curvature radius being infinitely large, so the additional pressure of a plane surface $p_s = 0$. This explains why no additional pressure exists on a plane surface of liquid. A soap bubble has two spherical surfaces with the inner and outer gas phases respectively. Since the thickness of liquid film is ignorable, the curvature radii of the two surfaces are approximately equal. As a result, the additional pressure for a soap bubble is double of that of a droplet with the same curvature radius, i.e.

$$p_s = \frac{4\sigma}{r} \tag{6-18}$$

3.2　Effect of high dispersion on vapor pressure

Under conditions of certain temperature and pressure, any pure liquid has a specific saturated vapor pressure. However, this is not the case for curved liquid. For example, experiments showed that the vapor pressure of liquid droplets is related not only to the nature of substance, temperature and pressure, but also to the size of droplets. The relationship between vapor pressure and radius of liquid droplet is described by Kelvin equation, which can be derived as the following.

Suppose plane liquid and its vapor are in equilibrium at constant temperature and pressure, the chemical potential of the two phases are equal, that is,

$$u_l(T,p) = u_g(T,p^*) = u_g^\ominus(T,p) + RT\ln\frac{p^*}{p^\ominus}$$

where p is the pressure exerted on the liquid and p^* is the saturated vapor pressure at temperature T.

If the plane liquid is dispersed into tiny droplets with radius r, correspondingly the saturated vapor pressure will change. To rebuild the phase equilibrium after dispersion, the changes in chemical potential must be equal, i.e.

$$du_l(T,p) = du_g(T,p^*) \tag{6-19}$$

The change in potential energy of the pure liquid caused by the variation in pressure under the condition of constant temperature ($dT = 0$) can be further expressed as

$$du_l(T,p) = dG_{l,m}^* = -S_{l,m}^* dT + V_{l,m}^* dp = V^* dp$$

According to equation (6-18), at constant temperature, the change in the chemical potential of the vapor can be expressed as

$$du_g(T,p^*) = RT \ln p^*$$

Substitute the above two equation into equation (6-19), we can get

$$V_{l,m}^* dp = RT \ln p^*$$

Assume that when the plane liquid is dispersed into tiny droplet, the pressure exerted on the liquid is changed from p to $p+p_r$, correspondingly the saturated vapor pressure is changed from p^* to p_r^*. We can integrate the above formula to get

$$V_{l,m}^* \int_p^{p+p_s} dp = \int_{p_0^*}^{p_r^*} RT d\ln p^*$$

$$V_{l,m}^* p_s = RT \ln \frac{p_r^*}{p_0^*} \tag{6-20}$$

where $V_{l,m}^*$ is the molar volume of pure liquid, which can be expressed as the ratio of the molecular weight M over the density ρ of the liquid, i.e.

$$V_{l,m}^* = \frac{M}{\rho}$$

p_s is the additional pressure of the spherical droplet with radius r, which equals

$$p_s = \frac{2\sigma}{r}$$

Substituting the above formula $V_{l,m}^*$ and p_s into equation (6–20), we can get

$$\frac{M}{\rho} \cdot \frac{2\sigma}{r} = RT\ln\frac{p_r^*}{p_0^*}$$

which can be rewritten as

$$\ln\frac{p_r^*}{p_0^*} = \frac{2\sigma M}{RT\rho r} \tag{6–21}$$

This expression is known as the Kelvin equation, indicating that the smaller a liquid droplet is, the larger its vapor pressure (Table 6–3). When the radius of the droplet reduces to 10^{-9} m, its saturated vapor pressure is triple of that of plane water, which makes it evaporate fast. This is the theoretical basis of spray drying method commonly used in pharmaceutical industry. It can also be applied to predict the vapor pressure of a bubble in a liquid. In this case, the curvature radius is negative and a vapor pressure lowering is predicted. That is, for a bubble in a liquid the smaller a bubble is, the smaller the saturated vapor pressure.

Table 6–3 The relationship of the radius of a liquid droplet or bubble to the ratio of vapor pressure $\frac{p_r^*}{p_0^*}$

r/m	10^{-5}	10^{-6}	10^{-7}	10^{-8}	10^{-9}
Droplet	1.0001	1.001	1.011	1.114	2.937
Bubble	0.9999	0.9989	0.9897	0.8977	0.3405

[Example 6–2] At 298.15K, the density of water is $1000kg \cdot m^{-3}$, surface tension is $72.75 \times 10^{-3}kg \cdot m^{-3}$, the molar mass is $0.01805kg \cdot m^{-3}$. For a spherical liquid droplet and a bubble in a liquid with radius of $10^{-9}m$, calculate their relative vapor pressures p_r/p_0 respectively.

Solution:

For a spherical liquid droplet, the sign of curvature radius is positive. According to Kelvin formula

$$\ln\frac{p_r}{p_0} = \frac{2\sigma M}{RT\rho r} = \frac{2\times72.75\times10^{-3}\times18.05\times10^{-3}}{8.314\times298.15\times10^3\times10^{-9}} = 1.0595$$

$$\frac{p_r}{p_0} = 2.8849$$

For a bubble in a liquid, the sign of curvature radius is negative

$$\ln\frac{p_r}{p_0} = \frac{2\sigma M}{RT\rho r} = \frac{2\times72.75\times10^{-3}\times18.05\times10^{-3}}{8.314\times298.15\times10^3\times(-10^{-9})} = -1.0595$$

$$\frac{p_r}{p_0} = 0.3466$$

3.3 Effect of high dispersion on solubility

The Kelvin formula also applies to crystal materials, which means that the vapor pressure of microcrystals is always greater than the common crystals due to their relative small size. According to the law of Henry, the partial pressure of any solute shall be direct ratio with its solubility in the solution. Specifically, for particles with different sizes, their partial pressures can be expressed as

$$p_r = kx_r, p_0 = kx_0$$

where p_r and x_r refer to the partial pressure and solubility of small particle respectively, p_0 and x_0 are the counterparts of large particles. Substituting the two expressions into Kelvin equation leads to the following formula

$$\ln \frac{x_r}{x_0} = \frac{2\sigma M}{RT\rho r} \tag{6-22}$$

where r is the radius of small particle. The formula indicates that the solubility of a small particle is dependent on its radius. The smaller the radius of a particle is, the larger its solubility.

For a crystal grain, because its curvature radius is positive, the right side of equation (6-21) is always positive. This implies that the solubility of any tiny crystal will greater than normal solubility, which is the reason for the formation of **supersaturated solution**(过饱和溶液). Leave a cup of hot solution in a cold environment and let it cool down naturally. When its temperature drops below the saturation point, crystals should have started to precipitate. However, it is not the case. The newly solidified grains are very tiny, so they have a high solubility. As a result, even though the concentration has reached the saturation point of large crystals, it is still lower than that of tiny crystal grains. So the solution contains more dissolved solute than the solvent would normally dissolve under the same conditions, so it is named supersaturated solution. Supersaturated solutions are extremely unstable. Triggering events such as addition of crystal seeds, stirring, scrubbing the vessel wall and so on, all can accelerate the formation of crystals.

In the crystallization operation, if the degree of the supersaturation of the solution is too high, the resulting crystal will be very fine, which is unfavorable for the following filtration and washing. In order to obtain large crystal particles, crystal seeds should be introduced into the solution to trigger the crystallization before the degree of supersaturation gets too high. Another problem arising from supersaturation state is that the newly crystallized grains from the solution are various in sizes. In this situation, the solution is unsaturated for small crystal grains, but supersaturated for large crystal grains. Prolonging the crystallization time can make the small crystal particles gradually dissolve until they disappear, while the large crystal particles continually grow bigger. Finally, the remained crystal grains will be large and uniform in size. The process is called **aging**(陈化) of precipitation.

3.4 Metastable state

Normally, surface phenomena such as increase in saturated vapor pressure and crystal solubility are ignorable for a system with low degree of dispersion. However, with the increase in the dispersion degree, the surface phenomena will become too significant to ignore. One example is the formation of a new phase from a bulk parent phase, which requires the creation of an interface between two phases. The newly formed phase is usually very tiny, thus generating a high interface Gibbs function. So the systems are in energetically unstable state which is called **metastable state(介稳状态)**, such as supersatureated vapor, superheated liquid and supercooled liquid, as discussed below.

3.4.1 Supersaturated vapor

The saturation vapor pressure is the partial pressure of the water vapor in equilibrium with bulk water liquid. At certain temperature, if the vapor pressure reaches the saturation point, but still no condensation occurs. Such vapor is called **supersaturated vapor(过饱和蒸气)**. According to Kelvin equation, the vapor pressure of newly formed tiny droplets is much larger than that of bulk water. Even though the vapor may be saturated for bulk water, it is still unsaturated for the newly formed tiny droplets. So supersaturated vapor can exist stably, though be in a metastable state. In fact, in pure water vapor the relative humidity can reach several hundred percent without condensation. However, if there is dust in the vapor or inner surface of container is rough, these substances can serve as the condensation nuclei of the vapor, making the condensation easy to occur. Artificial precipitation is achieved by spaying tiny AgI particles into the cloud, which provides condensation nuclei for water vapor, making the condensation occurred at relatively low humidity.

3.4.2 Superheated liquid

To make vapor bubbles form and expand in a bulk liquid, the vapor pressure inside the vapor bubble must exceed that outside the bubble. During heating process, when the liquid is about to boiling, the newly formed vapor bubble in the bulk liquid must be very tiny. Such tiny vapor bubble with a highly curved surface will produce additional vapor pressure on the surface. Suppose that at 101.325kPa and 100 ℃, there is a vapor bubble with a radius of 10^{-8}m in the water, as shown in Fig. 6-8. The surface tension of water is 5.885×10^{-2}N·m^{-1}, the additional pressure on the bubble generated by the curved surface is

$$p_s = \frac{2\sigma}{r} = \frac{2 \times 5.885 \times 10^{-2}}{10^{-8}} = 1.177 \times 10^4 \, kPa$$

Suppose that the static pressure of water is negligible, the total pressure that the bubble needs to resist is

$$p_t = p_{air} + p_s = 101.325 + 1.177 \times 10^4 = 1.187 \times 10^4 \, kPa$$

However, under the current condition the vapor pressure inside the bubble is only 94.34kPa, which is far less than the total pressure p_t that it needs to resist. So the bubble is impossible to exist. Such liquid that is heated above its boiling point, but still in a liquid state, is called **superheated liquid(过热液体)**. To make the bubble exist, the liquid must be heated further to increase the vapor pressure inside it. Only when the vapor pressure is equal to or greater than the pressure p_t, can the liquid begin to boil. Once the superheated liquid begins to boil, the high temperature may cause it to boil violently. To prevent the liquid from bumping, some materials such as zeolites, sintered ceramic chips and capillaries are often put into the liquid. These porous materials contain gas in their pores, which may serve as the nuclei of gas phase upon being heated, thereby helping the liquid bypass the difficult stage of generating extremely fine bubbles. Consequently, liquid boiling can occur at low degree of superheating.

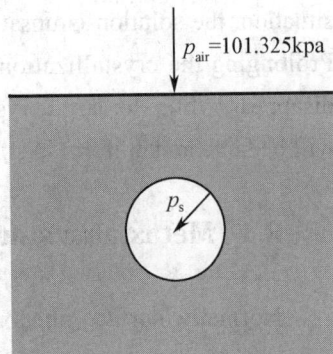

Fig. 6-7 Schematic diagram of generating superheated liquid

3.4.3 Supercooled liquid

Cooling down a liquid at constant pressure, if the liquid still does not freeze even at a temperature below its freezing point, the liquid is called **supercooled liquid(过冷液体)**. Why does supercooled liquid exist? When a liquid begins to freeze, the new-formed solid grain is very tiny, whose saturation vapor pressure is greatly larger than that of the bulk solid, as indicated by Kelvin equation. When the temperature drops to the freezing point of the liquid, the vapor pressure of the liquid is equal to the vapor pressure, but lower than that tiny solid grain. As a result, no freezing occurs. The temperature must be lowered further to make the vapor pressure of tiny crystal equal to that of the liquid, i.e. to the freezing point of tiny crystal grains, which is usually much lower than the freezing point of the bulk liquid. For example, pure liquid water may stay liquid at -40°C without freezing.

Recrystallization is a commonly used method for purifying substances. To avoid the formation of supercooled liquid, tiny crystals of this substance are usually introduced into the liquid as the nuclei of condensation, which makes the freezing take place at a temperature close to the normal freezing point. This method is particularly effective for the extraction and purification of volatile, low-boiling components.

Section 4   Adsorption on the Surface of Solution

4.1 Adsorption phenomena on the surface of solution

The surface tension of the solution is influenced by chemical nature and concentration of the solute for a given solvent. According to the specific effect of solute on the surface tension of aqueous solution, the solutes can be roughly divided into three classes, as demonstrated in Fig. 6–8. Plot I showed that for this kind of solutes, the surface tension of the solution gradually increase as the solution concentration increases. For aqueous solution, this type of solutes includes inorganic salt (e.g. NaCl), non-volatile acid (e.g. H_2SO_4) and alkali (e.g. KOH), organic compounds containing multiple —OH groups (e.g. sucrose, glycerin). Plots II showed that for some solutes, the surface tension

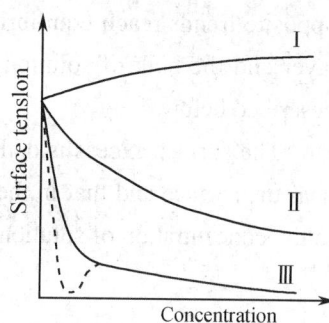

Fig. 6–8   Isothermal curve of surface tension

tends to decrease slowly with the increase in the concentration of solution. Most soluble organic compounds including short-chain fatty acids, alcohol and aldehyde belong to this class. Plot III showed that there are some solutes which can evidently reduce the surface tension even at very low concentration. After reaching a certain concentration, the surface tension of the solution does not change with the concentration of the solution any more. Compounds belonging to this class can be expressed as RX, where R represents an alkyl group containing 10 or more carbon atoms and X represents polar group such as —OH, —COOH, —CN, —CONH$_2$, —COOR′ or ionic group such —SO$_3^-$, —NH$_3^+$, —COO$^-$, etc. Sometime, part of the curve appears as dotted line in Fig. 6–8, which may be caused by the presence of certain impurities.

Experiments showed that the concentration of solute at the surface layer is different from that in the main body of a solution, which is named **adsorption phenomenon(吸附现象)**. If the concentration of solute at the surface layer is greater than that in the bulk solution, it is named positive adsorption. Otherwise, it is named negative adsorption.

The adsorption phenomena on the solution surface can be explained by requirement to minimize the Gibbs function of a system in a spontaneous process. According to equation (6–8), under the condition of constant temperature, pressure and surface area, the only way to decrease surface Gibbs function of the system is to reduce the surface tension.

If the addition of a solute reduces the surface tension, the increase in the surface concentration will make the system more stable. In this case, the solute tends to concentrate on the surface rather than stay in the solution, resulting in positive adsorption. Oppositely, if the addition a solute increases the surface tension, the increase in the surface concentration will make the system less stable. The solute prefers to stay in the solution rather on the surface, resulting in negative adsorption. Generally speaking, any solute that can increase the surface tension is named **surface inert agent(表面惰性物质)**. Any solute that can reduce the surface tension is named **surface active agent(表面活性物质)**. However, customarily only those agents that can reduce the surface tension significantly at very low concentration are named surface active agent or surfactant.

4.2 Gibbs adsorption isotherm formula and its application

Adsorption process leads to difference in the concentration of solute at the solution surface and that in the solution. Such concentration difference will in turn cause the solute to diffuse between the surface layer and the bulk of the solution, making the solution concentration uniform throughout. When the two opposite trends reach equilibrium, there will be definite concentration distribution between the surface layer and the bulk of solution, which can be quantitatively measured by **surface excess(表面过剩)** as described below.

The surface excess is defined as the difference between the amount per unit area of the solute at or near the surface and that in the bulk solution. At constant temperature, the relationship of surface excess to the concentration of solution and surface tension can be expressed as

$$\Gamma = -\frac{c}{RT}\left(\frac{d\sigma}{dc}\right)_T \tag{6–23}$$

where Γ is the surface excess of solute, c is the equilibrium concentration of the bulk solution, σ is the surface tension of the solution. The formula was firstly derived by Gibbs with thermaldynamic method, so it is named Gibbs adsorption isotherm formula.

The Gibbs adsorption isotherm formula indicates that at a given temperature, if the change rate of surface tension with concentration, $\frac{d\sigma}{dc} < 0$, then $\Gamma > 0$, that is, if the increase in the concentration of the solute reduces the surface tension, positive adsorption will take place at the surface layer. Otherwise, if the change rate of surface tension with concentration, $\frac{d\sigma}{dc} > 0$, then $\Gamma < 0$, that is, if the increase in the concentration of the solute increases the surface tension, negative adsorption will take place at the surface layer.

To calculate the surface excess with the Gibbs adsorption isotherm formula, it is necessary to determine the value of $\dfrac{d\sigma}{dc}$. If the functional relationship between σ and c is known, the derivative can be obtained directly by applying differentiation operation.

[Example 6-3] At 298.15K, the surface tension of butyric acid can be expressed as $\sigma = \sigma_0 + a\ln(1 + bc)$, where σ_0 is surface tension of pure water, c is the equilibrium concentration of butyric acid in the water, $a = 0.0131\text{N} \cdot \text{m}^{-1}$, $b = 19.62\text{dm}^3 \cdot \text{mol}^{-1}$.

(1) Try to calculate the value of Γ, when $c = 0.20\text{mol} \cdot \text{dm}^{-3}$

(2) If the concentration of butyric acid is large enough that $bc \geqslant 1$, how much is the saturation adsorption?

Soluton:

(1) $\sigma = \sigma_0 + a\ln(1 + bc)$

The derivative of the above formula is

$$\frac{d\sigma}{dc} = -\frac{abc}{1+bc}$$

Substituting the equation into Gibbs adsorption isotherm formula, yield

$$\Gamma = -\frac{c}{RT}\left(\frac{d\sigma}{dc}\right)_T = \frac{abc}{RT(1+bc)}$$
$$= \frac{0.0131\times19.62\times0.20}{8.314\times291.15\times(1+19.62\times0.20)} = 4.31\times10^{-6}\text{mol} \cdot \text{m}^{-2}$$

(2) If $bc \geqslant 1$, then $1+bc \approx bc$

$$\Gamma_\infty = \frac{abc}{RT(1+bc)} = \frac{a}{RT} = \frac{0.0131}{8.314\times291.5} = 5.411\times10^{-6}\text{mol} \cdot \text{m}^{-2}$$

Section 5　Surfactants

5.1　Classification of surfactants

Surfactant (表面活性剂) is a kind of substances that can significantly reduce the surface tension of a liquid when added to the liquid. Surfactants are **amphiphilic (双亲性)** molecules that have both **hydrophilic (亲水性)** groups and **lipophilic (亲脂性)** groups. For example, the sodium stearate (the main ingredient of soap), as an amphipathic surfactant, it contains a long hydrophobic(lipophilic) C17 alky chain and a hydrophilic carboxyl group. Usually, the symbol "○" is used to represent the hydrophilic head group and the symbol "□" is used to represent lipophilic tail. So the schematic diagram of a surfactant molecule looks like a match stick, as shown in Fig. 6-9.

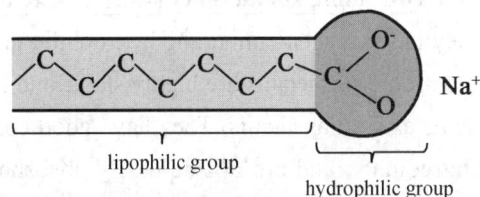

lipophilic group

hydrophilic group

Fig. 6-9　Schematic diagram of a surfactant molecule

PPT

微课

The lipophilic moieties are fairly similar among different surfactants, which can be liner, branched or aromatic hydrocarbon chains. They have a little influence on the property of surfactants. In contrast, the hydrophilic group has a huge effect on the property of surfactants. Based on whether the hydrophilic group can be ionized or not after being dissolved in water, surfactants are usually classified as ionic or nonionic ones.

5.1.1 Ionic surfactants

Ionic surfactant (离子型表面活性剂) is made up of molecules that have charged groups, which can be further classified as anionic, cationic or zwitterionic surfactants, according to the characteristic of the charged groups.

(1) Anionic surfactants   An **anionic surfactant** (阴离子型表面活性剂) carries an negatively charged hydrophilic group after being ionized in water, typically including carboxylate, sulfonate, sulfate, phosphate salt etc. Sodium stearate ($C_{17}H_{35}COONa$) and sodium lauryl sulphate ($C_{12}H_{25}SO_4 Na$) are the two representatives of anionic surfactants, which are widely used in soaps, shampoos and detergents.

(2) Cationic surfactants   An **cationic surfactants** (阳离子型表面活性剂) carries a positively charged hydrophilic group, which is mainly composed of ammonium salts. Since the primary, secondary and tertiary amine salts are almost not soluable in water, they are not suitable for use as surfactant. While the quaternary ammonium salts which is soluable in water, are most commonly used as surfactant, such as benzalkonium bromide, domiphen bromide etc. These surfactants pharmaceutically used as bactericide for they readily absorbed on the cell membrane. The advantage of cationic surfactants is that their antibacterial activity is affected by the pH value of the solution. However, it is worth noting that cationic surfactants should not be used in combination with anionic ones. Otherwise, they will combine with anionic surfactants and precipitate out, thus losing their surface activity.

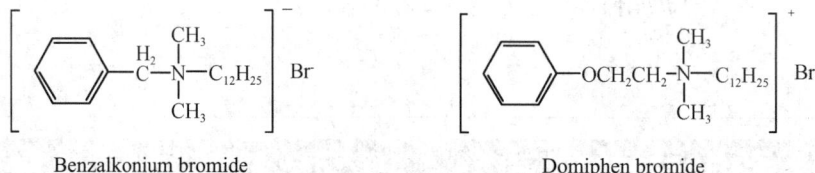

Benzalkonium bromide   Domiphen bromide

(3) Zwitterionic surfactants   For the **zwitterionic surfactants** (两性型表面活性剂), their hydrophilic part carries both positive charge and negative charge at the same time. The most commonly seen zwitterionic surfactants are betaines ($R—N^+(CH_3)_2—CH_2COO^-$) and amino acids ($R—NHCH_2—CH_2COOH$).

5.1.2 Non-ionic surfactants

Non-ionic surfactants (非离子型表面活性剂) could not be ionized when dissolved in water. But they have oxygen-containing hydrophilic group, which could form hydrogen bond with water molecules. Non-ionic surfactants are highly stable and less sensitive to water hardness, pH, additional inorganic salts, acids as well as alkalis. They have good compatibility with various ionic surfactants and pharmaceutical ingredients, and are not be easily absorbed onto the solid surface, so they are widely used in food, cosmetics and pharmacy industry.

The non-ionic surfactants, although not ionized in water, typically contain hydroxyl (—OH) or ether group (—O—) as their hydrophilic groups. For ionic surfactants, one single hydrophilic group is enough to make the molecule soluble in water. However, for non-ionic surfactants, the hydrophilicity of these two groups is comparably weak, so there should be at least several such groups in the chemical structure in order to make the whole surfactant molecule dissolvable in water.

According to the hydrophilic part, non-ionic surfactants are categorized into **polyoxyethylene type** (聚氧乙烯型) or **polyhydric alcohol type** (多羟基型). The polyoxyethylene type has high water solubility while the polyhydric alcohol type is less soluble in water. Due to the disparity of their physiochemical property, they are used for different purposes.

(1) Poly(oxyethylene) type non-ionic surfactants   The poly(oxyethylene) type non-ionic surfactants are synthesized by the addition reaction between the active hydrogen containing compounds with ethylene oxide. Usually, the hydrogen containing compounds are fatty alcohols (ROH), alkylphenols, fatty carboxy (RCOOH), fatty amine (RNH_2), fatty amide ($RCONH_2$), polyhydric alcohols, fatty acid esters, lipid, sorbitol and so on. These compounds are highly reactive and can easily react with poly(oxyethylene) to form the amphiphilic structure of the surfactants with molecular formula expressed as alkyl—$(CH_2CH_2O)_n$— poly(oxyethylene). To understand the chemical structure of this type of surfactants, please refers to chemical structure of Tween.

① Adducts of fatty alcohol and ethylene oxide

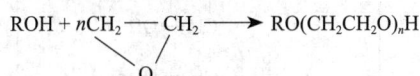

$$ROH + nCH_2\!\!-\!\!CH_2 \xrightarrow{\quad} RO(CH_2CH_2O)_nH$$
(with O bridging CH_2—CH_2)

The fatty alcohols can be lauryl alcohol, cetyl alcohol, oleyl alcohol and so on.

② Adducts of alkylphenols and ethylene oxide

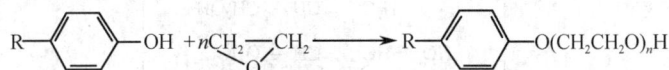

$$R\!-\!\!\!\bigcirc\!\!\!-\!OH + nCH_2\!\!-\!\!CH_2 \xrightarrow{\quad} R\!-\!\!\!\bigcirc\!\!\!-\!O(CH_2CH_2O)_nH$$

The most commonly used alkylphenols are nonylphenol and octylphenol.

③ Adducts of fatty acids and ethylene oxide

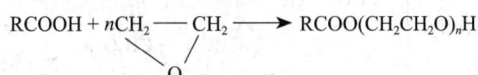

$$RCOOH + nCH_2\!\!-\!\!CH_2 \xrightarrow{\quad} RCOO(CH_2CH_2O)_nH$$

The fatty acids could be stearic acid, lauryl acid and oleyl acid.

④ Adducts of fatty amine and ethylene oxide

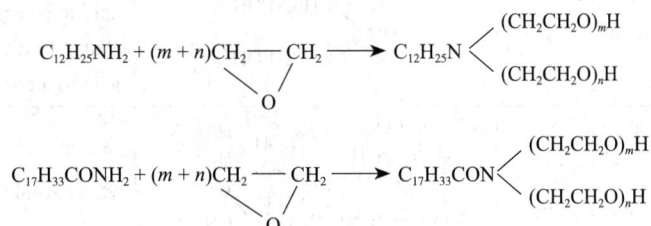

$$C_{12}H_{25}NH_2 + (m+n)CH_2\!\!-\!\!CH_2 \xrightarrow{\quad} C_{12}H_{25}N \!\!<^{(CH_2CH_2O)_mH}_{(CH_2CH_2O)_nH}$$

$$C_{17}H_{33}CONH_2 + (m+n)CH_2\!\!-\!\!CH_2 \xrightarrow{\quad} C_{17}H_{33}CON \!\!<^{(CH_2CH_2O)_mH}_{(CH_2CH_2O)_nH}$$

⑤ Adducts of polypropylene glycol and ethylene oxide

Addition reaction could happen between polypropylene glycol and ethylene oxide to form the polyoxypropylene chain. However, the steric hindrance of methyl groups prohibits the formation of hydrogen bonds, resulting in the low water solubility of the products. So the polyoxypropylene chain can be used as the hydrophobic part of a surfactant.

(2) Polyol type nonionic surfactants   The polyol type nonionic surfactants are synthesized via the reaction between poly-hydroxyl compounds with fatty acid. The commonly used poly-hydroxyl compounds are listed in Table 6-4, including polyhydric alcohols, amino alcohol and hydroxyl rich sugars.

Table 6-4   Hydrophilic groups of the poly-hydroxyl type non-ionic surfactants

Type	Poly-hydroxyl compounds	Chemical formula	Water solubility after forming ester or amide with fatty acids
Polyhydric alcohols	Glycerol with 3 hydroxyl groups	CH_2-OH — $CH-OH$ — CH_2-OH	Water insoluble with self-emulsifying effect
	Pentaerythritol with 4 hydroxyl groups	$HOH_2C-\overset{\overset{CH_2OH}{\mid}}{\underset{\underset{CH_2OH}{\mid}}{C}}-CH_2OH$	Water insoluble with self-emulsifying effect
	Sorbitol[①] with 6 hydroxyl groups	CH_2OH — $CH-OH$ — $HO-CH$ — $CH-OH$ — $CH-OH$ — CH_2OH	Water insoluble with self-emulsifying effect
	Sorbitan with 4 hydroxyl groups	$HO-HC-CH-OH$ / $H_2C\ \ CHCH-CH_2OH$ / $O\ \ \ OH$	Water insoluble with self-emulsifying effect
Amino alcohols	Monoethanolamine Diethanolamine	$H_2NCH_2CH_2OH$ — $HN\big\langle\ ^{CH_2CH_2OH}_{CH_2CH_2OH}$	Water insoluble Water soluble when molar ratio of acid to alcohol is 1 : 2[②] Water insoluble when molar ratio of acid to alcohol is 1 : 1[②]
Sugars	Sucrose With 6 hydroxyl groups	(sucrose ring structure)	Water soluble or insoluble

① Sugars could be L-isomers or D-isomers, the commercial available sorbitol is obtained via reduction of L-glucose, hence sobitols are L-isomers.

② Molar ratio of acid to alcohol is 1 : 2.

$$C_{11}H_{23}CON \begin{cases} CH_2CH_2OH \\ CH_2CH_2OH \end{cases} \qquad HN \begin{cases} CH_2CH_2OH \\ CH_2CH_2OH \end{cases}$$

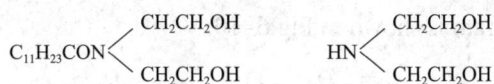

Molar ratio of acid to alcohol is 1 : 1

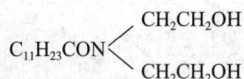

$$C_{11}H_{23}CON \begin{cases} CH_2CH_2OH \\ CH_2CH_2OH \end{cases}$$

Polyhydric alcohols like glycerol and pentaerythritol could be esterified with fatty acids or palmitic acids. These kinds of nonionic surfactants are harmless to human body, and can be applied as emulsifiers or softener of fiber in the food or cosmetics industries.

Sugar like sucrose which has 8 hydroxyl groups makes it an ideal hydrophilic group. Since sucrose and fatty acids (the lipophilic group) come from natural sources, non-ionic surfactants derived from sucrose esterified with fatty acids are normally safe, non-toxic, non-irritating, environmental friendly and biodegradable. Thereby, they have wide application in chemical, food and pharmaceutical industries.

Sorbitol is a kind of hexahydric alcohol made by hydrogenation of glucose and it has 6 hydroxyl groups. Under certain circumstances, it may dehydrate from its structure and becomes mono-anhydrides (sorbitan) or di-anhydrides. Polysorbate-type nonionic surfactants, which are esters formed by sorbitan with fatty acids are commercially supplied as Spans. Based on the type of fatty acids, there are different kinds of Spans as listed in Table 6–5.

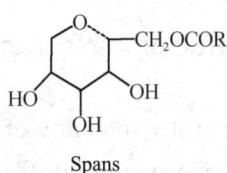

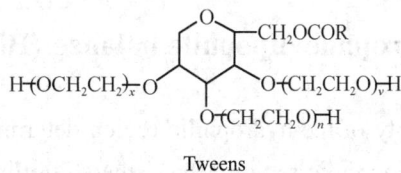

Spans　　　　　　　　　　　Tweens

Table 6–5　Esters of sorbitan or ethoxylated sorbitan with different acids

	Lauric acid (R=C$_{11}$H$_{23}$)	Pamitic acid (R=C$_{15}$H$_{31}$)	Stearic acid (R=C$_{17}$H$_{35}$)	Oleic acid (R=C$_{17}$H$_{33}$)
Sorbitan	Span 20	Span 40	Span 60	Span 80
Ethoxylated sorbitan	Tween 20	Tween 40	Tween 60	Tween 80

Span(司盘) can be used as emulsifiers. Because of being generally insoluble in water, Span is rarely used alone, but usually used in combination with other water soluble surfactants in order to obtain better emulsifying effect.

Tween(吐温) is another type of non-ionic surfactants which is obtained by linking the hydrophilic poly(oxyethylene) (HO(CH$_2$CH$_2$O)$_n$H) with the hydroxyl group on a Span by ether bond. It can also be synthesized by the addition of ethylene oxides to Span. Just like Spans, there are also different types of Tweens.

Since Tween contains poly(oxyethylene) in its structure, it is more hydrophilic compared to Span. And the hydrophilicity will be further enhanced with increasing amount of poly(oxyethylene) in its structure. Moreover, the oxygen contained in poly(oxyethylene) could also improve the solubility of Tween by forming hydrogen bond with the water molecules. Once Tween is dissolved in water, the conformation of the hydrophilic group will change from jag-like to curve-like where the hydrophobic hydrocarbon (—CH$_2$—) turns inwards and the hydrophilic oxygen turns outwards to interact with water molecules. The schematic diagram is shown in Fig.6-10.

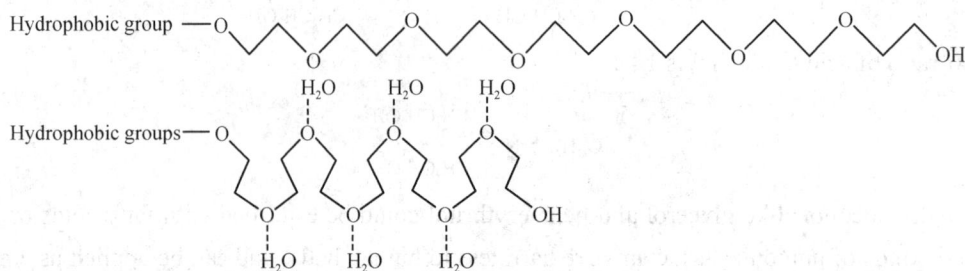

Fig. 6-10   The two possible conformations of Tween: jag-like(top);curve-like(bottom)

As the temperature rises, the molecules will move more violently, which may break the hydrogen bonds between Tweens and water molecules. Therefore, the water solubility of nonionic surfactants decreases with increasing temperature. As a result, the surfactants will precipitate out and the transparent solution will turn cloudy. And when this phenomenon appears, the corresponding temperature is called "cloud point". For example, the cloud point for Tween 80 is 93℃, which means that Tween 80 will no longer be soluble in water when the temperature rises above 93℃. Generally, this phenomenon is reversible. When the temperature decreases, the cloudy solution will become clear again. Cloud points are characteristic for all the poly(oxyethylene) containing non-ionic surfactants.

5.2   The hydrophile-lipophile balance (HLB) value of surfactants

The hydrophilicity of the hydrophilic region determines the water solubility of surfactants, and the lipophilicity of the lipophilic region affects the solubility of surfactants in oil. If the hydrophilicity is too strong, the whole surfactant molecule will enter the water phase. Otherwise, the surfactant molecule will distribute mainly in the oil phase. The balance between hydrophilic group and lipophilic group has a significant influence on the property of surfactants. Therefore, Griffin proposed to use the **hydrophile-lipophile balance value (HLB, 亲水-亲油平衡值)** to reflect the hydrophilicity of surfactants. Surfactants with higher HLB values are considered to be more hydrophilic, while those with lower HLB values tend to be more lipophilic.

The lipophilicity of surfactants is related with the chemical structure of the lipophilic group. Usually the lipophilicity becomes stronger with increasing length or molecular mass of the alky chains. For example, surfactants containing octadecyl chains in the lipophilic group are less water soluble compared to those containing dodecyl chains. Similarly, the larger molecular mass of the hydrophilic groups, the more hydrophilic the non-ionic surfactants will be. The HLB value of nonionic surfactants could be calculated using the equation as below

$$\text{HLB of non-ionic surfactants} = \frac{\text{molecular mass of the hydrophilic group}}{\text{molecular mass of the hydrophobic group}} \times 20 \tag{6-24}$$

Paraffin as a completely lipophilic molecule has an HLB value of 0. And polyethylene glycol as a completely hydrophilic molecule has an HLB value of 20. Usually, the HLB value of non-ionic surfactants is within the range of 0~20.

For most fatty acid esters of polyol, the HLB value is calculated using following equation.

$$HLB = 20\left(1-\frac{S}{A}\right) \tag{6-25}$$

where S is the saponification number, the number of milligrams of potassium hydroxide needed to saponify the esters contained in 1g of the substance, and A is the acid number, usually the weight of potassium hydroxide needed in milligrams to neutralize the free fatty acids present in 1g of oil.

For instance, glyceryl monostearate has an S value of 161 and A value of 198. Therefore $HLB = 20\left(1-\frac{161}{198}\right) = 3.74$.

The above equation can not apply to the anionic or cationic surfactants. The reason is that for ionic surfactants, the hydrophilicity of the hydrophilic groups per unit mass is much stronger than that of the non-ionic surfactants. Alternatively, the HLB value for the ionic surfactants is determined based on the HLB value of chemical groups, which is calculated as the sum of the HLB values of all the chemical groups contained in the structure plus 7. The HLB values of various chemical groups are listed in Table 6-6.

Table 6-6　The HLB values of various functional groups

Hydrophilic chemical group	HLB	Lipophilic chemical group	HLB
— SO₄Na	38.7		
— COOK	21.1	— CH —	
— COONa	19.1	— CH₂ —	
Sulfonate salt	11.0	— CH₃	−0.475
— N (tertiary amine R₃N)	9.4	— CH =	
Ester (sorbitan ring)	6.8		
Ester (free)	2.4		
— COOH	2.1		
— OH (free)	1.9	— (CH₂CH₂CH₂O) —	−0.15
— O —	1.3		
— OH (sorbitan ring)	0.5		

To obtain the HLB value of sodium dodecyl sulfate, the calculation based on the above method is as follows: 38.7 + 12 × (−0.475) + 7 = 40.0.

The advantage of this method is that it takes into account of the effect of different chemical groups, thus making the HLB value additive.

If two surfactants with different HLB values are mixed with each other, the HLB value of the mixture can be calculated as follows.

$$HLB = \frac{[HLB]_A \times m_A + [HLB]_B \times m_B}{m_A + m_B} \tag{6-26}$$

where $[HLB]_A$ and $[HLB]_B$ are the HLB value of surfactant A and surfactant B, m_A and m_B are the mass of surfactant A and surfactant B respectively.

For instance, if there is a mixture contains 40% of Span 20 (HLB value=8.6) and 60% of Tween 80 (HLB value=14.9), the HLB value of the mixture =8.6 × 0.4+14.9 × 0.6=12.3. But this method does not apply to all the surfactants, and the obtained result should be confirmed by experiments. As shown in Table 6-7 and Table 6-8, the HLB values of surfactants could predict their water solubility and potential applications.

Table 6-7 Relationship between HLB value of surfactants and water dispersity

HLB	Water dispersity
1 to 3	Non-dispersible
3 to 6	Not well dispersed
6 to 8	Unstable and milky-like dispersion
8 to 10	Stable milky-like dispersion
10 to 13	Translucent to transparent dispersion
>13	Transparent dispersion

Table 6-8 Applications of surfactants with different HLB values

HLB	Application	Examples
1 to 3	Anti-foaming agent	Paraffin (0), Oleic acid (1), Span 65 (2.1)
3 to 6	W/O (water in oil) emulsifier	Span 80 (4.7), Span 40 (6.7), Span 20 (8.6), Acacia (8.0)
7 to 9	Wetting and spreading agent	Acacia (8.0), Gelatin (9.8)
8 to 18	O/W (oil in water) emulsifier	Acacia (8.0), Gelatin (9.8), Tween 80 (15), Tween 20 (16.7)
13 to 15	Detergent	Triethanolamine oleate (12)
15 to 18	Solubilizer	Tween 20 (16.7), Sodium oleate (18), Potassium oleate (20)

5.3 Diverse applications of surfactants

The surface tension of a solution could be significantly lowered by the ordered arrangement of surfactant at the surface. For example, when surfactants are dissolved in water, they orientate at the surface with the hydrophobic regions exposed outside the aqueous environment to avoid contact with water. And the reduction in surface tension is because that some water molecules at the interface are replaced by the surfactant molecules and the attractive forces between surfactant molecules are less than that between water molecules. Therefore, the contraction force, nature of surface tension is reduced.

Surfactants have multiple functions and are widely used in industrial manufacture, scientific research and daily lives. Generally, surfactants can be used as solubilizers, emulsifiers or demulsifiers, wetting and dispersing agents, foaming or anti-foaming agents and grinding-aid agents. They could also be used for rust protection, sterilization, and elimination of static electricity. This section mainly focuses on their application in the pharmaceutical fields.

5.3.1 Solubilizing effect of surfactants

(1) **Formation of micelles (胶束)** When surfactants are dissolved in water, they are initially absorbed on the surface forming a monolayer to decrease the surface tension or the surface free energy. With the increasing addition of surfactants, they begin to enter the aqueous phase by forming aggregates which is called micelles. The lowest concentration of surfactants needed in a bulk solution to form micelles is called critical micelle **concentration (CMC, 临界胶束浓度)**. In the structure of micelles, the hydrophilic groups form an outer shell and the lipophilic groups assemble into a hydrophobic core, as shown in Fig. 6-11. The formation of micelles can reduce the contact area of the lipophilic groups with water solution, thereby reducing the surface free energy of the solution and stabilizing the system.

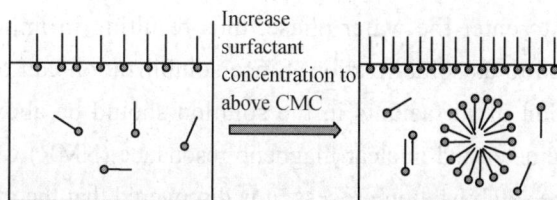

Fig. 6–11　Formation of micelles

Most micelles are around several nanometers in size and contain around 60 to 100 surfactant molecules. Usually, the CMC is a narrow range of concentration below which micelles cannot form, but there are also rare cases where several (less than ten) surfactant molecules firstly form assemblies, also called tiny micelles. With increasing concentration of surfactants, the size of these tiny micelles gradually increases, and upon reaching the CMC, spherical micelles will be formed. And upon further addition of surfactants, the spherical micelles will transform to layered micelles with the hydrophilic groups facing outwards and the lipophilic groups hided inside according to the result given by X-ray diffraction. And if the concentration continues to increase, the micelle will become rod-shaped based on the result of light scattering. Fig. 6–12 shows the micelles of various shapes.

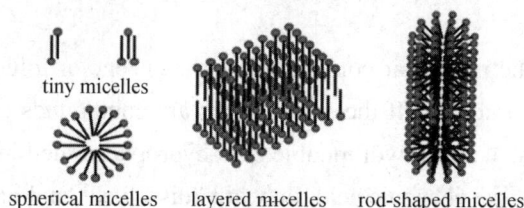

Fig. 6–12　various shapes of micelles

The CMC value varies depending on the type of surfactants and environmental conditions, such as temperature, pressure and the presence of other surfacants. For surfactants with long and liner hydrocarbon chains, since the attractive force between molecules is strong, they are more likely to form micelles and thereby have lower CMC value. By contrast, for surfactants with short and branched hydrocarbon chains, micelles cannot be easily formed due to steric hindrance and weak intermolecular attractive force, and thereby have a high CMC value. Usually, the CMC value for most surfactants is around 0.001 to 0.02mol $\cdot$ L^{-1}, or 0.02% to 0.4% in mass ratio. For instance, the CMC value of sodium dodecyl sulfonate in water at 298K is 1.2×10^{-3}mol $\cdot$ L^{-1} measured by a conductivity meter.

Around the CMC, the distribution of surfactant molecules and the number of particulate matters in the bulk solution change greatly, thereby significantly affecting the physical properties of the solution, including surface tension, solubility, osmotic pressure, conductivity and detergency as shown in Fig. 6–13.

(2) Solubilization　For pharmaceutical ingredients with low water solubility, once they are added into the micelle containing solution, the molecules could diffuse into the micelles and distribute within the core or the shell of the micelle. With the aid of micelles, those water insoluble

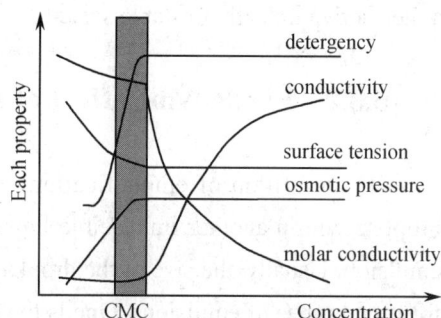

Fig. 6–13　Effects of surfactant concentration on the properties of the solution

molecules are more likely to enter the water phase, thus resulting in improved solubility in water. This phenomenon is referred to as solubilization. Since solubilization can only occur in the presence of micelles, the concentration of surfactants in the solution should be above the CMC value. X-ray diffraction, UV spectrophotometer and nuclear magnetic resonance (NMR) were used to investigate the change of micelles during the solubilization process, it is discovered that the mechanism of solubilization differs based on the type of surfactants and solubilisate. Take Tween, a nonionic surfactant, as an example, the solubilization process of various solubilisate are shown in Fig. 6–14.

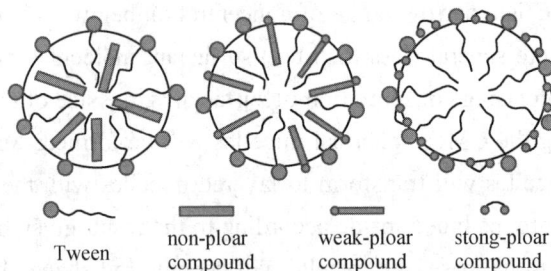

Tween   non-ploar compound   weak-ploar compound   stong-ploar compound

**Fig. 6–14 Solubilization mechanism of compounds
with different polarity**

    If the solubilisates are the non-polar compounds, like benzene or toluene, they are "dissolved" in the hydrophobic cores of the micelles. If the solubilisates are compounds containing polar groups, like salicylic acid, they are orientated at the hydrophobic core-hydrophilic shell interface. For the solubilisates with strong polarity, like p-hydroxybenzoic acid, they are "dissolved" and dispersed in the palisade layer (the hydrophilic shell, like poly-oxyethylene). Therefore, for the water insoluble substance, the first step of the solubilization process is being absorbed or "dissolved" in the micelle, then being transported to water phase together with micelles. If judged by appearance, the original aggregates of the water insoluble substance will gradually disappear and turn into a clear colloidal system, just like they are "dissolved".

    It should be noted that solubilization is different from dissolution. Dissolution means the solute is dispersed in the solution as molecules or ions, the concentration of the solute will affect the colligative properties of the solution. However, in the case of solubilization, many molecules of the solubilisates enter into micelles instead of the bulk solution. Therefore, they have little effect on the colligative properties of the solution which is in fact determined by the original micelle concentration.

    Also, solubilization is different from emulsification. Solubilization is a process of reduction in free energy, so a stable colloidal system is obtained eventually. While emulsions prepared by emulsification is a thermodynamically unstable system.

5.3.2 Emulsifying effect of surfactants

    (1) Definition of emulsification   The process of making one kind of liquid dispersed as small droplets within another immiscible liquid is called emulsification and the obtained dispersing system is emulsion. Usually, the size of the droplet is within the range from 1 to 50μm. Two immiscible liquids can form two types of emulsions. One is the oil-in-water emulsions, wherein oil (organic solvents immiscible with water) is dispersed in water, which is denoted as O/W. The other is water-in-oil emulsions, wherein water is dispersed in oil, which is denoted as W/O.

Generally, emulsions could be produced by certain mechanical methods, like shaking, stirring, homogenizing and exposure to ultra-sonication. Regardless of the production method, the obtained emulsion is highly dispersed and has high surface free energy due to large surface area. Therefore, emulsions are considered to be thermodynamically unstable and surfactants are needed in order to obtain emulsion with good stability.

To prepare the emulsion, firstly, the surfactants are put into the dispersing medium, then the dispersed phase is gradually add into the medium under vigorous stirring, finally emulsions could thereby be formed.

(2) Types of emulsion   To identify the type of emulsions, methods listed below could be used.

① Dilution

Adding a few drops of an emulsion into the water, if there is no phase separation, it means that the emulsion could be diluted with water, thus it is O/W type of emulsions. By contrast, if there is phase separation, it means that the emulsion could not be diluted with water, thus it is W/O type of emusion.

② Staining

Adding trace amount of hydrophilic dye like potassium permanganate into the emulsion, then taking some samples under the microscope for observation, if the droplet is stained while the dispersing medium is not, it means that this is O/W type of emulsions. If lipophilic dyes like Sudan Ⅲ is added to the emulsion and only droplets are found being stained, then it is W/O type of emulsions.

③ Conductivity measurement

Inserting two electrodes into the emulsion and measuring the conductivity. Usually emulsions with high conductivity are O/W type of emulsions, while emulsions with low conductivity are W/O type of emulsions.

Since emulsions are highly unstable systems, emulsifying agents or emulsifiers are required to prepare emulsion with good stability. Surfactants which could decrease the surface free energy are most commonly seen emulsifiers. There are two types of emulsifier: hydrophilic emulsifier and hydrophobic emulsifier. The hydrophilic emulsifiers could be used to prepare the O/W type of emulsions. Examples include water soluble monovalent metal soaps (sodium, potassium and lithium soaps), chemically synthesized soaps ($ROSO_3Na$ and RSO_3Na), egg yolk, casein, starch, silica gel, natural gums, magnesium carbonate and clay. The lipophilic emulsifiers could be used to prepare the W/O type of emulsions. Examples include divalent and trivalent metal soaps (calcium and magnesium), esters of fatty acids, fatty alcohol, graphite, lanolin and rosin.

According to the Bancroft rule, emulsifiers tend to promote dispersion of the phase in which they do not dissolve very well. And the reason for this is that at the interface between two distinct liquid phases, there are two corresponding surface tensions, σ_{oil} and σ_{water}. The interface film will bend towards the side with higher surface tension in order to reduce the surface area of that phase. As a consequence, the liquid phase with higher surface tension will be wrapped up and thus becoming the dispersed droplets. Since the hydrophilic emulsifiers could greatly reduce σ_{water}, making it lower than σ_{oil}, the interface film will therefore bend towards the oil phase. Consequently, the oil phase will become droplets wrapped up by water and form the O/W type of emulsion. In contrast, the lipophilic emulsifiers could significantly lower σ_{oil}, making it lower than σ_{water}. So in this case, the water phase will be dispersed in oil and the W/O type of emulsions could be obtained, as shown in Fig. 6–15.

(3) How can emulsifiers make the emulsion stable?

① Reduction of surface tension

Most of the emulsifiers are surfactants. Surfactants could be absorbed on the interface and decrease the interfacial tension between two phases, thereby, keeping the dispersed droplets from coalescing and improving the stability of the emulsion. But reducing the surface tension alone is not enough to maintain long term stability of the emulsion, and it cannot explain that why some non-surfactant materials, like solid particles also have stabilizing effect on the emulsions.

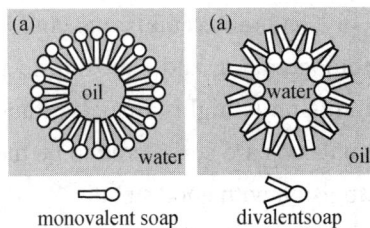

Fig. 6–15　Two types of emulsions:
A. O/W; B.W/O

② Formation of interfacial films

The interfacial films formed by emulsifiers could provide physical barriers to prevent the coalescence of dispersed droplets and maintain the stability of emulsion. And this is considered to be the most important stabilizing mechanism for the emulsifiers. There are three types of protective films:

a. Monolayer interfacial film

When surfactants are absorbed at the surface of droplets, they will orientate at the interface and form a monolayer to prevent the coalescence of droplets. If sufficient surfactants are added, the molecular arrangement will be tight and a strong film could be formed.

b. Multilayer interfacial film

If hydrophilic polymers are used as emulsifiers, they will be absorbed as multiple layers at the surface of the droplets to keep them stably dispersed. For example, acacia could act as emulsifiers and form multilayer interfacial film around the droplets. Such polymers could also increase the viscosity of the dispersing medium which further improves the stability of emulsion.

c. Interfacial film composed by solid particle

As non-surfactant substance, solid particles could also be absorbed at the oil-water interface and form protective films to make the droplets stably dispersed, The stabilizing effect depends on the mechanical strength of the film. If the solid particles are hydrophilic, they could be used to stabilize the O/W type emulsion. For solid particles that are lipophilic, they could be used as emulsifiers for the W/O type of emulsion.

③ Electrostatic repulsion

Emulsifiers could be positively or negatively charged in the emulsion. When the dispersed droplets are coated with these charged emulsifiers, there will be electrostatic repulsion between the droplets, which helps to keep them separated. For example, if soaps (like sodium soap RCOONa) are used as emulsifiers to prepare O/W type of emulsion, the hydrophilic group will be ionized and become $RCOO^-$, and the droplets will carry negative charges. The repulsive forces between two droplets could prevent them from coalescing.

There are also cases that the droplets in W/O type of emulsions could also become charged due to the friction between the droplets and dispersing medium. It is similar with the situation in which glass carries positive charges after being rubbed with furs. And the type of charges that the droplets would carry can be judged by the **Coehn principle(柯恩规则)**. When one substance is dispersed into another, the one with higher dielectric constant values tends to carry positive charge and the one with lower dielectric constant values usually carries negative charges. Since water has a dielectric constant value higher than that of most organic solvents, in the case of O/W type of emulsion, the oil droplets would carry negative charges.

While, for the W/O type of emulsion, the water droplets will be positively charged instead. Therefore, when droplets carrying same charges come close to each other, the electrostatic repulsion will keep them apart.

The volume fraction of two phases also plays a key role in determining the type of emulsion. For spheres of the same radius, there are either hexagonal or cubic ways for closest packing. No matter which way is chosen, the volume ratio of spheres accounts for 74.2% of the total volume, and the porosity has a volume ratio of 25.98%. If the volume ratio of the dispersed phase exceeds 74%, the emulsions may collapse and even undergoes phase inversion. When the volume fraction of the one phase is between 0.26 and 0.74, either O/W type or W/O type of emulsion could be formed. And if the volume fraction of one phase is below 0.26 or exceeds 0.74, only one type of emulsion could be obtained. This theory is based experimental results, but it does not apply to all the cases of phase inversion.

(4) Demulsification　In the manufacturing process of the pharmaceutical products, the formation of emulsions sometimes causes operational difficulties. Therefore, **demulsification(破乳)** is required in this case. Demulsification refers to the destruction of the protective effect of emulsifiers and separation of the emulsion into separated water phase and oil phase. There are several ways that can be used to destabilize an emulsion. The physical ways include increasing temperature or pressure, centrifugation and applying electrical fields to promote coalescence. And the chemical ways involves the addition of demulsifiers which could migrate to the interface and neutralize the effect of emulsifiers.

5.3.3　Wetting and dewetting

The wettability of solid surface means its ability to be wetted by liquids. Usually, wettability alteration is needed for various purposes. Sometimes we need to change the surface from wettable to non-wettable, and sometimes otherwise. With the aid of surfactants, we can adjust the contact angle between the liquid and solid according to the practical needs.

The wetting agents could facilitate the spreading of liquids on the solid surfaces by reducing the surface tension. Oppositely, the dewetting agents prevent the spreading of liquids on solid surfaces. Both of them are widely applied in fields such as pharmaceutics, oil extraction, ore flotation, welding, plating and transportation. For example, the inner glass wall of ampoules and syringes are purposely coated with dewetting agents to make them water unwettable, so that all the liquids could be taken out completely. Otherwise, there will be residues left in the container, causing inaccuracy in the given dosage, also a waste of pharmaceutical ingredients. In the preparation of topically used ointment, surfactants are used as wetting agents to improve the wettablity of the skin and so that the ointment could be evenly applied to the skin. Also, the surfactants here could also prevent the clothes from being contaminated and promote removal of the ointment after use.

Similarly, by turning the inner wall of the heat exchanger hydrophobic, the flow resistance of water could also be reduced and thermal efficiency could be improved. When it comes to welding, plating and printing, wetting agents are frequently added to the paints to make sure the well spreading and firm adherence of paints on the interface.

For insects like mosquitoes, hairs on their legs are cannot be wetted by water, therefore, there will be a contact angle greater than $90°$ between their legs and water. And the existence of surface tension makes them able to stand and glide, even lay their eggs on the water. And it is not difficult to eliminate these creatures, simply by spraying the soapy water with concentration from 0.1% to 0.25% (by mass ratio) to the surface, they will be devastated. The reason is that the soaps could decrease the surface tension and the contact angle making their legs wetted by water, as a consequence, they can no longer stand on the water surface.

5.3.4 Foaming and defoaming

(1) Foaming agents   Foams are formed when gas is dispersed in liquids. Since these systems are thermodynamically unstable, foaming agents such as saponins, proteins, surfactants and solid powders e.g. graphite should be added in order to maintain the stability of foams. After being absorbed at the interface, the foaming agents could reduce the surface tension and form a film with considerable strength preventing the foams from rupture due to mechanical collision. Moreover, to make the foams stable, liquids should have proper viscosity so that the evaporation could be reduced，because evaporation could cause the thinning of liquid film and eventually leads to the rupture of foams. Usually, a little amount of addictives such as glycerin help to increase the viscosity of the liquids. Foaming agents with larger molecular weight have stronger intermolecular attraction force, so they could form films with higher mechanical strength and stabilize the foams more efficiently. The stabilizing mechanism of solid powders for the foams is similar to that of the emulsion.

(2) Anti-foaming agents   In pharmaceutical production process such as fermentation and extraction of herbal medicine, defoaming is much more important than foaming. The reason is that the formation of foams may bring about serious problems in the industrial process. For instance，foams can cause defects on surface coating, overflow of liquids and non-efficient filling of a container. Therefore, anti-foaming agents are usually added to eliminate the foams. There are mainly three types of anti-foaming agents.

① Oil based anti-foaming agents

The oil could be vegetable oil, mineral oil, or any other oil that is insoluble in the foaming medium and cannot spread on the surface of foaming medium. Usually, oils are less effective in preventing the formation of foams, but given their low toxicity, they are still widely used.

② Alcohols, esters and ethers

Alcohols, esters and ethers containing hydrocarbon chains with at least 5 to 8 carbon atoms such as octanol and tributyl phosphate could be used as defoaming agents. Since they are also surface active, they could replace the original foaming agents at the interface. But due to comparably short hydrocarbon chains, they cannot form a strong film and foams will rupture consequently. They are the best at quickly breaking the foams on small scale.

③ EO/PO based anti-foaming agents

This type of anti-foaming agents includes polyoxypropylene-polyoxyethylene copolymers (Pluronic L61 or L81). Their chemical structure may be expressed as below.

$$H-(OC_3H_6)_m-(OC_2H_4)_n-(OC_3H_6)_m-(OC_2H_4)_m-(OC_3H_6)_n-H$$

The hydrophilic polyoxyethylene regions and the hydrophobic polyoxypropylene regions appear repeatedly in the structure. Pluronics with PO : EO ratio between 4 : 1 and 9 : 1 are widely used as antifoams.

5.3.5 Grinding aid

During the grinding process of solids, if surfactants as one type of grinding aids are added, the grinding will be more thorough and more efficient. If no grinding aids are involved, when the substance is grinded into fine particles with size less than tens of microns, the surface area will increase significantly. Consequently, the system will become thermodynamically unstable due to tremendous Gibbs free energy. Generally, systems have a natural tendency to decrease the Gibbs free energy. Without the presence of surfactants, particles tend to reduce their surface area or Gibbs free energy by aggregation into larger particles. Therefore, in order to improve the grinding efficiency and obtain stably dispersed particles with small size, it is necessary to add some grinding aids. In the grinding process, surfactants are widely used as grinding aids. They could orderly orientate at the particle surface and reduce the surface tension of solid particles, thereby decreasing the tendency of aggregation. Surfactants are also able to penetrate deep into the crevices of the particles, just like wedges being inserted into the cracks, which further helps to cleave the particles. As is shown in Fig. 6–16a, with the aid of surfactants, the cracks on the particles will expand and tend to split into smaller particles under external forces. And the additional surfactants will be readily absorbed onto those newly formed surfaces to prevent the cracks from healing and avoid cohesion between particles. Moreover, the surfactants arrange orderly at the particle surface with the hydrophobic hydrocarbon chains facing outwards, as shown in Fig. 6–16b, which makes the particles less likely to contact with each other, and easy to roll with the resulting smooth surface. All these factors contribute to the improvement of grinding efficiency.

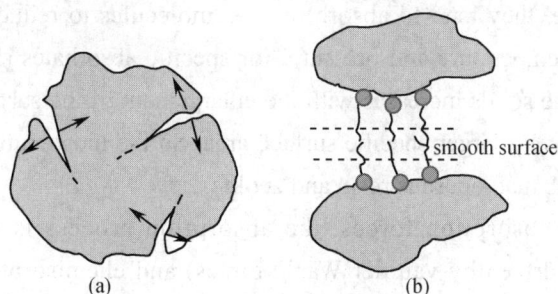

(a) (b)

smooth surface

Fig. 6–16　Grinding aid of surfactant

5.3.6　Suspending effect

Suspension (混悬剂) is a mixture of insoluble solid particles (diameter>100nm) dispersed in certain aqueous medium. Just like emulsion, suspension is also thermodynamically unstable, and the particles tend to aggregate and sediment which is driven by the reduction in Gibbs free energy. Stabilizers such as surfactants and polymers should be added to maintain the stability of suspension. When stabilizers such as proteins, acacia or starch are added, these macromolecules will be absorbed onto the particle surface and form a hydration layer which prevents the particles from aggregation. While, when surfactants are used as stabilizers, they could lower the surface tension and the Gibbs free energy are reduced by absorption onto the interface, thereby reducing the tendency of aggregation and making particles well suspended. For sulfa containing drugs and sulfur powders, these substances are hydrophobic with contact angle larger than $90°$, and cannot be wetted by water. When being prepared into suspension, particles made of hydrophobic substance cannot be well dispersed and easily aggregate in water. If surfactants are added to the suspension, surfactants will be orientated on the particle surface with lipophilic groups contacting the hydrophobic surface and hydrophilic groups facing towards the water. As a result, the particle surface is turned from hydrophobic to hydrophilic, thereby improving the stability of the suspension.

Section 6　Absorption at the Solid-Gas Interface

Absorption (吸附) is the adherence of gas molecules on solid surfaces. The gas being absorbed is referred to as **absorbate** (吸附质), and the solids here are denoted as **absorbents** (吸附剂). If charcoal is added to a container filled with bromine vapor, the red bromine vapor with red color will gradually disappears as it is absorbed by charcoal.

Absorption of solids is also a consequence of reduction in surface free energy. Due to the imbalanced attractive forces existing on the surface molecules, solids especially those with porosity possess high surface free energy. Since solids are immobile, they cannot reduce the free energy by decreasing the surface area. Therefore, they tend to absorb the gas molecules to reduce the surface free energy. Apparently, under certain temperature and pressure, for specific absorbates and absorbents, the amount of gas being absorbed by the solids increases with the enlargement of the surface area of the absorbents. An ideal absorbent must have a larger specific surface area. So the most commonly seen absorbents are activated charcoal, silica gel, macroporous resin and zeolites.

Base on the type of absorption forces, the absorption process is generally classified into physisorption (absorption driven by van der Waals forces) and chemisorption (absorption driven by covalent bonding).

6.1　Physisorption and chemisorption

Physisorption (物理吸附) is driven by the **Van der Waals forces** (范德华力) which are non-specific and relatively weak. Gases that can be liquefied easily are more likely to be absorbed, since the absorption process is just like the liquefaction of gases on solids. The physisorption process is exothermic, and the heat given out in this process is called enthalpy of adsorption, denoted as ΔH_{ads}. The ΔH_{ads} of a physisorption is relatively low, usually within the range of 20 to 40kJ · mol^{-1}, similar with the heat of condensation. In the physisorption process, gas molecules could be absorbed on to the solid surface as monolayer and/or multiple layers. Since the gas molecules are loosely bound to the solid surface, they are easily desorbed from the surface. Either absorption or desorption happens quickly and equilibrium between them could be rapidly established. And physisorption usually take places under low temperature condition.

In the **chemisorption** (化学吸附) process, there are chemical reactions going on between the solids and the absorbates, including electron transfer, atomic rearrangement, breaking or formation of covalent bond. Chemisorption is highly selective, and can only occur between certain solids and absorptive species. For instance, hydrogen could be chemically absorbed on the surface of tungsten or nickel, but cannot be absorbed on copper or aluminum. The heat given out for chemisorption is much greater than that for physisorption. The ΔH_{ads} of chemisorption is in the range of 40 to 400kJ · mol^{-1}, similar to the heat released during a chemical reaction. Since chemical bond formation is involved between the absorbates and solids, the absorptive gases are usually absorbed on the surface in the form of monolayer and cannot be desorbed easily due to the bond strength. Chemisorption is difficult to reverse and needs a long time to reach equilibrium. In contrast with the physisorption, chemisorption usually occurs under relatively high temperature condition.

Though physisorption and chemisorptions differs greatly, it does not mean they are incompatible with each other, they could coexist under certain conditions. For example, oxygen could be absorbed on tungsten as both atoms and molecules, some oxygen molecules could even be further absorbed on the pre-absorbed oxygen atoms to form multiple-layered structure.

6.2   Soild-Gas surface absorption isotherms

To investigate the absorption process, the amount of the gas being absorbed should be quantified. The amount of gas being absorbed (denoted as Γ) is defined as the moles (mol) or volumes (STP) of gas being absorbed by solids per unit mass. If solids with m kg absorbs x moles or V m^3 of gas, then $\Gamma = \dfrac{x}{m}$ or $\Gamma = \dfrac{V}{m}$. For certain amount of absorbents, when the absorption equilibrium is reached, the amount of gas being absorbed depends on the pressure and temperature, so $\Gamma = f\,(T,\,p)$. By keeping the temperature or pressure constant, the relationship between Γ and the other parameter could be obtained. When the pressure is fixed, measuring Γ under various temperatures gives a graph of Γ versus T, which is called **adsorption isobaric** (吸附等压线). If the temperature is constant, the graph of Γ versus p is called **adsorption isotherm** (吸附等温线). When ammonium is absorbed on charcoal, the adsorption isotherm is shown in Fig. 6-17. In the graph, the pressure has a significant impact on the Γ within the region of low pressure, where Γ grows linearly with the increasing pressure. By further increasing the pressure, the rise of Γ gradually slows down, and a plateau is reached at high gas pressures (most obviously seen under -23.5℃). The graph also tells us that the Γ decreases with the increasing temperature. There are mainly 5 types of isotherms based on the experimental measurement, and these isotherms are shown in Fig.6-18.

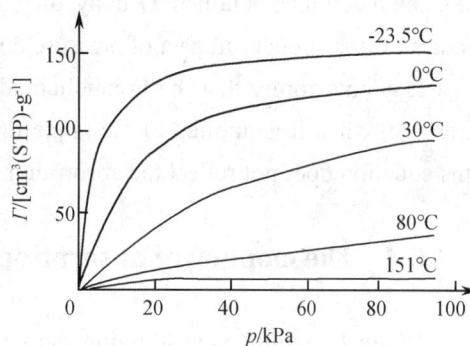

Fig. 6-17   Adsorption isotherms of ammonia on charcoal

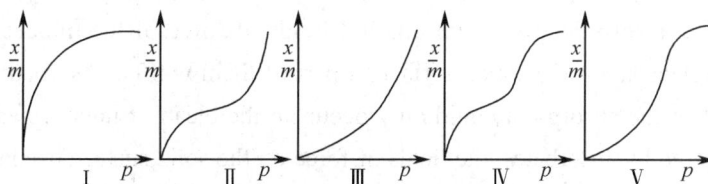

Fig. 6-18   Five types of adsorption isotherm.

Type Ⅰ isotherms are obtained when the gas is absorbed as monolayer and Γ reaches a plateau when the solid surface is fully covered or saturated by the absorbates.

Type Ⅱ isotherms are encountered under two cases. For the non-porous solid, this means multilayer absorption of gas on the solid surface. While, for solids with porosity, this might remind the capillary condensation of gases in the pores.

Type Ⅲ and type Ⅴ isotherms occur when the absorption forces in the first monolayer is relatively small, gases cannot be easily absorbed to the solid surface.

Type Ⅳ isotherms indicate the capillary condensation of gases in the pores of solids, and the upper limit is determined by the pore volume of the solids.

6.3 Freundlich adsorption isotherm

To obtain the functional relationship between Γ and the pressure under constant temperature, an equation was proposed by Freundlich in 1907, expressed as below

$$\frac{x}{m} = kp^{1/n} \tag{6-27}$$

where p (with unit of Pa) is the pressure of gas, k and n are constants related with the temperature and species of absorbates and absorbents. The value of k which could be seen as the amount of gas being absorbed under unit pressure ($p=100kPa$) decreases with the increasing temperature.

Taking logarithms

$$\lg \frac{x}{m} = \lg k + \frac{1}{n}\lg p \tag{6-28}$$

A plot of $\lg \frac{x}{m}$ versus $\lg p$ should give a straight line, and based on the slope and intercept, the value of k and n could be obtained. Usually, the value of slope is within the range from 0 to 1, slope with higher values means stronger impact of pressure on the gas absorption.

It is noteworthy that the Freundlich adsorption isotherm is only applicable to the range of medium pressure, when it is applied to the range low or high pressure, there will be significant deviations. And this equation does not reflect the absorption mechanisms.

6.4 The monolayer absorption theory—the Langmuir adsorption isotherm

When Langmuir was studying the gas absorption on gold at low pressures, he discovered some regular patterns by analyzing the data. Then he proposed a **monolayer absorption theory (单分子层吸附理论)** and developed the **Langmuir adsorption isotherm(朗缪尔等温吸附)** from kinetic considerations. His theory is based on several assumptions.

(1) Solids tend to absorb due to the unsatisfied fields of force of the molecules or atoms at the surface. When gas molecules hit the solids surface, a part of them will be absorbed with heat given out during this process. But the absorption could only occur on the clean or unoccupied surface of solids. After being fully covered by absorbates, the fields of force on the solid surface become saturated and the absorption ceases, therefore a monolayer of absorbates is formed.

(2) The absorption is in dynamic equilibrium. When the equilibrium is established, the velocity of absorption (similar to condensing) is equal to that of desorption (similar to evaporation) under specific temperatures.

(3) There are no interactive forces between the absorbed molecules or atoms.

(4) The solid surface is homogeneous, and the heat of absorption is independent of the degree of coverage.

At specific time point, if the fraction of surface area covered with absorbates is referred to as θ, the fraction of the unoccupied surface area will be $1-\theta$. Within every second, the amount of gas molecules hit onto the solid surface per unit area is proportional to the pressure of gas. Therefore, the velocity of absorption denoted as v_2 could be expressed as

$$v_2 = k_2 p\,(1-\theta) \tag{6-29}$$

where k_2 is the rate constant of absorption.

Meanwhile, the velocity of desorption denoted as v_1 is expressed as

$$v_1 = k_1 \theta \tag{6-30}$$

where k_1 is the rate constant of desorption.

When the absorption equilibrium is established, the velocity of absorption and that of desorption equals with each other.

$$k_2 p\,(1-\theta) = k_1 \theta \tag{6-31}$$

$$\theta = \frac{k_2 p}{k_1 + k_2 p} \tag{6-32a}$$

By defining $b = \dfrac{k_2}{k_1}$, the above equation could be changed into

$$\theta = \frac{bp}{1+bp} \tag{6-32b}$$

where b is called the absorption constant or equilibrium constant which is related with the temperature and the properties of the absorbates and absorbents. The higher the b value is, the stronger the absorption ability. High temperature facilitates desorption, but is unfavorable for absorption, thus the value of b is relatively small at high temperature.

For certain amount of absorbents, the θ increases linearly with the pressure within the low pressure range. When the pressure reaches certain value, the θ gets close to 1, and the Γ no longer increases with the rise in pressure. The Γ_∞ is the maximum amount of gas being absorbed when the solid surface is fully covered by a monolayer of absorbates. At any point in time during absorption, θ could be written as

$$\theta = \frac{\Gamma}{\Gamma_\infty} \tag{6-33}$$

$$\frac{\Gamma}{\Gamma_\infty} = \frac{bp}{1+bp} \tag{6-34}$$

Equation above could well describe the absorption isotherm in Fig. 6–19. When the pressure is low, $bp \ll 1$, $1 + bp \approx 1$, then $\Gamma = \Gamma_\infty bp$. Since the Γ_∞ and b could be seen as constant for given absorbates and absorbents at specific temperature, Γ is proportional to the p. If the pressure is within the medium range, this equation could be changed into $\Gamma = \Gamma_\infty bp^n$, which well fits the curve of absorption isotherm. When the pressure is high, $bp \gg 1$, $1 + bp \approx bp$, then $\Gamma = \Gamma_\infty$, indicating that the solid surface has been almost completely covered by the absorbents.

$$\Gamma = \Gamma_\infty \frac{bp}{1+bp}$$

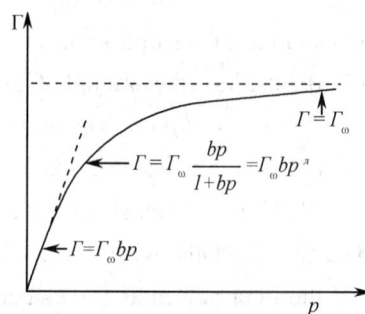

Fig. 6–19　Schema illustration of the Langmuir adsorption isotherm

After rearrangement, the equation turns into

$$\frac{p}{\Gamma} = \frac{1}{\Gamma_\infty b} + \frac{p}{\Gamma_\infty} \tag{6-35}$$

A plot of $\frac{p}{\Gamma}$ versus p gives a straight line of slope $\left(\frac{1}{\Gamma_\infty}\right)$ and intercept $\left(\frac{1}{\Gamma_\infty b}\right)$. And the Γ_∞ and b can be determined by the slope and intercept. Derived from enormous experimental data, the Langmuir adsorption isotherm applies for the monolayer absorption, and could well fit the Type I isotherms. However, the Langmuir equation does not work for the multilayer absorption.

6.5 Multilayer absorption theory—BET absorption isotherms

The **multilayer absorption theory (多层吸附理论)** was proposed by Brunauer, Emmett and Teller in 1938. They believe that the van der Waals forces exist not only between the gas and solids but also between gas molecules. Therefore, if the free gas molecules hit a layer of absorbates that already have been absorbed, these free molecules are still likely to be absorbed. This means that there could be multilayer absorption of gas on solids. Dynamic equilibrium is established between different layers, and a new layer could start to form before previous layer is fully covered. The absorption of the first layer is driven by the intermolecular forces between gas and solids. And the absorption of the second and above layers is due to the intermolecular forces between the absorbate molecules. Usually, the enthalpy of absorption for the first layer is greater than that for the second and above layers.

The BET model is shown in Fig. 6-20. The area of clean solid surface is referred to as S_0, the area of the first and second absorption layers are referred to as S_1 and S_2 respectively. During the absorption process, parts of S_0 will turn to S_1, if the gas molecules detach from solid surface, S_1 changes back to S_0. When the rate of absorption and desorption equals, the equilibrium is reached. Similarly, S_1 and S_2 will transform into each other and

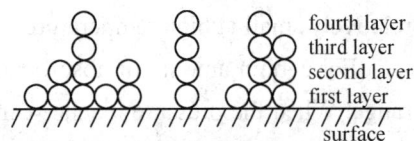

Fig. 6-20　The model of BET Multilayer absorption

establish a dynamic equilibrium eventually. Gas molecules could be absorbed as infinite layers and such equilibrium always exists between two adjacent layers. The resulting BET equation is expressed as

$$\frac{p}{\Gamma(p_0-p)} = \frac{1}{\Gamma_\infty C} + \frac{C-1}{\Gamma_\infty C} \cdot \frac{p}{p_0} \tag{6-36}$$

where p_0 and p refers to the saturation pressure and the equilibrium partial pressure of gas at the temperature of adsorption. C is a constant related with the temperature and properties of absorbates and absorbents. Γ_∞ is the amount of gas absorbed as monolayer.

A plot of $p/(p_0-p)$ versus p/p_0 gives a straight line. The slope is $(C-1)/\Gamma_\infty C$, and the intercept is $1/\Gamma_\infty C$. And the constant C and Γ_∞ could be calculated via the value of the slope and intercept.

The liner relationship of this plot could be well maintained only when the value of p_0/p ranges from 0.05 to 0.35. Otherwise, there will be large deviation due to the heterogeneous nature of solid surface and the intermolecular forces between the absorbed gas molecules. Some researchers believe that the deviation might also be related with the capillary condensation which usually occurs under high pressure. The capillary condensation is a phenomenon where the absorbed gas will condense into liquids within the pores of solids when multilayer absorption proceeds to a specific point. Therefore, the Γ grows rapidly with the increasing pressure due to the capillary condensation, which could explain the steep rise on the isotherms when the value of p_0/p exceeds 0.4.

The BET isotherm is an extension of Langmuir isotherm from monolayer absorption to multilayer absorption. And the BET equation is widely used to calculate the surface area of solid materials.

Section 7   Absorption at the Solid-Liquid Interface

Absorption happens when the solids is added to a solution. Absorption in the solution differs from that in the gas phase. Firstly, both the solute and solvent molecules could be absorbed by the absorbents. The solutes and solvents are competing for the solid surface. Secondly, most of the absorbents are solids with porosity, it is time taking for the absorbate molecules to diffuse into the pores. Hence, it is much slower to reach the absorption equilibrium in the solution than in the gas phase. Thirdly, the absorbates could be either molecules or ions, so the absorption on the solid-liquid interface could be the **absorption of molecules (分子吸附)** or the **absorption of ions(离子吸附)**.

7.1   Absorption of molecules

For solutes that are non-electrolyte or weak electrolyte, they will be absorbed as molecules by the solids in the solution. If m(kg) of absorbents is introduced to a solution with volume of V and mass density of ρ_{B_1} in a container, when the equilibrium is reached after a period of shaking, the density of the solution is measured to be ρ_{B_2} after filtration, then the apparent absorption amount of solutes (Γ_{app}) could be calculated as

$$\Gamma_{app} = V \frac{\rho_{B1} - \rho_{B2}}{m} \tag{6-37}$$

In reality, the absorption of solutes is inevitably accompanied by the absorption of solvents. Since the absorption of solvents is less considered in this equation, the Γ obtained by calculation is usually lower than the actual Γ in the experiment. Therefore, the absorption amount of solutes obtained by this equation is called Γ_{app}.

For the solids in dilute solution, there are mainly four types of absorption isotherms, as shown in Fig. 6-21. The "L" type (Langmuir type) and "S" type isotherms are most commonly seen, while the "Ln" and "HA" type isotherms are rarely seen. For the "S" type isotherm, the solutes could not be easily absorbed when the concentration of is low, but the absorption will become easy to proceed when the concentration increases to a certain point. The "L" type isotherm indicates that the solutes have a strong tendency to be absorbed, and the solute molecules could easily replace the solvent molecules absorbed on the solid surface. If the solids prefer the solutes to the solvents, solutes could be completely absorbed by the solids even in a dilute solution, which leads to the "HA" type isotherm. If the solutes penetrate into the solid structure during the absorption process and cause the swelling of solid matrix, the corresponding isotherm will be the "Ln" type.

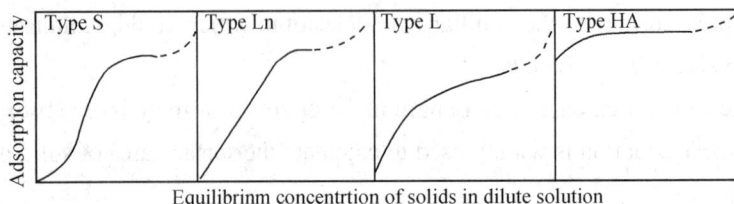

Fig. 6–21　**Adsorption isothermals of solids on dilute solution**

Absorption in a solution could also be expressed by the Freundlich, Langmuir and BET isotherm after replacing the pressure (p) with concentration C. Then the equation will change into

$$\frac{x}{m} = kc^{1/n} \tag{6-38}$$

And the equation will become

$$\Gamma = \Gamma_\infty \frac{bc}{1+bc} \tag{6-39}$$

where, these equations are empirical and the constants have no specific meaning. Since the absorption in solution is complicated and is affected by various factors, the absorption mechanism is still unclear. But there are several empirical laws could be followed.

(1) Solutes which could reduce the Gibbs free energy of solids to the greatest extent are the most preferentially absorbed.

(2) Polar absorbents prefer to absorb the polar absorbates and vice versa. For example, charcoal as a non-polar absorbent does not absorb water, while silica gel which is a polar absorbent could absorb water efficiently. Therefore, charcoal is suitable for the absorption of organic molecules in water, and silica gel performs well in absorbing the polar solutes in a non-polar organic solvent.

(3) Solutes with lower solubility are the more likely to be absorbed.

(4) Temperature has an impact on the exothermic absorption process. Generally, the absorption amount of solutes decreases with the increase in temperature.

7.2　Absorption of ions

After being ionized in the solution, electrolyte solutes are absorbed as ions by the solids. There are **ion exchange absorption**(离子交换吸附) and **ion exclusive absorption**(离子选择吸附).

7.2.1　Ion exclusive absorption

Absorption of ions could be selective. Sometimes solids may absorb a specific kind of ion, either anionic or cationic. Then part of the counter ions will be attracted due to the electrostatic interaction and form a surrounding rigid layer. There are also a few counter ions distributing loosely around the rigid layer forming a diffuse layer.

7.2.2　Ion exchange absorption

During the absorption process of ions, if the solids release dissimilar ions carrying similar charges into the solution, this phenomenon is called ion exchange absorption. So the ion exchange absorption is a process where the ions in the solution replace the ions with the same charge in the solid. Such solid absorbents are also called ion exchangers. Typical ion exchangers are ion exchange resins with porous structure in the form of microbeads. They are made of cross-linked polystyrene with different functional groups.

Ion exchangers are classified into four main types based on their functional group as follows.

Strong acidic, those contain sulfonic acid groups ($-SO_3H$).

Strong basic, those contain quaternary amine groups ($-CH_2N(CH_3)_2OH$).

Weak acidic, those contain carboxylic acid ($-COOH$).

Weak basic, those contain primary, secondary, and/or tertiary amine groups ($-NH_2$, $-CH_2NHCH_2$, $-CH_2N(CH_3)_2$).

Generally, cationic resins absorb ions with negative charge and anionic resins absorb ions with positive charge. For the absorption of strongly alkaline solutes, the weak acidic rather than the strong acidic resins should be selected. Otherwise, desorption of solutes will be difficult. For the absorption of alkaline solutes, the strong acidic resins are recommended, since the absorption forces are insufficient when using the weak acidic resins.

7.3   Solid absorbents

Solid absorbents have gained widely application in the pharmaceutical fields. Here is a brief introduction of several frequently used solid absorbents.

7.3.1   Activated carbon

Activated carbon (活性炭) is often used for discoloration, purification, absorption and extraction of active ingredients, like atropine sulfate and coenzyme A. And it is characterized by its porosity and capability for gas absorption. Activated charcoal could be produced from any carbonaceous materials derived from plant, animal and mineral. The plant-derived charcoal which is suitable for pharmaceutical use could be obtained by carbonization of wood, bamboo and rice hull at high temperatures around 600℃ in an inert atmosphere. Sometimes trace amount of silica or zinc oxide were added for providing porous structure for the deposition of carbon particles. Activation is necessary for any carbon-based materials to become the activated carbon. The purposes of this activation process include the removal of impurities, increasing of surface area, clearance of the pore channel, causing defects and dislocations in the crystal lattice and making the crystal imperfect.

The most commonly used method for activation is heating in which materials are exposed to oxidized atmospheres at high temperatures ranging from 500℃ to 1000℃. After the activation process, the amount of CCl_4 absorbed by 1kg of charcoal could increase from 0.001kg to 1.48kg. Activated carbon is a non-polar absorbent suitable for the absorption of non-polar solutes in water. Generally, the less soluble solutes are more likely to be absorbed. And the absorption ability of activated carbon will be compromised with increasing water content.

7.3.2   Silica gel

Silica gels (硅胶) are white or transparent powders with water content of 3% to 7%. It is composed of silicon dioxide with chemical formula expressed as $xSiO_2 \cdot yH_2O$. Silica gel has a porous structure and it is a polar absorbent with rich hydroxyl groups on the surface. It has strong affinity for water molecules and could absorb moisture up to 40% by mass ratio. Therefore, it is widely used as desiccant.

To prepare silica gel, Na_2SiO_3 solution is mixed with sulfuric acid and sprayed as droplets from a nozzle, after solidification and aging in which the net-like structure is strengthened, these droplets will turn to solid microbeads. The obtained products are further washed off additional salts and kept under

400℃ for 4h for drying. Before use, silica gel should be kept at 120℃ for another 24h for activation.

The absorption ability of silica gel will be attenuated with increasing water content. Based on the water content, silica gels are classified into five levels, those with water content of 0%, 5%, 15%, 25% and 35% are referred to as level I to V, respectively. Silica gel is frequently used in moisture absorption and chromatography. And it could be used to extract cardiac glycoside, alkaloids and steroids from traditional Chinese medicine.

7.3.3 Aluminum oxide

Aluminum oxide (氧化铝) also known as alumina is a porous absorbents with strong absorption ability. In the preparation process of alumina, the first step is to obtain alkali alumina by dehydration of aluminum hydroxide via heating at 400℃. Then the alkali alumina is mixed with twice amount of 5% HCl, heated to boiling and washed to neutral with water. And the neutral alumina could be obtained through heating induced activation. After further acidification by acetic acid and activation by heating, the acidic alumina is eventually obtained.

Similar to silica gel, alumina is also a polar absorbent. And its absorption ability will be impeded with the increasing water content. Based on the water content, there are five types of alumina. They are type I, II, III, IV and V with corresponding water content of 0%, 3%, 6%, 10% and 15%. When the alumina are saturated with water, they could be regenerated by dehydration through heating at temperature range of 275℃ to 315℃. Alumina is usually used as desiccant, catalyst and carrier of catalyst, and absorbent in chromatography to separate different chemical compounds extracted from Chinese herbs.

7.3.4 Molecular sieves

Molecular sieves (分子筛), also called zeolites, are crystalline metal aluminosilicates mainly composed of SiO_2 and Al_2O_3. They could be natural or synthesized with chemical formula usually expressed as $M_{2/n} \cdot Al_2O_3 \cdot xSiO_2 \cdot yH_2O$, where M represents metal ion (e.g. sodium, potassium, calcium). Molecular sieves have gained widely application in the absorption and separation of substances based on their pore sizes which are determined by particular metal ions during formation. For the molecular sieves, the molar ratio of SiO_2 to Al_2O_3 is referred to as Si/Al ratio, the greater value of the ratio means the molecular sieves are more resistant to heat and acid.

There are various types of sieves with crystal lattice mainly composed of SiO_4 and AlO_4 tetrahedra. By changing the Si/Al ratio, synthetic condition and the spatial arrangements of these two tetrahedras, various types of sieves which differ in pore size and structure could be obtained. The SiO_4 group is electrically neutral due to sharing of its oxygen atoms, while the AlO_4 group has a single negative charge, which is generally compensated by a cation (Na^+, K^+, Ca^{2+}, etc.). Even one type of molecular sieve could be further divided into several subtypes. Each type of sieve has particular pore sizes, molecules have comparable or smaller sizes could diffuse into the pores and being absorbed, while molecules with larger sizes could not. Therefore, the molecular sieves could be used to sieve and separate molecules based on their sizes.

Till 2004, there are more than 150 types of synthetic molecular sieves. And the most commonly used are type A, X, Y, M and ZSM. The type A sieves, characterized by small pore sizes, include 3A, 4A and 5A with corresponding pore size of about 3, 4 and 5 Angstroms. The ZSM-5 type with the Si/Al ratio greater than 40 is the most thermal stable and has become one of the most promising sieves in practical application. For natural porous zeolites, when the porosity accounts for more than 50% of the total volume, they could also be used to prevent bumping, i.e. irregular boiling of liquids.

Molecular sieves offer several advantages over other absorbents.

(1) Selectivity   Molecular sieves only allow the passage of molecules smaller than the pore size and absorb them once they enter the cavities. While larger molecules are too big to enter the pores and they are less likely to be absorbed, thus resulting in different retention behaviors. So a mixture of molecules with different sizes could be well separated by the sieving effect. For example, the 5A type molecular sieves with pore size of 0.5nm could be used to separate n-butane from isobutane and benzene in a liquid mixture. The molecular diameter of n-butane is smaller than 0.5nm, while those of isobutane and benzene are greater than 0.5nm, therefore, n-butane could be absorbed by the molecular sieves while the isobutane and benzene could not. Due to their absorption selectivity based on molecular size, molecular sieves are widely used for separation of mixtures.

(2) Strong absorption ability at low concentration of absorbents   Regular absorbents are less efficient when the concentration of absorbates is relatively low. While for the molecular sieves, as long as the molecular size of absorbates is smaller than the pore channel, they could still exhibit strong absorption ability even at low concentrations.

(3)Strong absorption ability at high temperatures   For the regular absorbents, the absorption amount decreases with increasing temperature. While the molecular sieves could maintain high absorption efficiency at temperatures as high as 800℃.

7.3.5 Macroporous resins

Macroporous resins (大孔树脂) are polymer based porous absorbents without ion exchanging groups. Resins could be synthesized by polymerization of raw materials like styrene and divinylbenzene in water containing 0.5% gelatin with the presence of pore directing agents. Generally, they are white in granular form with size around 0.45~0.85mm. Resins have network structure, high surface area of around 100 to 700m² per gram and pore sizes of 5 to 300nm. These characteristics make them able to absorb certain organic compounds from the aqueous solution with high selectivity. Therefore, they are a new type of resin developed after the ion exchange resin and now widely used as absorbents for separation and purification.

There are different types of resins based on the raw materials, like the styrene type, 2-methacrylate type, acrylonitrile type and divinylbenzene type resins, etc. By altering the basic chemical structure, resins could be synthesized with or without functional groups. They could be polar, weakly polar or non-polar and the pore sizes are adjustable during preparation.

Macroporous resins are physicochemical stable, and do not dissolve in acid, base and organic solvent. The absorption behavior of resins relies on the van der Waals forces and hydrogen bonding, and the sieving effect of resins is achieved via their porous structure. Separation techniques based on resins are fast, efficient, sensitive and highly selective. For natural compounds with high molecular weight which cannot be well separated by common methods, macroporous resins greatly simplified the separation and purification process own to their unique characteristics. With the application of new techniques based on macroporous resins, it becomes much more efficient to obtain a specific active ingredient from Chinese herbs. Resins are classified into various types based on their porosity, pore size, surface area and chemical structure, and they differ greatly in properties. And the type of resin to be used should be chosen according to the practical needs.

重 点 小 结

表面现象是物理化学的重要概念之一。 本章讨论了表面现象的物理本质， 即表面层分子所受的非平衡力。 提出了研究表面现象的热力学准则即表面吉布斯自由能和表面张力。 以此为基础，进一步探讨了不同表面现象的判据和相关应用。 具体包括如下几点： ①铺展和润湿现象及其对应判据， 分别为铺展系数和杨氏公式； ②依据拉普拉斯方程和开尔文公式， 探讨附加压力和饱和蒸气压的大小， 以及其对高分散系统对物理性质的影响； ③溶液表面的吸附分类及定量描述——吉布斯等温式； ④表面活性剂的分类及应用； ⑤固气、固液表面的吸附规律和特点及常见吸附剂的应用。 本章的知识内容对于药学专业在药物制剂、 药物有效成分的提取和纯化及药物在体内吸收分布等方面有广泛的应用， 要求学生能够利用本章的基础知识， 解决药学领域的相关问题。

Object detection

I. Select the correct option for the following problems (one option for each problem).

1. Which liquid do you think has the strongest surface tension?

    A. clean water   B. soapy water   C. NaCl solution   D. alcohol solution

2. The direction of surface tension is always

    A. along the normal of liquid surface, towards the interior of the liquid

    B. along the normal of liquid surface, towards the interior of the gas

    C. along the tangent of the liquid surface

    D. no definite direction

3. At constant temperature and composition, the factors affecting the surface Gibbs function include

    A. only surface area   B. only surface tension

    C. both surface area and surface tension   D. on definite function relation

4. Inject a small amount of water into a horizontal glass capillary. Both ends of the water column in the capillary are concave. When heating the concave surface of the right end, which end the the water will move to?

    A. left end   B. right end

    C. being stationary   D. difficult to determine

5. If a liquid can spread on a given solid, then the corresponding spreading factor S should be

    A. >0   B. <0

    C. = 0   D. can not be determined

6. At constant temperature and pressure, for a given substance, the relationship between the saturation solubility of its coarse grain c_1 and that of its tiny grain c_2 is

    A. $c_1 > c_2$ B. $c_1 < c_2$ C. $c_1 = c_2$ D. unable to determine

7. At constant temperature, a give volume of water is dispersed into tiny liquid drops, which of the following property remain unchanged?

    A. saturation vapor pressure   B. surface Gibbs function

    C. surface tension   D. surface area

8. The purpose of adding surfactant to pesticides is

    A. to improve pesticide's insecticidal ability

    B. prevent pesticide volatilization

    C. to improve the wetting ability of pesticides on plant leaves

    D. make pesticides more volatile

9. If a solid cannot be wetted by water, the contact angle of water with the solid surface should be

    A. $\theta = 0°$ B. $\theta > 90°$ C. $\theta < 90°$ D. $\theta = 180°$

10. If water can spread on a solid surface, then which of the following relationship among the three surface tensions $\sigma_{l,g}$, $\sigma_{l,g}$ and $\sigma_{s,g}$ is correct?

    A. $\sigma_{l,s} - \sigma_{l,g} > \sigma_{s,g}$ B. $\sigma_{l,s} + \sigma_{s,g} > \sigma_{l,g}$ C. $\sigma_{l,s} + \sigma_{s,g} > \sigma_{l,g}$ D. $\sigma_{l,s} + \sigma_{l,g} < \sigma_{s,g}$

II. Select the correct options for the following problem (at least two options for each problem).

1. Which of the following description about the physical adsorption is correct?

    A. no selectivity

    B. the adsorption layer can be either a single or multiple molecular layers

    C. the adsorption rate is high

    D. the adsorption is stable, difficult to desorb

    E. the adsorption rate is low

2. Which of the following options belongs to the basic properties of the oil-in-water emulsion(O/W)?

    A. easily dispersed in water   B. easily dispersed in oil

    C. high conductivity   D. low conductivity

    E. the droplets can be stained with organic dye

III. Try to answer the following problem.

According to theory about surface tension, try to determine if a pure-water bubble or a soap bubble evaporates faster.

Reference answers

I. 1. C;   2. B;   3. A;   4. A;   5. A;   6. B;   7. C;   8. C;   9. B;   10. D.

II. 1. ABC;   2. ACE.

III. According to the Kelvin formula, the vapor pressure of a liquid droplet increases with its surface tension, but decreases with the increase in radius of the droplet. So if the pure-water bubble and the soap bubble are of the same size, the water bubble will evaporate faster than the soap bubble does, due the former has a larger surface tension than the latter.

Chapter 7　Sol

知识要求

1. 掌握

（1）分散系统的基本概念。

（2）溶胶的基本特征。

（3）溶胶的电学性质。

（4）溶胶胶团结构式。

2. 熟悉

（1）溶胶的净化方法。

（2）溶胶的动力学性质。

（3）溶胶的光学性质。

（4）溶胶的聚沉和舒尔茨 – 哈迪规则。

3. 了解

（1）溶胶的制备与净化。

（2）溶胶的双电层结构。

能力要求

1. 能掌握溶胶的基本特征和三大基本性质，并判断溶胶表面电荷的来源、带电性强弱、溶胶稳定性大小，并能表述溶胶的双电层结构。

2. 能选择溶胶的制备方法并掌握稳定溶胶的方式，判断溶胶的散射光强弱、电解质对溶胶稳定性的作用大小。

3. 能运用所学溶胶的知识应解决生活和科学研究中有关胶体的问题，并能解释跟胶体相关的现象。

Section 1　Introduction of Colloidal Chemistry

Thomas Graham (1861) studied the ability of dissolved substances to diffuse into water across a permeable membrane. He observed that crystalline substances such as sugar, urea, and sodium chloride passed through the membrane, while others like glue, gelatin and gum Arabic did not. The former he called crystalloids and the latter colloids. Graham thought that the difference in the behavior of "crystalloids" and "colloids" was due to the particle size. Later it was realized that any substance, regardless of its nature, could be converted into a colloid by subdividing it into particles of colloidal size.

Now, **colloid (胶体)** is an important branch of physical chemistry, which studies the intersection and overlap of chemistry, physics, biochemistry, materials science and so on, and has become the theoretical basis for these subjects. Colloid is a kind of highly dispersed system and widely exists in living bodies, such as human blood, cells and cartilage. Many physiological and pathological changes in organisms and the efficacy of drugs are related to the properties of the colloid system. In pharmaceutical engineering, separation and extraction of effective components of traditional Chinese medicine, drug identification and other work, we often need to use the theoretical and practical guidance of colloidal chemistry. So it is very important and absolutely necessary for pharmaceutical workers to master the basic concepts, theories and skills of colloidal science. In addition, colloidal chemistry is widely used not only in medicine but also in materials, food, energy, environment and other fields.

Section 2   Dispersion System

2.1   Concept of dispersion system

A system in which one or more substances are highly dispersed in another medium is called a **dispersion system (分散系统)**. The dispersed material is called a dispersed phase or discontinuous phase, and the uniform medium in which the dispersed phase is dispersed is called a dispersion medium or continuous phase. The dispersion system with the same particle size of dispersed phase is called mono-dispersion system, while the dispersion system with different size of dispersed phase is called poly-dispersion system.

2.2   Classification of dispersion system

In a **true solution (真溶液)** as sugar or salt in water, the solute particles are dispersed in the solvent as single molecules or ions. Thus the diameter of the dispersed particles ranges from 1Å to 1nm.

On the other hand, in a **suspension(悬浊液)** or a **emulsion (乳浊液)**, as sand stirred into water, the dispersed particles are aggregates of millions of molecules. The diameter of these particles is greater than 100nm.

The **colloidal solutions** or **colloidal dispersions (胶体)** are intermediate between the true solutions and the suspensions. In other words, the diameter of the dispersed particles in a colloidal dispersion is more than that of the solute particles in a true solution and smaller than that of a suspension. When the diameters of the dispersed particles in a solvent range from 1nm to 100nm, the system is termed a **colloidal solution**, **colloidal dispersion**, or a **colloid**. The material with particle size in the colloidal range is said to be in the **colloidal state**.

The size and characteristics of the dispersed phase in the three dispersion systems are shown in the Table 7-1.

PPT

Table 7–1 Size and characteristics of the dispersed phase in dispersion systems

Type name	Size of dispersed phase	Main characteristics
Suspension Emulsion	$>10^{-7}$m （>100nm）	Not pass through the filter paper and semi-permeable membrane, non-diffusion, visible under the ordinary microscope
Colloid	$10^{-7}\sim10^{-9}$m （1~100nm）	Pass through the filter paper but not through the semi-permeable membrane, slow diffusion, visible under the ultramicroscope
True solution	$<10^{-9}$m （<1nm）	Pass through the filter paper and the semi-permeable membrane, fast diffusion, invisible under the ultramicroscope

2.3 Colloidal dispersion

The colloidal particles are not necessarily corpuscular in shape. In fact, these may be rod-like, disc-like, thin films, or long filaments. For matter in the form of corpuscles, the diameter gives a measure of the particle size. However, in other cases one of the dimensions (length, width and thickness) has to be in the colloidal range for the material to be classed as colloidal. Thus, in a broader context we can say: A system with at least one dimension (length, width, or thickness) of the dispersed particles in the range 1nm to 100nm, is classed as a colloidal dispersion.

Section 3　Types of Colloidal System and Characteristics of Sol

3.1 Types of colloidal system

The colloidal system consists of the **dispersed phase (分散相)** and **dispersion medium (分散介质)** or continuous phase in which the colloidal particles are dispersed. For example, for a colloidal solution of copper in water, copper particles constitute the dispersed phase and water is the dispersion medium (Fig. 7–1).

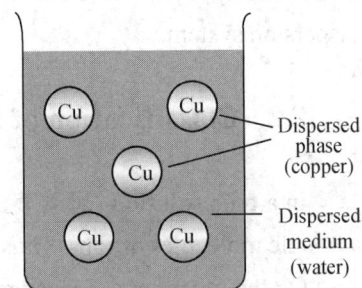

Fig. 7–1　A colloidal system of copper in water

Because either the dispersed phase or the dispersion medium can be a gas, liquid or solid, there are eight types of colloidal systems possible. A colloidal dispersion of one gas in another is not possible since the two gases would give a homogeneous molecular mixture. The various types of colloidal systems are listed in the Table 7–2.

In this chapter, we will restrict our study mainly to the colloidal systems which consist of a solid substance dispersed in a liquid. These are frequently referred to as sols or colloidal solution. The colloidal solutions in water as the dispersion medium are termed **hydrosols** or **aquasols(水溶胶)** . When the dispersion medium is alcohol or benzene, the sols are referred to as **alcosols (酒精溶胶)** and **benzosols (苯溶胶)** , respectively.

Table 7–2　Types of colloidal system

Type Name	Dispersed Phase	Dispersion medium	Examples
Foam	gas	liquid	whipped cream, shaving cream, soda-water
Solid foam	gas	solid	froth cork, pumice stone, foam rubber
Aeroso	liquid	gas	for, mist, clouds
Emulsion	liquid	liquid	milk, hair cream
Solid emulsion (gel)	liquid	solid	butter, cheese
Smoke	solid	gas	dust, soot in air
Sol	solid	liquid	paint, ink, colloidal gold
Solid sol	solid	solid	ruby glass (gold dispersed in glass), alloys

Sols are colloidal systems in which a solid is dispersed in a liquid. These can be subdivided into two classes.

Lyophilic sols (亲液溶胶) are those in which the dispersed phase exhibits a definite affinity for the medium or the solvent. The examples of lyophilic sols are dispersions of starch, gum, and protein in water.

Lyophobic sols (憎液溶胶) are those in which the dispersed phase has no attraction with the medium or the solvent. The examples of lyophobic sols are dispersion of gold, iron (Ⅲ) hydroxide and sulphur in water.

The affinity or attraction of the sol particles for the medium, in a lyophilic sol, is due to hydrogen bonding with water. If the dispersed phase is a protein (as in egg) hydrogen bonding takes place between water molecules and the amino groups (—NH—, —NH$_2$) of the protein molecule. In a dispersion of starch in water, hydrogen bonding occurs between water molecules and the —OH groups of the starch molecule. There are no similar forces of attraction when sulphur or gold is dispersed in water.

3.2　Characteristics of lyophilic and lyophobic sols

3.2.1　Heterogeneity

The dispersed phase particles of sol are composed of a large number of atoms or molecules. There is an obvious phase interface between particles of dispersed sol phase and medium, so sol is a superfine heterogeneous system. For example, the dispersed phase particles in ferric hydroxide sol are composed of many ferric hydroxide molecules, which are much larger than the molecules in the surrounding medium.

3.2.2　High dispersity

The particle in the dispersed sol phase form their own phase in the system, so the dispersity of the sol is very high. Many properties of colloids, such as slow diffusion, impenetrable semi-permeable membrane, and dynamic stability, are related to its high dispersity.

3.2.3　Aggregation instability

Sol is a highly dispersed multi-phase system with large surface area and surface energy. Dispersed phase in sol will spontaneously gather to reduce the energy of the system and cause the particles to aggregate.

Section 4 Preparation and Purification of Sol

4.1 Preparation of sol

Lyophilic sols may be prepared by simply warming the solid with the liquid dispersion medium e.g., starch with water. But lyophobic sols have to be prepared by special methods. These methods fall into two categories:

(1) **Dispersion methods (分散法)** in which larger macro-sized particles are broken down to colloidal size.

(2) **Condensation methods (凝聚法)** in which colloidal size particles are built up by aggregating single ions or molecules.

4.1.1 Dispersion methods

In these methods, material in bulk is dispersed in another medium.

(1) Mechanical dispersion using colloid mill (胶体磨法) The solid along with the liquid dispersion medium is fed into a Colloid mill (Fig. 7–2). The mill consists of two steel plates nearly touching each other and rotating in opposite directions with high speed. The solid particles are ground down to colloidal size and are then dispersed in the liquid to give the sol.

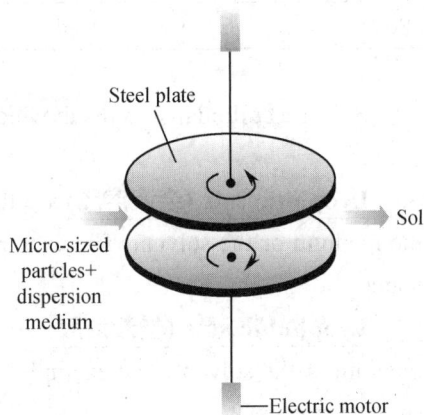

Fig. 7–2　A colloid mill

"Colloidal graphite" (a lubricant) and printing inks are made by this method. Recently, mercury sol has been prepared by disintegrating a layer of mercury into sol particles in water by means of ultrasonic vibrations.

(2) Bredig's arc method (电弧法)　It is used for preparing hydrosols of metals e.g., silver, gold and platinum. An arc is struck between the two metal electrodes held close together beneath de-ionized water. The water is kept cold by immersing the container in ice/water bath and a trace of alkali (KOH) is added. The intense heat of the spark across the electrodes vaporises some of the metal and the vapour condenses under water. Thus, the atoms of the metal present in the vapor aggregate to form colloidal particles in water. Since the metal has been ultimately converted into sol particles (*via* metal vapour), this method has been treated as of dispersion (Fig. 7–3).

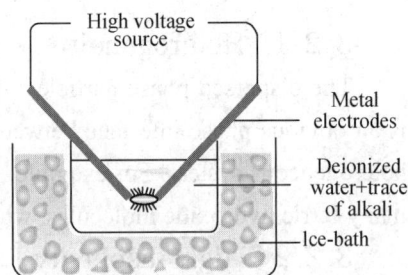

Fig. 7–3　Bredig's arc method

Non-metal sols can be made by suspending coarse particles of the substance in the dispersion medium and striking an arc between iron electrodes.

(3) Ultrasonic method (超声波法)　High frequency ultrasound has a great tearing force on the dispersed phase, to achieve the effect of dispersion. Ultrasonic dispersion method is also widely used in the preparation of emulsion. The hydrosol of sulfur and gypsum can be prepared by ultrasonic method.

(4) Peptizing method (胶溶法)　Some freshly precipitated ionic solids are dispersed into colloidal solution in water by the addition of small quantities of electrolytes, particularly those containing a common ion. The precipitate adsorbs the common ions and electrically charged particles then split from the precipitate as colloidal particles.

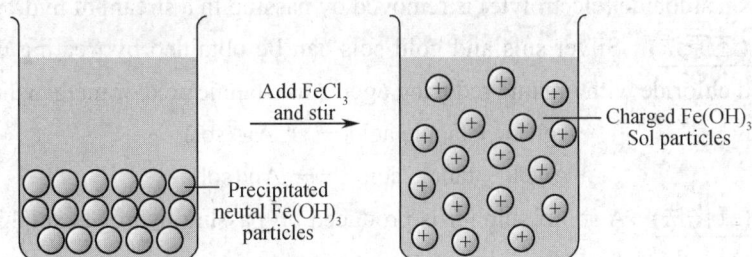

Fig. 7–4　Sol of ferric hydroxide is obtained by stirring fresh precipitate of ferric hydroxide with a small amount of FeCl₃

The dispersal of a precipitated material into colloidal solution by the action of an electrolyte in solution, is termed peptization. The electrolyte used is called a peptizing agent. Peptization is the reverse of coagulation of a sol.

Examples of preparation of sols by peptization.

(1) Silver chloride, AgCl, can be converted into a sol by adding hydrochloric acid (Cl^- being common ion.)

(2) Ferric hydroxide, $Fe(OH)_3$, yields a sol by adding ferric chloride (Fe^{3+} being common ion).

4.1.2　Condensation methods

These methods consist of chemical reactions or change of solvent whereby the atoms or molecules of the dispersed phase appearing first, coalesce or aggregate to form colloidal particles. The conditions (temperature, concentration, etc.) used are such as permit the formation of sol particles but prevent the particles becoming too large and forming precipitate. The unwanted ions (spectator ions) present in the sol are removed by dialysis as these ions may eventually coagulate the sol.

The more important methods for preparing hydrophobic sols are listed below.

(1) Physical condensation　The condensation of vapor or dissolved substances into colloids. For example, when mercury vapor is introduced into cold water, mercury hydrosol can be obtained, and a small amount of oxides generated during heating mercury can be used as stabilizers. **Solvent replacement method (溶剂更换法)** uses the different solubility of substances in different solvents to change the ordinary solution into supersaturated solution, and the solute can agglomerate into colloidal particles. When a solution of sulphur or resin in ethanol is added to an excess of water, the sulphur or resin sol is formed owing to decrease in solubility. The substance is present in molecular state in ethanol but on transference to water, the molecules precipitate out to form colloidal particles.

(2) Chemical condensation

a. **Hydrolysis (水解法)**　Sols of the hydroxides of iron, chromium and aluminium are readily prepared by the hydrolysis of salts of the respective metals. To obtain a red sol of ferric hydroxide, a few drops of 30% ferric chloride solution is added to a large volume of almost boiling water and stirred with a glass rod.

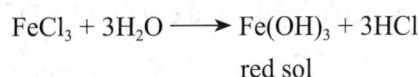

$$FeCl_3 + 3H_2O \longrightarrow Fe(OH)_3 + 3HCl$$

red sol

b. **Double decomposition (复分解法)**   An arsenic sulphide (As_2S_3) sol is prepared by passing a slow stream of hydrogen sulphide gas through a cold solution of arsenious oxide (As_2O_3). This is continued till the yellow colour of the sol attains maximum intensity.

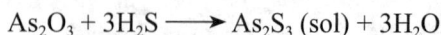

$$As_2O_3 + 3H_2S \longrightarrow As_2S_3 \text{ (sol)} + 3H_2O$$

Excess hydrogen sulphide (electrolyte) is removed by passing in a stream of hydrogen.

c. **Reduction (还原法)**   Silver sols and gold sols can be obtained by treating dilute solutions of silver nitrate or gold chloride with organic reducing agents like tannic acid or methanal (HCHO).

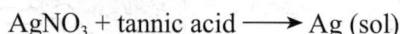

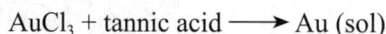

$$AgNO_3 + \text{tannic acid} \longrightarrow Ag \text{ (sol)}$$
$$AuCl_3 + \text{tannic acid} \longrightarrow Au \text{ (sol)}$$

d. **Oxidation (氧化法)**   A sol of sulphur is produced by passing hydrogen sulphide into a solution of sulphur dioxide.

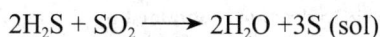

$$2H_2S + SO_2 \longrightarrow 2H_2O + 3S \text{ (sol)}$$

In qualitative analysis, sulphur sol is frequently encountered when H_2S is passed through the solution to precipitate group 2 metals if an oxidizing agent (chromate or ferric ions) happen to be present. It can be removed by boiling (to coagulate the sulphur) and filtering through two filter papers folded together.

4.2   Purification of sol

In the methods of preparation stated above, the resulting sol frequently contains besides colloidal particles appreciable amounts of electrolytes. To obtain the pure sol, these electrolytes have to be removed. This purification of sols can be accomplished by three methods: (a) Dialysis; (b) Electrodialysis; (c) Ultrafiltration.

4.2.1   Dialysis

Animal membranes (bladder) or those made of parchment paper and cellophane sheet, have very fine pores. These pores permit ions (or small molecules) to pass through but not the large colloidal particles. When a sol containing dissolved ions (electrolyte) or molecules is placed in a bag of permeable membrane dipping in pure water, the ions diffuse through the membrane. By using a continuous flow of fresh water, the concentration of the electrolyte outside the membrane tends to be zero. Thus, diffusion of the ions into pure water remains brisk all the time. In this way, practically all the electrolyte present in the sol can be removed easily. (Fig. 7-5)

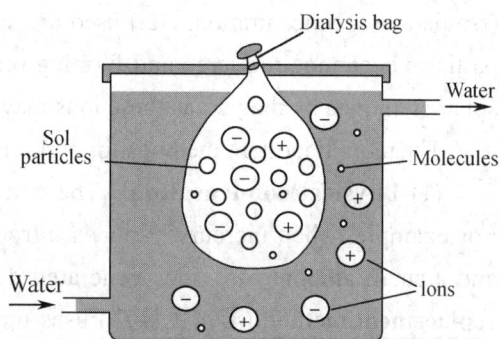

Fig. 7-5   Dialysis of a sol containing ions and molecules

The process of removing ions (or molecules) from a sol by diffusion through a permeable membrane is called dialysis. The apparatus used for dialysis is called a dialyser.

For example, A ferric hydroxide sol (red) made by the hydrolysis of ferric chloride will be mixed with some hydrochloric acid. If the impure sol is placed in the dialysis bag for some time, the outside water will give a white precipitate with silver nitrate. After a pretty long time, it will be found that almost the whole of hydrochloric acid has been removed and the pure red sol is left in the dialyser bag.

4.2.2   Electrodialysis

In this process, dialysis is carried under the influence of electric field (Fig. 7–6). Potential is applied between the metal screens supporting the membranes, which speeds up the migration of ions to the opposite electrode. Hence dialysis is greatly accelerated. Evidently, electrodialysis is not meant for nonelectrolyte impurities like sugar and urea.

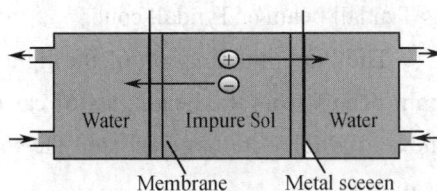

Fig. 7–6   Electrodialysis

4.2.3   Ultrafiltration

Sols can pass through an ordinary filter paper, because its pores are too large to retain the colloidal particles. However, if the filter paper is impregnated with collodion or a regenerated cellulose such as cellophane or visking, their pore size is much reduced. Such a modified filter paper is called an ultrafilter. (Fig. 7–7)

The separation of the sol particles from the liquid medium and electrolytes by filtration through an ultrafilter is called ultrafiltration.

Ultrafiltration is a slow process. Gas pressure (or suction) can be applied to speed it up. The colloidal particles are left on the ultrafilter in the form of slime. The slime may be stirred into fresh medium to get back the pure sol. By using graded ultrafilters, the technique of ultrafiltration can be employed to separate sol particles of different sizes.

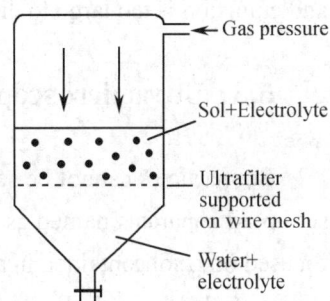

Fig. 7–7   Ultrafiltration

Section 5   Optical Properties of Sol

In general, when the frequency of incident light is the same as the natural frequency of molecules, absorption of light occurs. Light reflection occurs when the wavelength of incident light is smaller than the size of dispersed particles. Light scattering occurs when the wavelength of incident light is larger than the size of dispersed particles. The visible light wavelength is in the range of about 400~800nm, which is larger than the size 1~100nm of common colloidal particles, and light scattering can occur.

5.1   Tyndall effect

When a strong beam of light is passed through a sol and viewed at right angles, the path of light shows up as a hazy beam or cone. This is because sol particles absorb light energy and then emit it in all directions in space. This "scattering of light", as it is called, illuminates the path of the beam in the colloidal dispersion. The phenomenon of the **light scattering (光散射)** by the sol particles is called **Tyndall effect (丁达尔效应)** (Fig. 7–8).

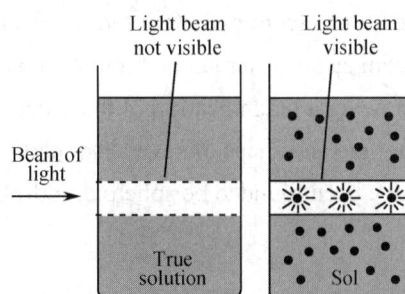

Fig. 7–8   Tyndall effect (Illustration)

The illuminated beam or cone formed by the scattering of light by the sol particles is often referred as Tyndall beam or Tyndall cone.

The hazy illumination of the light beam from the film projector in a smoke-filled theatre or the light beams from the headlights of car on a dusty road, are familiar examples of the Tyndall effect. If the sol particles are large enough, the sol may even appear turbid in ordinary light as a result of Tyndall scattering.

True solutions do not show Tyndall effect. Since ions or solute molecules are too small to scatter light, the beam of light passing through a true solution is not visible when viewed from the side. Thus, Tyndall effect can be used to distinguish a colloidal solution from a true solution.

Suspension and emulsion do not show Tyndall effect, too. The size of dispersed phase in suspension and emulsion is too large to directly reflect the light back without allowing light to pass.

5.2 Ultramicroscope shows up the presence of individual particles

Sol particles cannot be seen with a microscope. Zsigmondy (1903) used the Tyndall phenomenon to set up an apparatus named as the **ultramicroscope (超显微镜)**（Fig. 7–9）. An intense beam of light is focused on a sol contained in a glass vessel. The focus of light is then observed with a microscope at right angles to the beam. Individual sol particles appear as bright specks of light against a dark background (dispersion medium). It may be noted that under the ultramicroscope, the actual particles are not visible. It is the larger halos of scattered light around the particles that are visible. Thus, an ultramicroscope does not provide accurate information about the shape and size of sol particles.

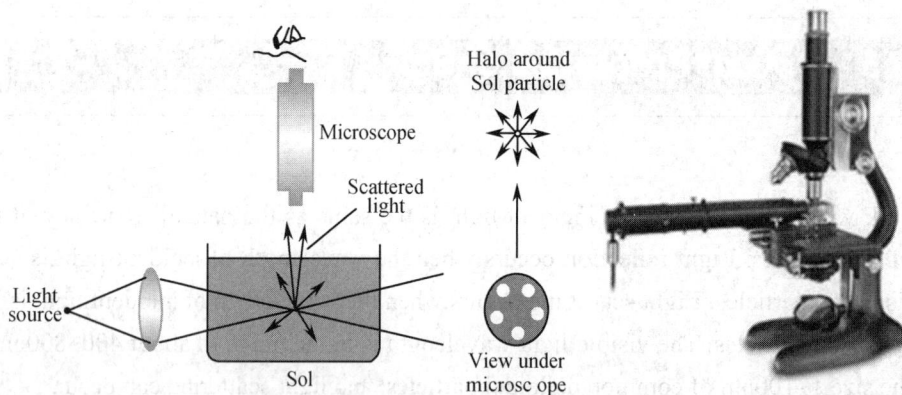

Fig. 7–9　Principle of the Ultramicroscope

Sol particles can be seen with an **Electron microscope (电子显微镜):** In an electron microscope, beam of electrons is focused by electric and magnetic fields on to a photographic plate. This focused beam can pass through a film of sol particles. Thus, it is possible to get a picture of the individual particles showing a magnification of the order of 10,000. With the help of this instrument, we can have an idea of the size and shape of several sol particles, including paint pigments, viruses, and bacteria. These particles have been found to be spheroid, rod-like, disc-like, or long filaments.

5.3　Rayleigh Scattering Formula

Lord Rayleigh studied the scattering of light with the electromagnetic theory and found the relationship between the emission intensity (I) of the sol system and the monochromatic incident light intensity (I_0), as shown in the following **Rayleigh scattering formula (瑞利散射公式)**.

$$I=\frac{24\pi^3\nu V^2}{\lambda^4}\left(\frac{n_2^2-n_1^2}{n_2^2+2n_1^2}\right)I_0 \tag{7-1}$$

where ν is the number of particles per unit volume, V is the volume per particle, λ is the wavelength of incident light, and n_2 and n_1 are the refractive index of dispersed phase and disperse medium, respectively. To illustrate the factors on opalescence intensity, the following analysis provides a clear explanation.

The opalescence intensity is inversely proportional to the fourth power of the wavelength. When the intensity of incident light remains constant, the shorter the wavelength of incident light is, the stronger the corresponding opalescence intensity will be. When the light is white, blue, and purple light scatter strongly. If white light is used to illuminate the sol, the scattered light seen from the side is blue or purple, while the penetrating light is orange red, which can be clearly seen in the sol of sulfur or frankincense. In signal equipment, for example, red is chosen as a danger signal because it is weak in scattering and strong in transmission, so it can be seen far away. In the same way, infrared and shortwave radio are used for positioning and tracking in communications and detection because of their weak scattering and strong penetration. Similarly, clear skies are blue, and the sun is red at sunrise and sunset.

The scattering intensity is proportional to the concentration of particles, that is, the more particles per unit volume, the stronger the opalescence intensity.

When all other conditions are equal, the Rayleigh formula is simplified as follows.

$$I=k\nu V^2 \tag{7-2}$$

If C represents the mass concentration of particles in the sol, and ρ represents the density of particles, then $\nu V\rho=C$, we have

$$I=k\frac{CV}{\rho} \tag{7-3}$$

For the same kind of sol with the same particle size but different concentration, k, V, and ρ are constant, then the emulsion intensity is proportional to the mass concentration of sol,

$$\frac{I_1}{I_2}=\frac{C_1}{C_2} \tag{7-4}$$

Under the same light source, this formula can be used to calculate the concentration of the unknown sol (C_2) by measuring the scattering intensity of the standard sol (I_1) with known concentration (C_1) and the unknown sol (I_2). This is the basic principle of **turbidimetric analysis（浊度分析）**.

The scattering intensity of the sol is proportional to the square of the particle volume. In the size range of colloidal particles, the larger the dispersion, that is, the smaller the volume of particles, the weaker the opalescence. The molecules of the solution are so small that the opalescence of the solution is weak or even imperceptible. Therefore, the Tyndall effect can be used to identify sol and solution.

The larger the refractive index difference (n_2-n_1) between the dispersed phase and the dispersion medium, the stronger the scattering intensity. When $n_1=n_2$, no opalescence occurs. Since the refractive index of the dispersed sol particles differs greatly from that of the dispersed medium, sol opalescence is obvious. However, the refractive index of the macromolecular compound is very little different from that of the dispersion medium, the opalescence of the macromolecular solution is very weak.

It is important to note that Rayleigh's formula applies only to extremely dilute colorless nonmetallic sol, not to metallic sol and suspension.

5.4   The color of sol

The color of a hydrophobic sol depends on the wavelength of the light scattered by the dispersed particles. The wavelength of the scattered light again depends on the size and the nature of the particles. This is fully borne out from the following data in the case of silver sol (Table 7–3).

Table 7–3   Color of Ag-sol

Color of Ag-sol	Particle diameter / mm
Orange-yellow	6×10^{-5}
Orange-red	9×10^{-5}
Purple	13×10^{-5}
Violet	15×10^{-5}

The color changes produced by varying particles size have been observed in many other cases.

Section 6   Dynamic Properties of Sol

6.1   Brownian movement

When a sol is examined with an ultramicroscope, the suspended particles are shining specks of light. By observing an individual particle, it is found that the particle is undergoing a constant rapid motion. It moves in a series of short straight-line paths in the medium, changing directions abruptly.

The continuous rapid zig-zag movement executed by a colloidal particle in the dispersion medium is called Brownian movement or motion (Fig. 7–10).

In a suspension, the suspended particles being very large the probability of unequal bombardments diminishes. The force of the molecules hitting the particle on one side is canceled by the force of collisions occurring on the other side. Hence, they do not exhibit Brownian movement.

The phenomenon of Brownian movement is an excellent proof of the existence of molecules and their ceaseless motion in liquids. It also explains how the action of gravity, which would ordinarily cause the settling of colloidal particles, is counteracted. The constant pushing of the particles by the molecules of the dispersion medium has a stirring effect which does not permit the particles to settle.

Influencing factors: the smaller the particles, the higher the temperature, the smaller the viscosity of the medium, the more intense the Brownian motion.

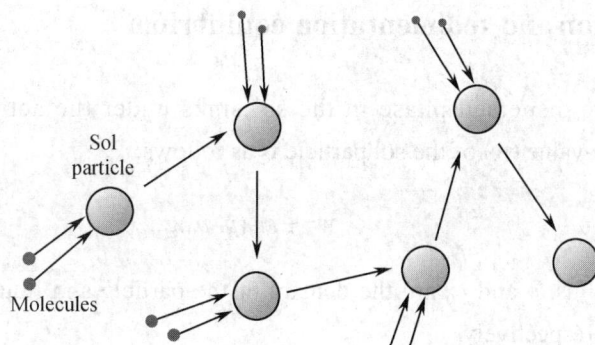

Fig. 7–10   The bombardment on the sides of the colloidal particles by molecules of dispersion medium causes the random movement of the particle

Around 1905, Einstein established Brownian motion theory with the concept of probability and molecular motility, the Einstein Brownian average displacement formula is obtained.

$$\bar{x} = \left(\frac{RTt}{3\,N_{A}\pi r\eta}\right)^{1/2} \tag{7–5}$$

where $\bar{x}$ is the average displacement of particles in the x-axis direction over time t; r is the particle radius; η is the medium viscosity; N_{A} is the Avogadro constant.

Svedberg performed photographic experiments on gold sols with a certain particle size using a super microscope. The results confirmed the accuracy of the above formula, and strongly proved that molecular kinematics can be used in colloidal dispersion systems. Using this formula to determine the size of the dispersed phase particles and Avogadro's constant yielded equally satisfactory results.

6.2   Diffusion

Diffusion is the phenomenon that the dispersed particles of the sol flow automatically from the high concentration area to the low concentration area due to Brownian motion. In 1885, Fick found that when the particle diffused along the X-axis, its diffusion velocity (dn/dt) was proportional to the cross-sectional area (A) and the concentration gradient (dc/dx), and the corresponding relationship was as follows.

$$\frac{dn}{dt} = -DA\frac{dc}{dx} \tag{7–6}$$

This is the **Fick's first law of diffusion (费克扩散第一定律)**, which states that the concentration gradient is driving the diffusion. Here, dn/dt is the amount of particle diffusion over area A per unit time at certain concentration gradient dC/dx. The coefficient D is called diffusion coefficient, which represents the unit concentration gradient, the number of particles passing through the unit cross-sectional area per unit time, meaning the diffusion capacity of particles in the medium.

$$D = \frac{RT}{L}\frac{1}{6\pi\eta r} \tag{7–7}$$

Equation (7–6) indicates that the smaller the radius of the particle, the smaller the viscosity of the medium and the higher the temperature, the larger the value of D, meaning that the particle is more prone to diffusion.

6.3　Sedimentation and sedimentation equilibrium

The process that the dispersed phase in the sol sinks under the action of gravity is called sedimentation. The gravity value (w) of the sol particle is as follows.

$$w=\frac{4}{3}\pi r^3(p-p_0)g \tag{7-8}$$

where r is the particle radius, ρ and ρ_0 are the density of the particle and liquid medium, and g is the gravitational acceleration, respectively.

At the same time, the dispersed particles are also subjected to a certain resistance (f) during the sedimentation process, and its value (f) is shown in equation (7–8).

$$f=6\pi\eta ru \tag{7-9}$$

where η is the viscosity of the liquid medium, and u is the settling velocity of dispersed particles.

Before sedimentation, u is equal to 0. As the settlement begins, the settlement of sol particles will accelerate under the action of gravity, so the value of u will become larger and the resistance (f) also increases. When the value of resistance (f) is equal to the gravity of the particles (w), the dispersed particles are in the equilibrium state of force, meaning the value of w and f are the same, resulting in constant settlement. We have

$$u=\frac{2r^2g(\rho-\rho_0)}{9\eta} \tag{7-10}$$

From this equation, the larger the particle radius, the larger the density difference between the dispersed phase and the dispersed medium, and the larger the settlement velocity will be. At the same time, the higher the viscosity of the dispersion medium, the lower the settling speed. The dynamic stability of sol is marked by the settlement velocity. The smaller the settlement velocity is, the more the dynamic stability of sol will be. In a highly dispersed sol system, the particles fall by the gravity, and the Brownian motion tends to homogenize the concentration. When these opposite forces are equal, the distribution of dispersed particles reaches equilibrium and a certain concentration gradient is formed. This state is called sedimentation equilibrium, as shown in Fig. 7–11.

The smaller the dispersed particles are, the longer it takes to establish the sedimentary equilibrium, and the better the dynamic stability of the sol system is. When dispersed particles are extremely small, the time required to settle by gravity alone is so long that it is virtually impossible to observe. The supercentrifuge with more than one million times the gravity can shorten

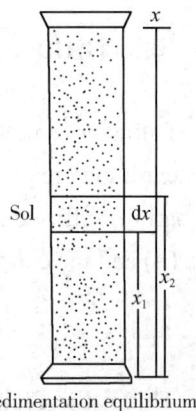

Sedimentation equilibrium

Fig. 7–11　Sedimentation equilibrium of sol

the settling time and make it possible to see the settling phenomenon, which expands the application of settlement measurement. Settlement analysis is to find the particle radius according to Stokes' law and further calculate the molar mass M of the colloidal particles.

$$M=\frac{4}{3}\pi r^3\rho N_A \tag{7-11}$$

Sedimentation equilibrium refers to the state where the dispersion rate of the dispersed phase particles is equal to the settling rate. Settling and diffusion are two opposite competing processes. Large mass particles are easy to settle and vice versa. When diffusion and sedimentation cancel each other out, the particles form a stable concentration gradient with height distribution. This state is called sedimentation equilibrium. Distribution of sol concentration with height after reaching settlement equilibrium can be expressed by the law of height distribution.

$$\ln \frac{c_1}{c_2} = \frac{N_A}{RT} \cdot \frac{4}{3}\pi r^3 (\rho - \rho_0)r(x_2 - x_1) \tag{7-12}$$

The larger the particle, the larger its equilibrium concentration gradient. c_1 and c_2 are the particles concentration at height x_1 and x_2 respectively; ρ and ρ_0 are the density of particles and medium respectively; r is the radius of colloidal particles; N_A is Avogadro's constant. By measuring the concentration of particles at different heights, the radius of the particles can be obtained, and the molar mass M of the particles can be calculated using equation (7-11).

Section 7 Electrical Properties of Sol

7.1 Electric phenomenon

The most important property of colloidal dispersions is that all the dispersed particles possess either positive or negative charge. The mutual forces of repulsion between similarly charged particles prevent them from aggregating and settling under the action of gravity. This gives stability to the sol. The sol particles acquire positive or negative charge by preferential adsorption of positive or negative ions from the dispersion medium. For example, ferric hydroxide sol particles are positively charged because these adsorb Fe^{3+} ions from ferric chloride ($FeCl_3$) used in the preparation of the sol. As a whole, sol is electrically

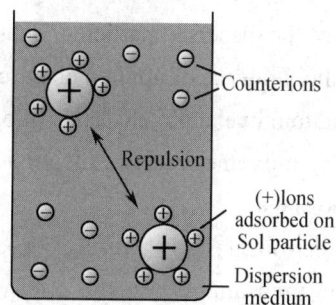

Fig. 7-12 Adsorption of ions from dispersion medium gives charge to Sol particles which do not settle on account of mutual repulsions

neutral, so the charge on the particle is counterbalanced by oppositely charged ions termed counterions (in this case Cl⁻) furnished by the electrolyte in dispersion medium. (Fig. 7-12)

Electric phenomenon refers to the relationship between the motion of sol particles and electrical properties, including electrophoresis, electroosmosis, flow potential, and sedimentation potential.

7.1.1 Electrophoresis

If electric potential is applied across two platinum electrodes dipping in a hydrophilic sol, the dispersed particles move toward one or the other electrode.

The movement of sol particles under an applied electric potential is called electrophoresis or cataphoresis.

If the sol particles migrate toward the positive electrode, they carry a negative charge. On the other hand, if they move toward the negative electrode, they are positively charged. Thus, by noting the direction of movement of the sol particles, we can determine whether they carry a positive or negative charge.

The phenomenon of electrophoresis can be demonstrated by placing a layer of As_2S_3 sol under two limbs of a U-tube. When a potential difference of about 100 volts is applied across the two platinum electrodes dipping in deionized water, it is observed that the level of the sol drops on the negative electrode side and rises on the positive electrode side (Fig. 7–13). This shows that As_2S_3 sol has migrated to the positive electrode, indicating that the particles are negatively charged. Similarly, a sol of ferric hydroxide will move to the negative electrode, showing that its particles carry positive charge. Using water as the dispersion medium, the charge on the

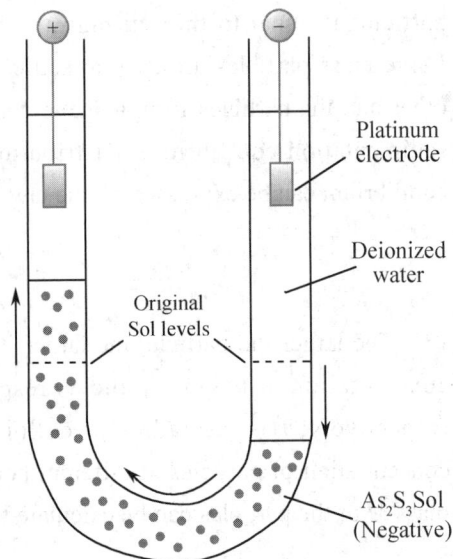

Fig. 7–13 Electrophoresis of a sol

particles of some common sols determined by electrophoresis is given below.

Some important applications of electrophoresis are : ① Removal of smoke from chimney gases; ② Removal of suspended impurities; ③ Electro-plating of rubber on metal surfaces from latex (a sol); ④ painting of metal parts of cars from colloidal pigments.

7.1.2 Electroosmosis

A sol is electrically neutral. Therefore, the dispersion medium carries an equal but opposite charge to that of the dispersed particles. Thus, the medium will move in opposite direction to the dispersed phase under the influence of applied electric potential. When the dispersed phase is kept, stationary, the medium is found to move to the electrode of opposite sign that its own.

The movement of the dispersion medium under the influence of applied potential is known as electroosmosis.

Electroosmosis is a direct consequence of the existence of zeta potential between the sol particles and the medium. When the applied pressure exceeds the zeta potential, the **diffuse layer (扩散层)** moves and causes electroosmosis.

The phenomenon of electroosmosis can be demonstrated by using a U-tube in which a plug of wet clay (a negative colloid) is fixed (Fig. 7–14). The two limbs of the tube are filled with water to the same level. The platinum electrodes are immersed in water and potential applied across them. It will be observed that water level rises on the cathode side and falls on anode side. This movement of the medium towards the negative electrode, shows that the charge on the medium is positive. Similarly, for a positively charged colloid electro-osmosis will take place in the reverse direction. Technically this phenomenon has been applied in the removal of water from peat, in dewatering of moist clay and in drying dye

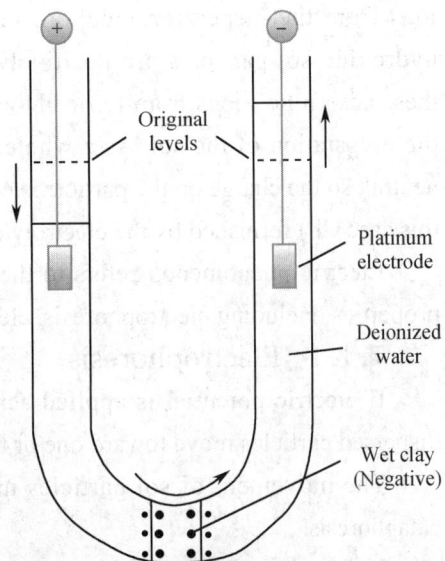

Fig. 7–14 Illustration of Electro-osmosis

pastes.

7.1.3 Flowing potential and sedimentation potential

Under the action of external force, the liquid is forced to flow through the porous membrane (or capillary) in a directional manner, and the potential difference generated at the two ends of the porous membrane (Fig. 7–15a). Flowing potential is an inverse phenomenon of electroosmosis.

When the dispersed phase particles move rapidly under the action of gravity or centrifugal force field, the potential difference generated at both ends of the moving direction (Fig. 7–15b). Sedimentation potential is the inverse phenomenon of electrophoresis.

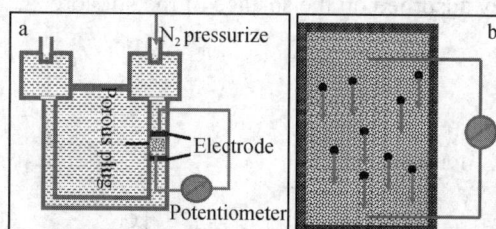

Fig. 7–15   Flow potential measurement diagram and sedimentation potential measurement diagram

7.2   Source of sol particle charge

All the dispersed particles of a sol carry a positive or a negative charge. They acquire this charge by ① Selective adsorption of ions from the aqueous medium; ② Ionization of surface groups; ③ Two-phase friction; ④ Isomorphous replacement.

7.2.1   Selective adsorption of ions

In most cases, the charge on the sol particles originates by the selective adsorption of ions common to the particles from the dispersion medium.

Examples:

(*i*) Ferric hydroxide sol particles are positive because they adsorb the common ion Fe^{3+} from the aqueous medium. (Fig. 7–16(a))

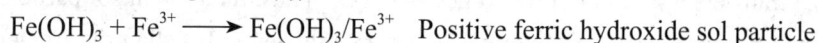

$Fe(OH)_3 + Fe^{3+} \longrightarrow Fe(OH)_3/Fe^{3+}$ Positive ferric hydroxide sol particle

(*ii*) Arsenic sulphide sol particles acquire a negative charge since they adsorb the common ion S^{2-} from the medium. (Fig. 7–16(b))

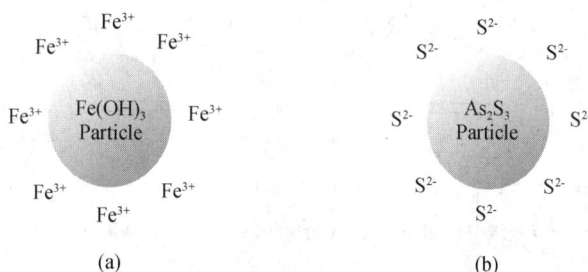

(a)   (b)

Fig. 7–16   (a) Fe(OH), sol particles adsorb Fe ions and become positive;
(b) As S sol particles adsorb S ions and acquire negative charge

$$As_2S_3 + S^{2-} \longrightarrow As_2S_3/S^{2-} \quad \text{Negative arsenic sulphide sol particle}$$

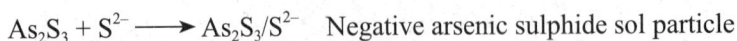

It is not necessary that a sol particle always adsorbs the same kind of ions. In fact, the particles may adsorb the anions or cations whichever are in excess and acquire the corresponding charge. According to Fajans rule of thumb, sol particles selectively adsorb ions with the same or similar composition, and the adsorbed ions are called potential-determining ions. For example, AgCl sol produced by the addition of $AgNO_3$ solution to sodium chloride solution, bears a positive charge if Ag^+ ions are in excess. On the other hand, if Cl^- ions are in excess, the AgCl sol particles acquire a negative charge. (Fig. 7–17)

The adsorption of electrolyte ions by the sol core is related to its hydration ability, and ions with weak hydration ability are easily adsorbed on the surface of the sol core.

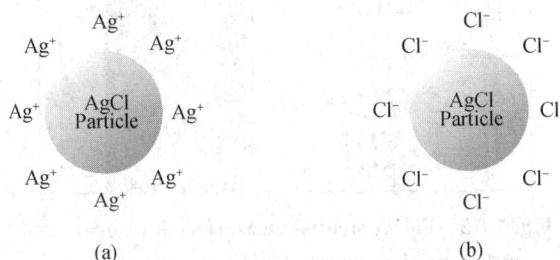

(a)　　　　　　　　　　　(b)

Fig. 7–17　(a) When Ag^+ ions are in excess, AgCl sol particle adsorbs these ions and becomes positive
(b) when Cl^- ions are in excess, the AgCl particle adsorbs these and acquires a negative charge

7.2.2　Ionization of Surface Groups

(1) Charge on soaps and detergent sols. Soaps and detergent sol particles are aggregates of many molecules. The hydrocarbons tails of the molecules are directed to the centre, while the groups $—COO^-$ Na^+ (or $—OSO_3Na^+$) constitute the surface in contact with water. As the ionization of the surface groups, the particle surface is now made of the anionic heads $—COO^-$ (or $—OSO_3^-$). This makes the sol particle negative.

(2) Charge on Protein Sols. Protein sol particles possess both acidic and basic functional groups. In aqueous solution at low pH, the $—NH_2$ group (basic) acquires a proton to get $—NH_3^+$, while at high pH, the $—COOH$ group (acidic) transfers a proton to OH^- to get $—COO^-$. Thus, the protein sol particle has positive charge at low pH and negative charge at high pH. At an intermediate pH called the **isoelectric point (等电点)**, the particles will be electrically neutral. The changes in the charge of the protein sol are shown by the direction of movement of the dispersed phase in electrophoresis. (Fig. 7–18)

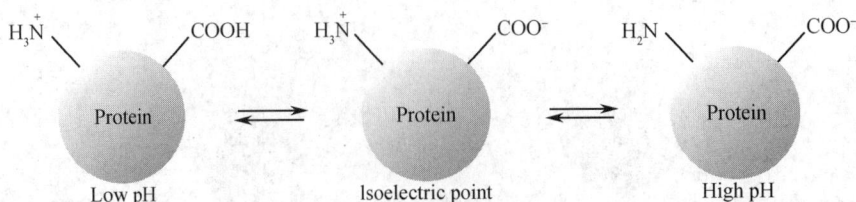

Low pH　　　　　　Isoelectric point　　　　　　High pH

Fig. 7–18　Charge on protein sol changes with pH

7.2.3　Two-phase friction charging

Cohen rule of thumb states that one phase with a large dielectric constant is positively charged and the other phase is negatively charged when two phases are in contact with friction.

7.3   Electrical double layer theory

If the surface of colloidal particle acquires a positive charge by selective adsorption of a layer of positive ions around it, this layer will attract counterions from the medium which form a second layer of negative charges. The combination of the two layer charges around the sol particle was called **Helmholtz double layer (亥姆霍兹双电层)**. Helmholtz thought that positive charges next to the particle surface were fixed, while the layer of negative charges along with the medium were mobile, as **Gouy** and **Chapman (古依-查普曼扩散双电层)** have proposed the diffuse layer. (Fig. 7–19)

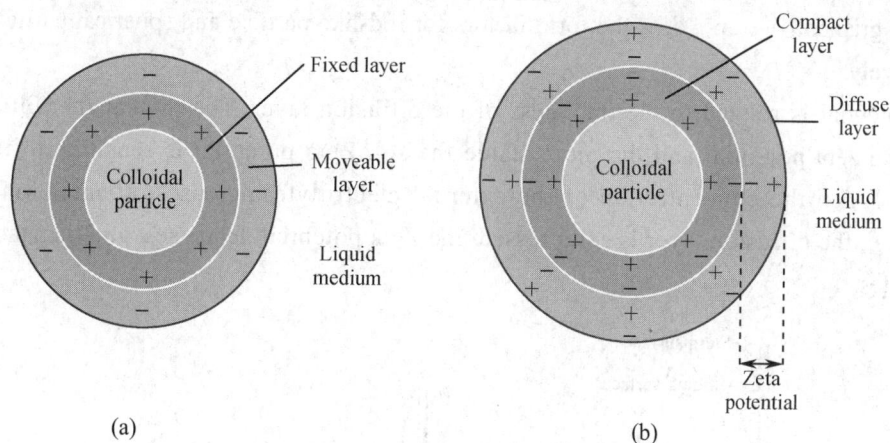

Fig. 7–19   Helmholtz double layer (a) and the
electrical double layer (Stern) (b)

More recent considerations have shown that the double layer is made of:

(a) A **compact layer (紧密层)** of positive and negative charges which are fixed firmly on the particle surface.

(b) A **diffusion layer (扩散层)** of counterions diffused into the medium containing positive ions.

The combination of the compact and diffuse layer is referred to as the **Stern Double layer (斯特恩双电层)** after the colloid chemist who first realized its significance. The diffusion layer is only loosely attached to the particle surface and moves in the opposite direction under an applied electric field. Because of the distribution of the charge around the particle, there is a difference in potential between the compact layer and the bulk of solution across the diffuse layer. The counter ions and solvent molecules in the solution are subjected to a sufficiently large electrostatic force, van der Waals force or characteristic adsorption force, and are tightly adsorbed on the solid surface to form a tight layer. The remaining counter ions constitute a diffusion layer. Here, sliding surface refers to the interface where the solid and liquid phases move relative to each other. It is an uneven surface outside the Stern surface. Under the action of an external electric field, the solid surface always moves with a thin layer of liquid, and the position where the solid and liquid are dislocated in the electric field is the relative sliding surface. The potential difference between the sliding surface and the solution body is called by **electrokinetic potential** or **Zeta potential (ζ-电势)**. The charged rubber particles only show a sliding surface when they are moving, so electric potential is also called electromotive potential.

So, the electric double layer includes two parts, a compact layer, and a diffusion layer, and includes three potentials (Fig. 7–20). Firstly, solid surface potential (φ_0) is the potential difference between the surface of the solid particles and the natural solution which can be measured electrochemically. Secondly, stern potential (φ_δ) is the potential difference between the Stern surface and the bulk solution. The third potential is electromotive potential (ζ) between the sliding surface and the bulk solution, which can be measured by electrodynamic phenomenon with equation (7–13).

$$\zeta = \frac{K\eta u}{\varepsilon_0 D_r E} \tag{7–13}$$

where η is the medium viscosity, Pa · s; u is the electrophoresis rate, m · s^{-1}; ε_0 is the dielectric constant of vacuum, $\varepsilon_0 = 8.85 \times 10^{-12}$ C · V^{-1} · m^{-1}; Dr is the dielectric constant of medium relative to vacuum; E is the potential gradient, V · m^{-1}. K is the form factors for rod-like particle and spherical particle are 1 and 1.5, respectively.

Zeta potential is related to the thickness of the diffusion layer. The thicker the diffusion layer, the larger the zeta potential and the more stable the sol. Zeta potential is sensitive to the external electrolyte. When the concentration of the external electrolyte increases, counter ions enter the compact layer, the diffusion layer is compressed, the Zeta potential decreases, and the stability of the sol deteriorates.

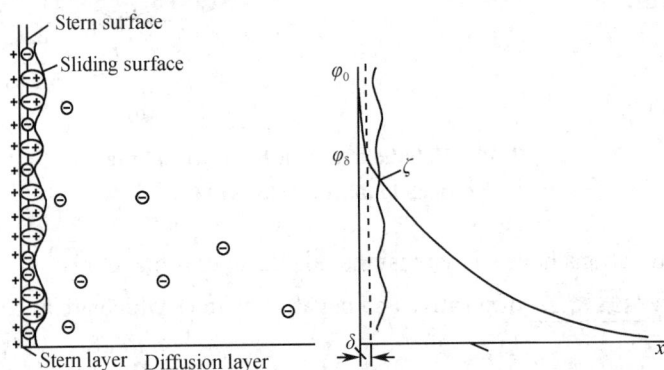

Fig. 7–20   The composition and three potentials of Stern Double layer

The presence of the double layer accounts for the electrical properties: (a) Cataphoresis; and (b) Electro-osmosis of colloids. It has been made possible to estimate the magnitude of the Zeta potential with the help of these properties. We have explained the theory of electrical double layer taking example of a positive sol. Our considerations could well be applied to a negative sol with the interchange of the disposition of positive and negative ions.

7.4 Structure of colloidal micelle

Based on the electrical double layer theory of sol, the internal structure and surface charge of sol particles can be understood. The center of a colloidal particle is called **colloidal nucleus (胶核)**, which is composed of a collection of atoms or molecules. Close to the colloidal nucleus, the ions adsorbed on the surface of the colloidal nucleus, known as potential-determining ions, and some of the negatively charged ions form the compact layer. The combination of colloidal nucleus and the compact layer is called **colloidal particle (胶粒)**. Outside the compact layer, the diffusion layer is made up of the ions with opposite charges. The whole of the colloidal nucleus, the compact layer and the diffusion layer is called

colloidal micelle (胶团) , which is electrically neutral.

For example, AgCl sol bears a positive charge when NaCl is in excess, and its colloidal structure is as follows (Fig.7–21).

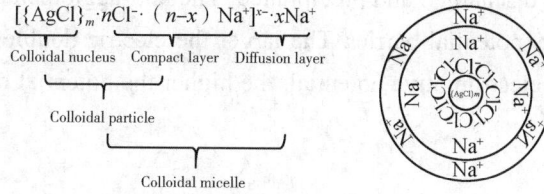

$$[\{AgCl\}_m \cdot nCl^- \cdot (n-x)\,Na^+]^{x-} \cdot xNa^+$$

Fig. 7–21 The composition and three potentials of Stern Double layer

Generally speaking, the charge of sol refers to the charge of colloidal particles. The electrical property of colloidal particles depends on the potential-determining ions adsorbed by the colloidal nucleus, and its charge amount depends on the difference between the charge of the potential-determining ions and the ions with an opposite charge in the compact layer. In the electric field, the movement of the colloidal particles is opposite to that of the diffuse layer.

Section 8　Stability and Condensation of Sol

8.1　Stability of sol

8.1.1　Kinetic stability and coalescence instability of sol

Sol is a thermodynamically unstable system. However, some sols can exist stably for a long time. For example, gold sols prepared by Faraday are left to settle on the tube wall for several decades. For this reason, various theories have been proposed, such as DLVO theory (proposed by Darjaguin, Landau, Verwey, and Overbeek in 1948), spatial stability theory and vacancy stability theory. DLVO theory holds that there are both repulsive potential energy and gravitational potential energy between sol particles.

The attractive force existing between the dispersed phase particles in the sol still has the van der Waals attractive nature in essence, but the range of this attractive force is thousands of times larger than that of ordinary molecules, so it is called remote van der Waals force. The potential energy is directly proportional to the first or second power of the distance between the particles and may be other more complex relationships. The relative stability or settling of colloidal systems depends on the relative magnitudes of the repulsive and suction potential energy. When the repulsive potential energy between particles is numerically greater than the suction potential energy, the colloid is in a relatively stable state. The particles will move closer to each other and aggregate together when the suction potential energy is numerically greater than the repulsive potential energy.

8.1.2　Factors of sol stability

The stability of sols is mainly due to three factors.

(1) Intense Brownian motion　The main factor affecting the dynamic stability of sol is dispersion. The greater the dispersion is, the more intense the Brownian motion is and the stronger the ability is.

(2) Presence of same charge on sol particles   The dispersed particles of a hydrophobic sol possess a like electrical charge (all positive or all negative) on their surface. Since like charges repel one another, the particles push away from one another and resist joining. However, when an electrolyte is added to a hydrophobic sol, the particles are discharged and precipitated. The anti-agglomeration stability of the sol depends mainly on the level of its potential barrier. The larger the electric double layer thickness of the colloidal particles, the higher the electromotive potential, the higher the potential barrier formed, and the more stable the sol (Fig.7–22).

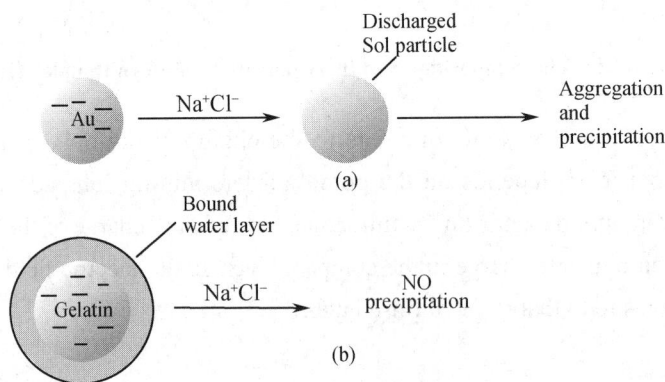

Fig. 7–22   (a) A negatively charged gold particle is precipitated by Na⁺ ions; (b) The water layer around gelatin particle does not allow Na⁺ ions to penetrate and discharge the particle

(3) Presence of Solvent layer around sol particle   The lyophilic sols are stable for two reasons. Their particles possess a charge and in addition have a layer of the solvent bound on the surface. For example, a sol particle of gelatin has a negative charge and a water layer envelope it. When sodium chloride is added to colloidal solution of gelatin, its particles are not precipitated. The water layer around the gelatin particle does not allow the Na^+ ions to penetrate it and discharge the particle. The gelatin sol is not precipitated by addition of sodium chloride solution. Evidently, lyophilic sols are more stable than lyophobic sols.

8.2   Coagulation or precipitation of sol

Sol is a highly dispersed, heterogeneous, thermodynamically unstable system with a large surface energy, so colloidal particles tend to coalesce with each other to reduce Gibbs free energy spontaneously. We know that the stability of a lyophobic sol is mainly due to the adsorption of positive or negative ions by the dispersed particles. The repulsive forces between the charged particles do not allow them to settle. If, somehow, the charge is removed, there is nothing to keep the particles apart from each other. They will aggregate (or flocculate) and settle down under the action of gravity.

The aggregation or settling down of the discharged sol particles is called coagulation or precipitation of the sol. How coagulation can be brought about? The coagulation or precipitation of a given sol can be brought about in four ways.

8.2.1   By addition of Electrolytes

When excess of an electrolyte is added to a sol, the dispersed particles are precipitated. The electrolyte furnishes both positive and negative ions in the medium. The sol particles adsorb the oppositely charged ions and get discharged. The electrically neutral particles then aggregate and settle down as precipitate (Fig. 7–23). The lowest concentration of electrolyte added when the sol begins to precipitate is called **coagulation value (聚沉值)**.The smaller the coagulation value of the electrolyte, the stronger the coagulation capacity of the electrolyte.

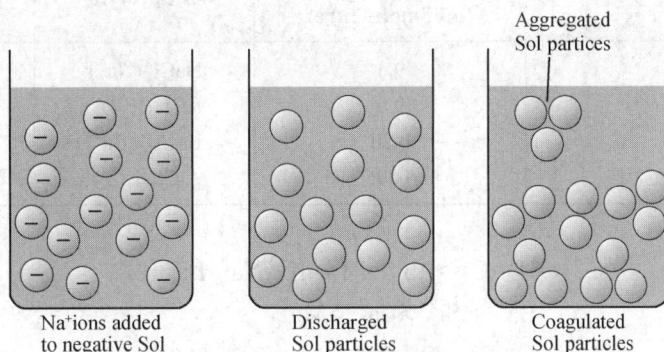

Fig. 7–23　Coagulation of a Sol (illustration)

A negative ion (anion) causes the precipitation of a positively charged sol, and *vice versa*. The effectiveness of an anion or cation to precipitate a sol, will naturally depend on the magnitude of the charge or valence of the effective ion. From a study of the precipitating action of various electrolytes on sol, Hardy and Schulze gave a general rule.

Schulze-Hardy Rule (舒尔茨–哈迪规则) states that the precipitating effect of an ion on dispersed phase of opposite charge increases with the valence of the ion. The higher the counter ion valence, the stronger the ability to settle. The coagulation ability is directly proportional to the sixth power of the valence Z of the ions with opposite sol electrical properties ($F \propto Z^6$).

The higher the valency of the effective ion, the greater is its precipitating power. Thus, for precipitating an As_2S_3 sol (negative), the precipitating power of Al^{3+}, Ba^{2+}, Na^+ ions is in the order

$$Al^{3+} > Ba^{2+} > Na^+$$

Similarly, for precipitating $Fe(OH)_3$ sol (positive), the precipitating power of cations $[Fe(CN)_6]^{3-}$, SO_4^{2-}, Cl^- is in the order.

$$[Fe(CN)_6]^{3-} > SO_4^{2-} > Cl^-$$

The precipitation power of an electrolyte or ion is experimentally determined by finding the minimum concentration in millimoles per liter required to cause the precipitation of a sol in 2 hours. This is called the flocculation value. The smaller the flocculation value, the higher the precipitating power of an ion.

It may be noted how rapidly the precipitation power increases with the increases of valence. The ratio for the mono-, di-, and trivalent anion or cation are approximately $1:40:90$ for $Fe(OH)_3$ sol and $1:70:500$ for the As_2S_3 sol (Table 7–4).

The coagulation ability of the same valence ions is also different. The order of the ions with the same charge according to the coagulation ability is called **the lyotropic series (感胶离子序)**. The coalescence ability of homologous positive ions on negatively charged sols increases with increasing atomic weight or ion radius, and the coalescence ability of homologous negative ions on positively charged sols decreases with increasing atomic weight or ion radius.

Table 7-4　Flocculation values

(Fe(OH)₃ Sol)		As₂S₃ Sol	
Electrolyte	Concentration (millimoles/litre)	Electrolyte	Concentration (millimoles/litre)
NaCl, (Cl⁻)	9.3	NaCl, (Na⁺)	51
KCl, (Cl⁻)	9.0	KCl, (K⁺)	50
K_2SO_4, $(SO_4)^{2-}$	0.20	$BaCl_2$, (Ba^{2+})	0.69
$K_3Fe(CN)_6$, $[Fe(CN)_6]^{3-}$	0.096	$AlCl_3$, (Al^{3+})	0.093

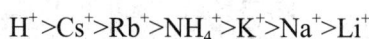

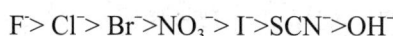

$$H^+ > Cs^+ > Rb^+ > NH_4^+ > K^+ > Na^+ > Li^+$$
$$Ba^{2+} > Sr^{2+} > Ca^{2+} > Mg^{2+}$$
$$F^- > Cl^- > Br^- > NO_3^- > I^- > SCN^- > OH^-$$

The ions with the same electrical properties as sol are helpful to the stability of the colloidal system, the higher the valence, the smaller the coalescence ability to the sol. In addition, some special effects of certain ions on sol agglomeration are described. The ability of H^+ to negatively charge sols and OH^- to positively charge sols is greater than the corresponding 1-1 valence salts. For the ions with opposite electrical properties to sols, if they can react with the ions on the colloidal particles and form insoluble substances, their coagulation abilities are particularly strong.

8.2.2　By mixing two oppositely charged sols

The mutual coagulation of two sols of opposite charge can be affected by mixing them. The positive particles of one sol are attracted by the negative particles of the second sol. This is followed by mutual adsorption and precipitation of both the sols. Ferric hydroxide (+ve sol) and arsenious sulphide (–ve sol) form such a pair. In the process of alum purification of water, the hydrolysis product ($Al(OH)_3$ sol) with positive charge mutually coagulates with the negatively charged suspended substances in the water.

8.2.3　By electrophoresis

In electrophoresis, the charged sol particles migrate to the electrode of opposite sign. As they encounter the electrode, the particles are discharged and precipitated.

8.2.4　Other factors on sol condensation

(1) Influence of physical factors, such as concentration, temperature, and external force field. Increasing concentration increases the chance of particle collisions and makes colloidal particles agglomerate more easily. With the increase of temperature, the sol condensation increases with the increase of the chance and strength of particle collision. Such as sulphur sol and silver halides sol dispersed in water, may be coagulated by boiling. Increased collisions between the sol particles and water molecules remove the adsorbed electrolyte and settle down. Because the density of colloidal particles and media is different, the sol will be precipitated under the action of centrifugal force.

(2) Effect of macromolecules on colloidal particles　The influence of macromolecular compounds on the stability of sol is related to its concentration. When a small number of macromolecules are added to the sol, macromolecules act as bridges to colloidal particles, which will reduce the stability of the sol and promote the aggregation of the sol. This is sensitization of macromolecules to sol (Fig. 7–24a).

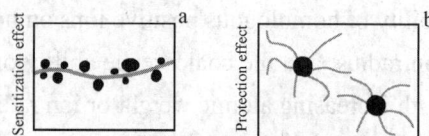

Fig. 7–24　Sensitization (a) and protection (b) of colloidal particles by macromolecule

Adding a larger number of macromolecules to the phobic sol can protect the sol from being settled. This phenomenon is called the protective effect of the macromolecular solution on the sol (Fig. 7–24b). The macromolecules are adsorbed around the colloidal particles of the hydrophobic sol, so that the colloidal particles cannot be directly contacted, which can prevent the sol particles being aggregated.

(3) Impact of organic matter and organic ions   Hydration film is one of the important factors for the stability of colloidal particles. Organic substances with strong hydrophilicity, such as ethanol, can easily take away the colloidal hydration film, causing the coagulation of sol.

Many organic ions are easily adsorbed by the colloidal particles and enter the compact layer, which has a relatively large settling capacity for the sol.

重 点 小 结

（1）溶胶的主要特征、制备方法和净化方法。
（2）溶胶体系的光学性质，特别是溶胶散射光强弱的影响因素分析。
（3）溶胶的动力性质，特别是有关扩散和沉降的现象分析和原因解释。
（4）溶胶的电学性质，特别是溶胶的电泳和电渗等电动现象。
（5）溶胶表面电荷的来源分析；溶胶的双电层理论和胶团结构式。
（6）溶胶稳定性和溶胶聚沉的因素分析。

Object detection

习题题库

I. Select the correct option for the following problems (one option for each problem).

1. The purpose of sol purification is to

    A. remove excess electrolyte   B. remove mechanical impurities

    C. increase of sol particles   D. infiltration stabilizer

2. Tyndall effect is caused by (   ) of colloidal particles on visible light.

    A. Diffraction   B. Reflection

    C. Scattering   D. Refraction

3. The coagulation values of $MgCl_2$ and $AlCl_3$ on AgI sol are 0.72 and 0.093 $mmol \cdot dm^{-3}$, respectively. Please judge the coagulation values of KCl on AgI sol.

    A. greater than 0.72 $mmol \cdot dm^{-3}$ B. less than 0.72 $mmol \cdot dm^{-3}$

    C. between 0.093 and 0.72 $mmol \cdot dm^{-3}$ D. less than 0.093 $mmol \cdot dm^{-3}$

4. Which of the following is the one that maintains the stability of the sol and easily destroys the sol?

    A. Brownian motion   B. Solvation

    C. Electrolyte   D. Scattering

5. Which of the following is not the origin of charge on colloidal particles?

A. Adsorption of ions from the aqueous medium

B. Ionisation of surface groups

C. Two-phase friction

D. Electrophoresis

II. Try to answer the following problem.

How does the electrophoresis provide information about the sign of charge on colloidal particles?

Reference answers

I. 1.A; 2.C; 3.A; 4.C; 5.D.

II. Omitted.

Chapter 8　Macromolecular Solution

学习目标

知识要求

1.掌握

（1）大分子化合物的结构特征。

（2）掌握大分子溶液的性质、大分子电解质溶液的性质。

2.熟悉

（1）大分子溶液的反常渗透压。

（2）大分子溶液黏度的几种表示方法。

（3）唐南膜平衡的概念及应用。

3.了解

（1）几种不同平均摩尔质量的定义与实验测定方法。

（2）凝胶的制备、分类和胶凝作用。

能力要求

1. 能够运用唐南膜平衡原理分析实际问题

2. 能够运用黏度法测定大分子化合物的摩尔质量

Macromolecules, also known as polymers, are very large molecules （"macro" is the Greek for large) built up of many molecular units which are linked together usually by covalent bonds. Their sizes range from 1 to 100nm and molecular weights excess $10000 \text{g} \cdot \text{mol}^{-1}$.

There are basically two types of macromolecules: natural and synthetic ones. Naturally occurring macromolecules include polysaccharides, proteins and nucleic acids, making up many of the materials in living organisms and playing highly specific roles in life. Synthetic macromolecules, which do not exist in nature, are man-made materials, such as plastics, rubbers and textiles, etc. Such macromolecules are indispensable in life and have a great industrial importance. Generally, the chains of natural macromolecules have more identical repeating units, more ordered, and more rigid than those of the synthetic ones.

Macromolecules are closely related to colloids. Historically colloids were known first, while macromolecules were recognized only in the early 1900s. Today, we realize that colloids and macromolecules are different entities but some of the same laws that govern colloids also govern macromolecules.

Section 1　Structure of Macromolecular Compound

1.1　Structural characteristics of macromolecular compound

Macromolecule consists of large number of repeating units, which are called of monomer units, structure units or simply monomers. For example, polyethylene (Fig. 8–1 (a)) is built up of the monomer unit of the methylene group and n is the degree of polymerization. The structures of another two common macromolecules are shown schematically in Fig. 8–1. The long macromolecular chain may take on many different configurations. Fig. 8–2 lists some typical architectures of the macromolecular chains.

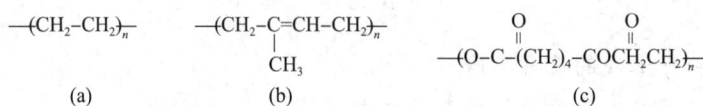

$$-(CH_2-CH_2)_n- \qquad -(CH_2-C=CH-CH_2)_n- \qquad -(O-C-(CH_2)_4-COCH_2CH_2)_n-$$
$$CH_3$$

(a) (b) (c)

Fig. 8–1　THE Chemical structures of some common macromolecules:
(a) Polyethylene; (b) Polyisoprene (rubber); (c) Polyester(fiber)

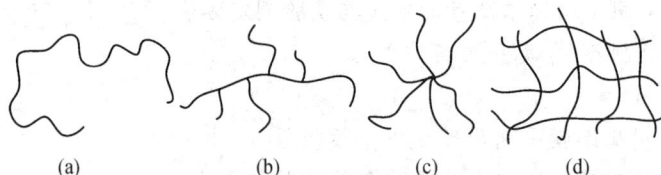

(a) (b) (c) (d)

Fig. 8–2　Some typical topological architectures of macromolecules:
(a) Linear; (b) Branched; (c) Star; (d) Cross-linked

Due to the large number of monomers, each macromolecule possesses a huge number of internal degrees of freedom as discussed in the following, presenting huge difference with that of low-molecular-weight compounds. In order to understand the properties of macromolecular solutions, it is necessary to start with a discussion of the conformational states of single chains. Here we may concentrate on the semi-flexibility of macromolecular chains. Many factors may determine macromolecular semi-flexibility, but the most common factor is the internal rotation. Let us choose polyethylene as an example and consider its full steric structure. The connection of monomers on a macromolecular chain has a restricted bond angle, however, the internal rotation of each bond around the previous bond on the chain is still possible even keeping this bond angle fixed. In real macromolecules, when the chains perform the internal rotation, the substituted side groups will interact with each other, causing a hindrance to the internal rotation, as illustrated in Fig. 8–3. There are three relatively stable conformations in the potential energy curve of the internal rotation of polyethylene, which can be regarded as the representative states in the statistics of macromolecule chain conformations. The potential energy difference $\Delta\varepsilon$ between the local minima in Fig. 8–3 (c) plays an important role on the flexibility of macromolecular chains. When $RT \gg \Delta\varepsilon$, the C—C bonds are quasi-free, these three states will occur with almost the same probabilities, and macromolecular chains possess high flexibilities and will exhibit random coils. When $RT << \Delta\varepsilon$, macromolecular chains will exhibit the fully extended conformation with a high rigidity due to the lowest-energy conformation dominating in the distribution. It is obvious that higher temperature will result in more flexible chains. For a flexible macromolecular chain, if the internal rotation around one bond of backbone chain produces three possible states, then one macromolecular chain with 500 such bonds, which is not very long compared to the real macromolecular chain, will possess theoretically $3^{500} \approx 3.6 \times 10^{238}$, an astronomical figures of conformations. Therefore, the statistical method has to be employed in order to learn the conformational properties.

We now consider the macromolecular chains on the basis of "coarse-grained" picture. The internal rotation of one bond around its neighbouring bonds will drive simultaneously the neibourghing monomers in motion. We may statistically merge these interacting monomers as an independent unit, defining them as one segment, which is called Kuhn segment, based on the freely jointed chain model. Thus, the macromolecular chain can be represented by many connected segments with each segment acting as an independently functional unit. As a result, one macromolecular chain may act like many small molecules, making macromolecular solutions having relatively high boiling points and osmotic pressures.

Besides the factors discussed above influencing the flexibility of macromolecular chain, solvents can also have an impact on the flexibility. There is a very strong attractive interaction between the solvent molecules and the macromolecular chains in good solvents. Solvent molecules can pass through the holes or cavities formed by a macromolecular chain and cause the chain to expand or swell. While in poor solvents, the attractive interaction between the solvent molecules and the macromolecular chain is much weaker than that between segments of the macromolecular molecules themselves. The macromolecular chain will be forced closer together in order to lower the energy of the system, leading to fewer interactions between the chain and the solvent molecules (Fig. 8–4).

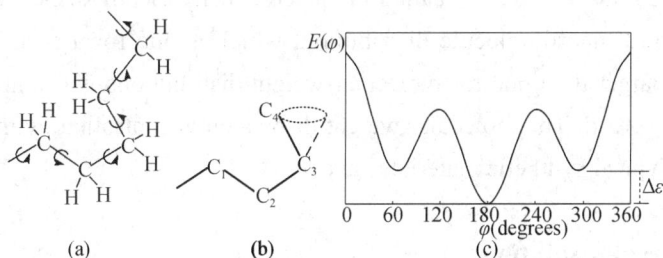

Fig. 8–3   Illustration of the internal rotation in polyethylene: (a) The general picture; (b) Internal rotation around previous bond with fixed bond angle; (c) The potential energy curve of the internal rotation of polyethylene

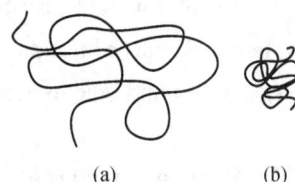

Fig. 8–4   Macromolecular configurations in solvents: (a) Expanded in a good solvent; (b) Coiled in a poor solvent

1.2   Average relative molecular mass of macromolecular compound

In contrast to small molecules and natural macromolecules with specific roles in biochemical processes, most macromolecules consist of similar molecules with different molecular weights. We can only obtain the average molecular weights and their distributions. Different experimental techniques provide different average molecular weights. There are four types of average molecular weight most frequently encountered in literature: number-average, weight-average, z-average, and viscosity-average. Assuming there are N_i macromolecular chains with molecular weight M_i, then the number-average molecular weight is defined by

$$M_n = \frac{\sum N_i M_i}{\sum N_i} = \frac{\sum c_i M_i}{\sum c_i} \tag{8-1}$$

where c_i represents the molecular concentration of the i-th macromolecular chain. Number-average molecular weight can be determined by osmotic pressure.

The weight-average and z-average molecular weights are defined as follows.

$$M_w = \frac{\sum W_i M_i}{\sum W_i} = \frac{\sum N_i M_i^2}{\sum N_i M_i} = \frac{\sum c_i M_i^2}{\sum c_i M_i} \tag{8-2}$$

$$M_z = \frac{\sum (W_i M_i) M_i}{\sum W_i M_i} = \frac{\sum N_i M_i^3}{\sum N_i M_i^2} = \frac{\sum c_i M_i^3}{\sum c_i M_i^2} \tag{8-3}$$

Here the molecular weight commonly means the molar mass of macromolecule and W_i is the molar mass of macromolecule of the i-th macromolecular chain. The weight-average and z-average molecular weights can be determined by light scattering and ultracentrifuge sedimentation methods, respectively.

Finally, the viscosity-average molecular weight is defined by

$$M_\eta = \left(\frac{\sum W_i M_i^\alpha}{\sum W_i} \right)^{\frac{1}{\alpha}} = \left(\frac{\sum N_i M_i^{\alpha+1}}{\sum N_i M_i} \right)^{\frac{1}{\alpha}} \tag{8-4}$$

which is obtained from the viscosity measurement of macromolecular dilute solutions. Here α is a constant and conventionally ranges from 0.5 to 1. We find that $M_\eta = M_n$ when $\alpha = -1$ and $M_\eta = M_w$ when $\alpha = 1$. In general, $M_n < M_\eta < M_w < M_z$. The ratio $d = M_w/M_n$, called the heterogeneity or polydispersity index, is a useful measure of the spread of a macromolecule distribution, which is one for a strictly uniform molecular-weight distribution and larger than one for molecular-weight distributions with finite widths. Larger values of d indicate a wider spread. The molecular-weight dispersion is controlled by the choice of catalyst and reaction conditions. Typical synthetic materials have $d \approx 4$.

1.3 Basic properties of macromolecular solution

Macromolecular solutions are normally homogeneous mixtures of macromolecules and small molecules. Macromolecular solutions have many similar properties to colloids, including:① the size of dispersed phase in the range of 1 to 100nm, ② inability to pass through semi-permeable membrane, and ③ slow diffusion velocity. However, they are different in essence. Macromolecular solutions are homogeneous solutions in thermodynamics equilibrium state with relatively high osmotic pressures and intrinsic viscosities, obeying the phase rule and relatively insusceptible to electrolyte. On the contrary, colloids are inhomogeneous systems in non-equilibrium with small osmotic pressures and viscosities, not obeying the phase rule and susceptible to electrolyte.

Macromolecules dissolve in solvents in several steps. Contrary to many low molecular weight substances initially diffusing into the solvent, the solvent will first wet the macromolecule and then diffuses into and swell it. Finally, the macromolecule diffuses out of the swollen mass into the solvent, completing the solution process. For macromolecules of high molecular weight, this process may take several hours or longer, depending on sample size, temperature, and so on. There are some macromolecules with cross-linked structure, that may only swell, reaching an equilibrium degree of swelling. Some macromolecules with high melting temperatures or strong internal secondary bonds cannot even be dissolved without degradation.

One of the simplest notions in chemistry is that "like dissolves like" , which is also applied to macromolecules. Here "like" may be defined variously in terms of similar chemical groups or similar polarities. Quantitatively, macromolecules are potentially mixed with solvents once the mixing free energy $\Delta G_{mix} = \Delta H_{mix} - T\Delta S_{mix} < 0$. The term $T\Delta S_{mix}$ is conventionally positive because there is an increase in the entropy on mixing, while the heat of mixing is usually positive, opposing mixing. Therefore the sign of ΔG_{mix} depends on the magnitude of ΔH_{mix}, ΔS_{mix}, and the temperature T. Thermodynamic properties of the macromolecular solution depend on how "good" the solvent is for the macromolecule as well as on the macromolecule itself.

Section 2   Macromolecular Electrolyte Solution

PPT

2.1   Significance of macromolecular electrolyte

Macromolecular electrolytes are macromolecular compounds bearing dissociated ionic groups, which is constructed by monomers containing charged chemical moieties. According to the charged state of dissociated macro-ions, macromolecular electrolytes can be classified into three types: cationic, anionic and amphoteric types, corresponding to dissociated macro-ions bearing positive, negative and both positive and negative charges. Macromolecular electrolyte often achieves a net charge from carboxylate group or from ammonium or protonated amines. For example, polyvinylamine is one of the cationic macromolecular electrolytes, while carboxymethyl cellulose and polyacrylic acid belong to the anionic macromolecular electrolytes. Proteins are typical amphoteric types. There are other counterions such as sulfate, hydrogen ions, and sodium ions in the solution of macromolecular electrolytes, which are evenly distributed around macro-ions or are surrounded in the cross-linked network formed by long chains of macro-ions. The macro-ions mixed with counterions make macromolecular electrolyte solutions exhibiting electrical properties such as conductivity and electrophoresis as well as the properties of acids, bases and salts. Natural and synthetic macromolecular electrolytes now have been widely applied in medicine, food industries, pharmacy and many other fields, which make the interest in the investigations of macromolecular electrolytes increase greatly.

2.2   Electrical properties of macromolecular electrolyte solution

The electrical properties of macromolecular electrolyte solution include weak conductivity, high charge density and high hydration. Firstly, the micro-ions dissociated from the macromolecular electrolyte move slowly and most of the counterions are bound in network formed from long chains, which makes the conductivity of the macromolecular electrolyte solution similar to that of the general weak electrolyte solution. Secondly the high charge density results from highly densely charged macromolecular electrolyte chains with the same kind charges mutually repelling each other. Thirdly in aqueous solutions, water molecules are closely arranged around the charged groups of macromolecular electrolyte, forming a special "electro-shrinking" hydration layer. In addition, there exist the hydrophobic layers formed from hydrophobic chains and water molecules. All these factors make macromolecular electrolytes highly hydrated. High charge density and high hydration make the molecular chains of macromolecular electrolytes repel each other in aqueous solution and easy to extend, increasing their stability and sensitive to small molecular electrolytes. The addition of acids, bases or salts, or the change of the pH value can cancel the interactions between the charges of the macromolecular electrolyte chains, making them behave like a macromolecular non-electrolyte.

2.3   Stability of macromolecular electrolyte solution

Benefiting from the high charge density and high hydration, macromolecular electrolyte solutions have good stability. In order to flocculate macromolecular electrolyte, large amount of electrolytes have to be added to the solution because they play roles of both neutralizing the charges and removing the solvated films of macro-ions. The addition of a large amount of electrolytes to the solution to make macromolecular electrolyte precipitate out of the solution is called salting out. The effect of salting out depends not on the valence of the ions but mainly on the ion species. When an electrolyte is added to the solution of a mixture of several macromolecular electrolytes, the macromolecular electrolytes with larger molecular weight precipitates first. Increasing the amount of electrolyte makes those of smaller molecular weight precipitate gradually. This process is called "fractional salting out", which is used widely by biochemists to isolate and purify proteins.

2.4   Buffering properties of protein

Proteins are polypeptides formed from different amino acids strung together by the peptide link, which are typical amphoteric macromolecular electrolytes. For simplicity, the structure of proteins may be described as $R\begin{smallmatrix} \diagup COOH \\ \diagdown NH_2 \end{smallmatrix}$, where —COOH, —NH$_2$ and R represent all carboxyl, amino groups and the remaining parts in the proteins, respectively. Proteins are amphoteric ions in solutions because of the following reactions.

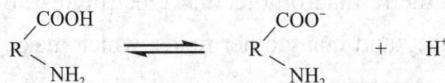

$$R\begin{smallmatrix} \diagup COOH \\ \diagdown NH_2 \end{smallmatrix} \rightleftharpoons R\begin{smallmatrix} \diagup COO^- \\ \diagdown NH_2 \end{smallmatrix} + H^+$$

where the carboxyl groups dissociate hydrogen ions to give proteins bearing negative charges, resulting in an acidic solution. On the other hand, the amino groups may obtain hydrogen ions to form protonated amines, leading to proteins bearing positive charges to obtain a basic solution.

$$R \diagup \overset{\text{COOH}}{\underset{\text{NH}_2}{}} + H^+ \rightleftharpoons R \diagup \overset{\text{COOH}}{\underset{\text{NH}_3^+}{}}$$

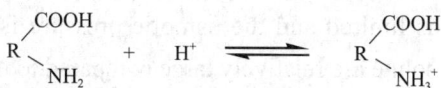

The amount of —COO⁻ and —NH$_3^+$ depends on the pH values. There exists a pH value, called **isoelectric point (pI)**(等电点), at which the amount of —COO⁻ and —NH$_3^+$ is equal and the protein is neutral. As the pH decreases, the amount of positive charge on the molecule increases by protonating a —COO⁻ or an —NH$_2$ group. When the pH is less than the pI, the molecule is positively charged. When the pH is greater than the pI, the molecule must be negatively charged. Each protein has its own pI, at which the properties of proteins have significant changes, making the viscosity, solubility, osmotic pressure and stability decrease to the minima (Fig. 8–5).

Many macromolecules, such as protein, are charged in the solution and move in response to an electric field. This motion is called electrophoresis. The electrophoretic mobility of a macromolecule in an electric field

Fig. 8–5   The illustration of the significant changes of the protein properties at the pI

depends on its net charge, size and shape. By using of the difference among the mobility of various macromolecules in an electric field, macromolecules can be separated from the mixtures. Generally protein electrophoresis is done in a buffer solution which guarantees the proteins in the mixture bearing the same charge and moving to the same direction in order to separate the proteins efficiently.

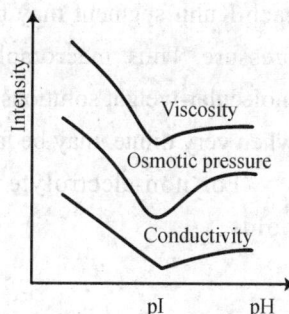

2.5   Interaction of macromolecular electrolytes

The macromolecular electrolytes may be flocculated in the solution by the addition of other macromolecular electrolytes of the opposite charge type. The mixture of macromolecular electrolytes of the same charge type does not flocculate. For example, for two proteins with pIs equal to 4.7 and 6.5, respectively, when the value of pH is in the range of about 5 to 6, then they have opposite charges and the mixture of these solutions will result in flocculation. When the pH is less than 4 or greater than 7, the mixture of the solutions will not result in flocculation because of the same charge type of the two charged proteins in this situation.

Section 3   Osmotic Pressure of Macromolecular Solution

PPT

3.1   Abnormal osmotic pressure of macromolecular solution

The osmotic pressure Π, one of the four well-known colligative properties of a non-electrolyte solution, is a property of primary interest in the discussion of macromolecular solution behavior. The thermodynamic basis of macromolecular solutions exhibiting osmotic pressures lies in the inequality between the chemical potentials of the pure solvent and the solvent in the solution. In the dilute solutions, the number of macromolecules is limited and the osmotic pressure is relatively small. However, the interactions between solvent and solute are relatively large compared to those between smaller molecules. As discussed in section 8.1, a real macromolecular chain may be divided into many Kuhn segments and each Kuhn segment may be viewed as an independent functional unit to have impact on the osmotic pressure. Thus, macromolecular solutions will have much more osmotic pressure than that of low-molecular-weight solutions with the same concentration. The behavior of macromolecular solutions, even when very dilute, may be far from ideal.

For non-electrolyte (electrically neutral molecules) of ideal solution, van't Hoff equation holds

$$\frac{\Pi}{c} = \frac{RT}{M} \tag{8-5}$$

where c, M and T are concentration, molecular weight and temperature, respectively. For non-electrolyte macromolecular solution, the deviation from ideal solution is large. Similar to the treatment of non-ideal gas, a Virial expansion can also be performed on the osmotic pressure of dilute macromolecular solutions

$$\frac{\Pi}{c} = RT(A_1 + A_2 c + A_3 c^2 + \cdots) \tag{8-6}$$

Here the A_i is the i-th Virial coefficients. The first Virial coefficient is

$$A_1 = \frac{1}{M_n} \tag{8-7}$$

which reflects the colligative property of ideal solutions. Interactions between one macromolecular molecule and the solvent result in the second Virial coefficient, A_2. Multiple macromolecule–solvent interactions produce higher Virial coefficients, A_3, A_4, and so on. For dilute macromolecular solutions, the series can be truncated from the second term and be simplified as

$$\frac{\Pi}{c} = \frac{RT}{M_n} + A_2 RT c \tag{8-8}$$

A_2 is a measure of the nonideality of the solution. A positive A_2 appearing in good solvents deviates upward compared with that of the ideal solution, while a negative value appearing in poor solvents deviates downward as shown in Fig. 8–6. There exists a temperature called Flory theta-temperature at which the second Virial coefficient vanishes and the solution becomes quasi-ideal and exhibits ideal chain behavior.

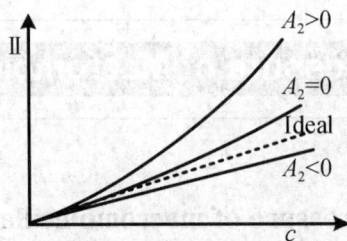

Fig. 8–6　The illustration of osmotic pressure deviation
from ideal solution depending on the sign of A_2

3.2　Determination of average relative molecular mass of macromolecules by osmotic pressure

According to equation (8-8), a straight line will be obtained by plotting osmotic pressure Π/RTc as a function of macromolecular concentration c. The number-average molecular weight and A_2 can be obtained from the slope and intercept of that line, respectively. This is the theoretical basis of the determination of number-average molecular weight by the osmotic pressure. It may be noticed that the limiting values $c \to 0$ change with the molecular weight.

$$\lim_{c \to 0} \frac{\Pi}{RTc} = \frac{1}{M} \tag{8-9}$$

Much larger M resulting in much smaller osmotic pressure, may cause the error of experiment too large. So only when M ranges from 1×10^4 to 5×10^5, the number-average molecular weights from osmotic pressure will be reliable.

3.3　Donnan membrane balance

Let us consider the equilibrium across a semi-permeable membrane between a solution containing macromolecular electrolyte and another solution containing small molecule salts as shown in Fig. 8-7. The semi-permeable membrane prevents macromolecular ions passing through, but allows solvent and other small ions, to pass through. In the final equilibrium small ions must be unequally distributed on the two sides of the membrane. This phenomenon, first pointed out by Donnan, is called **Donnan membrane balance (equilibrium)**（唐南平衡）.

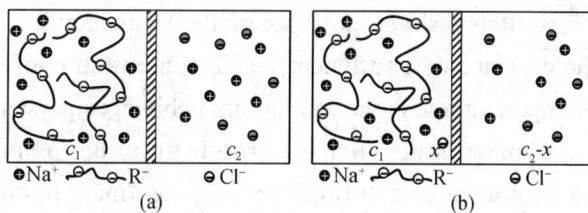

Fig. 8-7　Donnan equilibrium between a macromolecular electrolyte solution and small molecule salt: (a) Before equilibrium; (b) In equilibrium

Suppose a container is divided into two chambers by a semi-permeable membrane as shown in Fig. 8-7 (a) and the left chamber is filled with some macromolecular electrolyte solution NaR. If the right chamber is filled with pure water, the Na^+ ions dissociated from the macromolecular electrolyte in the left chamber will not diffuse into the right chamber due to the charge neutrality condition. Now if the right chamber is filled with NaCl solution, a portion of Na^+ ions and Cl^- ions can move to the left chamber. But their concentrations in the two chambers cannot be equal due to the charge neutrality condition.

The equilibrium distribution of small ions in the two chambers can be determined as follows. When the system is in equilibrium, the chemical potential of NaCl in both sides will be the same

$$\mu_{NaCl,left} = \mu_{NaCl,right} \tag{8-10}$$

thus,

$$RT\ln a_{\mathrm{NaCl,left}} = RT\ln a_{\mathrm{NaCl,right}} \tag{8-11}$$

$$a_{\mathrm{NaCl,left}} = a_{\mathrm{NaCl,right}} \tag{8-12}$$

The activity of an electrolyte is the product of the constituent ion activities, so we have

$$a_{\mathrm{Na^+,left}}a_{\mathrm{Cl^-,left}} = a_{\mathrm{Na^+,right}}a_{\mathrm{Cl^-,right}} \tag{8-13}$$

The ion activities in the dilute solution can be approximated by their concentrations,

$$c_{\mathrm{Na^+,left}}c_{\mathrm{Cl^-,left}} = c_{\mathrm{Na^+,right}}c_{\mathrm{Cl^-,right}} \tag{8-14}$$

According to equation (8–14), the products of the constituent ion concentrations of both sides are equal in Donnan membrane balance.

Suppose there are x mol $\cdot$ L^{-1} Na$^+$ ions and Cl$^-$ ions diffuse from the right chamber into the left chamber in reaching equilibrium. Substituting the concentrations of Na$^+$ ions and Cl$^-$ ions into equation (8–14), we have

$$(c_1+x)x = (c_2-x)^2 \tag{8-15}$$

$$x = \frac{c_2^2}{c_1+2c_2} \tag{8-16}$$

According to equation (8–16), the number of small-molecule electrolyte diffusing across semi-permeable membrane depends on the initial concentrations of macromolecular electrolyte and small-molecule electrolyte. When $c_1 \gg c_2$, $x \approx 0$, i.e., almost no small-molecule electrolyte diffuses into the left chamber across the semi-permeable membrane in equilibrium. However, when $c_1 \ll c_2$, $x \approx 1/2c_2$, which indicates that in this situation about one half of small-molecule electrolyte diffuse into macromolecular electrolyte solution and small-molecule electrolyte is distributed equally in both sides. This is a very important conclusion, for it is often desirable to suppress the Donnan effect, and we can see that this goal can be achieved in the presence of a sufficiently high concentration of neutral salt. The Donnan membrane balance plays an important role in the equilibrium in biological systems.

The osmotic pressure of macromolecular electrolyte solutions is much larger than that of usual non-electrolytic macromolecular solutions because one macromolecular electrolyte chain can dissociate much more small ions. However, we can still expand the osmotic pressure of macromolecular electrolyte solutions in the similar form as equation (8–6). Then the limit of Π/c at zero concentration can be used to determine the molecular weights of macromolecular electrolytes as well as of neutral macromolecules.

On the other hand, Donnan effect has great influence on the accurate determination of the osmotic pressure of macromolecular electrolyte solutions. In Fig. 8–7, if the right chamber is filled with pure water, small ions dissociated from the macromolecular electrolyte in the left chamber cannot diffuse into the right chamber. They are forced to stay in the left chamber to keep the solution neutral. The imbalance in the solute concentration between the two chambers then creates an osmotic pressure, which will overestimate the osmotic pressure of macromolecular electrolyte solution and underestimate the number-average molecular weight of macromolecular electrolyte as discussed in the following.

In displayed in Fig. 8–7, in Donnan equilibrium, the number-average molecular weight is determined by the osmotic pressures extrapolated to infinite dilution. The osmotic pressure Π of the system is the osmotic pressure difference of those of left and right chambers, we have

$$\Pi = \Pi_{\text{left}} - \Pi_{\text{right}} = 2(c_1 + x)\frac{RT}{M} - 2(c_2 - x)\frac{RT}{M} = \frac{RT}{M}\left(2c_1 \frac{c_1 + c_2}{c_1 + 2c_2}\right) \qquad (8\text{--}17)$$

Here equation (8–16) is used. Equation (8–17) is the formula of osmotic pressure of macromolecular electrolyte in Donnan equilibrium with small-molecule electrolyte. It is obvious that when $c_1 \gg c_2$, $\Pi = 2c_1 \frac{RT}{M}$, i.e., the osmotic pressure of macromolecular electrolyte is highly overestimated, making molecular weight underestimated. In contrast, when $c_1 \ll c_2$, $\Pi = 2c_1 \frac{RT}{M}$, just the formula of neutral macromolecule, i.e., in this situation macromolecular electrolyte does not dissociate and looks like a neutral macromolecule. So in the determination of the number-average molecular weight of macromolecular electrolyte, the addition of some electrolyte in excess is necessary in order to eliminate Donnan effect.

Section 4   Viscosity of Macromolecular Solution

PPT

4.1   Meaning and determination method of viscosity

When a fluid flows through a pipe, flow occurs only as a result of the application of a driving force to the fluid. The resistance to flow which this force overcomes depends on the viscosity of the fluid. The more viscous the fluid, the less fluid it is.

As shown in Fig. 8–8, there are two parallel plates filled with laminar fluid. When a constant external force is applied to the upper plate, causing it moves in a uniform straight line with velocity v in the y direction, and the lower plate is fixed. The liquid will move between the plates. The liquid attached to the moving plate has the same velocity as the moving plate. The liquid attached to the fixed plate is stationary. The liquid between the two plates can be regarded as composed of a number of fluid layers parallel to the plate, forming a flow velocity distribution of large up and small down.

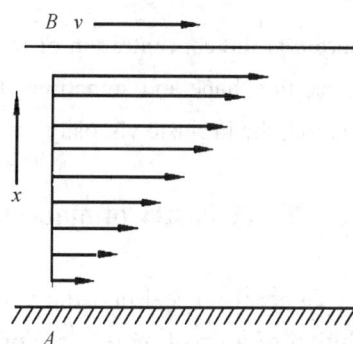

Fig. 8–8   The flow of fluid between two parallel plates

There is velocity difference between layers and relative motion between layers. As a result of the motion of the liquid molecules, the faster moving liquid layer has a force that pulls it in the direction of motion against the slower moving liquid layer next to it. At the same time, the slower moving liquid layer also acts on the faster moving liquid layer on the opposite direction of the force with the same magnitude to hinder its progress. The interaction force F between the two adjacent layers in the moving fluid due to relative movement is called shearing force of the fluid.

Suppose the contact area of the two liquid layers is A, the distance between them is dx, and the rate difference is dv. The research shows that for laminar flow, the shear force f per unit area between the two liquid layers is proportional to the rate of shear dv/dx

$$f = \frac{F}{A} = \eta \frac{dv}{dx} \qquad (8-18)$$

The coefficient η is called the viscosity coefficient or the viscosity (internal friction). It depends on the temperature and the identity of the substance.

The physical meaning of viscosity is the magnitude of the shear force generated per unit area when the velocity gradient is $1s^{-1}$. The relationship shown here is called Newton's law of viscosity.

Viscosity method:

The **relative viscosity (相对黏度)** of macromolecular solution, denoted by η_r, is given by the expression

$$\eta_r = \frac{\eta_0}{\eta} \qquad (8-19)$$

where η is viscosity of macromolecular solution and η_0 that of the solvent at the same temperature.

The **specific viscosity (增比黏度)**, denoted by η_{sp}, is given by

$$\eta_{sp} = \frac{\eta - \eta_0}{\eta_0} \qquad (8-20)$$

The **reduced viscosity (比浓黏度)**, denoted by η_c, is defined as

$$\eta_c = \frac{\eta_{sp}}{c} \qquad (8-21)$$

The intrinsic viscosity is defined as, the **intrinsic viscosity (特性黏度)** is defined as

$$[\eta] = \lim_{c \to 0} \frac{\eta_{sp}}{c} \qquad (8-22)$$

where c is the concentration of the solute. The intrinsic viscosity of macromolecule solution is used to deduce the shape and sometimes the viscosity-average molecular weight according to Mark-Houwink equation, the intrinsic viscosity $[\eta] = KM_\eta^\alpha$, where K and α are constants.

4.2　Viscosity of macromolecular solution

Generally speaking, the viscosity of macromolecular solution is much higher than that of a solution of a small molecule. For example, the viscosity of 1% rubber-benzene solution is about ten times that of pure benzene. Moreover, it does not obey Newton's law of viscosity. In a certain range, the viscosity varies with the shear force. The relationship between the shear force and the shear rate of the macromolecular solution is showed in Fig. 8–9 B. As seen from the figure, when the shear force on the macromolecular solution increases, the shear rate increases sharply, and there is no linear relationship between them. The non-horizontal segment of Fig. 8–10 B shows that its viscosity decreases with the increase of shear force. This is mainly due to the formation of a network of long chains of macromolecular solution. The higher the concentration of the solution, the longer the chains, the easier it is to form a network, and the greater the viscosity. A shear force is applied to the macromolecular solution so that the mesh structure is gradually destroyed and the viscosity is gradually reduced. When the shear force increases to a certain extent, the mesh structure is completely destroyed, and the viscosity is no longer affected by the shear force. In this case, the viscosity conforms to Newton's law of viscosity, as shown in the horizontal segment of curve B in Fig. 8–10. The viscosity resulting from the formation of a structure in solution is called structural viscosity, and its value is related to the shape of macromolecules, the concentration of the solution, the solvent used, and the temperature.

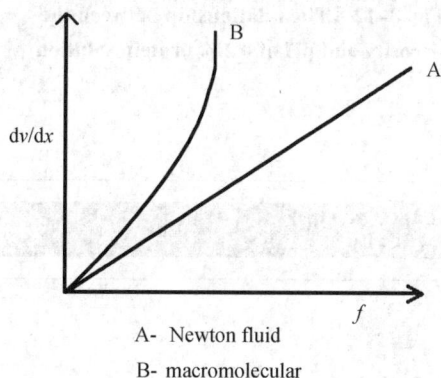

A- Newton fluid
B- macromolecular

Fig. 8–9   The relationship between dv/dx and f

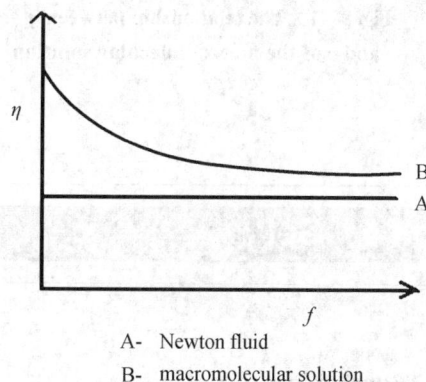

A- Newton fluid
B- macromolecular solution

Fig. 8–10   The relationship between η and f

4.3   Viscosity of macromolecular electrolyte solution

The main viscosity characteristic of macromolecular electrolyte solution is the presence of **electro-viscous effect**(电黏效应). When the concentration of the macromolecular electrolyte solution gradually becomes thinner, the ionization degree of the electrolyte solute in the water increases correspondingly, the charge density on the macromolecular chain increases, the repulsion between the chain segments increases, the molecular chain expands more, and the solution viscosity increases rapidly, which is called the electro-viscous effect. On the contrary, with the increase of solution concentration, the electro-viscous effect is reduced and the solution viscosity is decreased.

As shown in Fig. 8–11, the line a represented the relationship of η_{sp}/c and c for pectic acid aqueous solution of sodium. The results showed that addition of a certain amount of inorganic salts into macromolecule electrolyte solution (such as addition a large number of NaCl into the pectic acid sodium solution), small molecular electrolyte with sufficient ionic strength will appear around the chains of macromolecules. As a result, the ionization degree of macromolecules will be reduced with increasing the curling of molecular chain. The electro-viscosity effect is eliminated and the viscosity drops rapidly, which is attributed to make a linear relationship between η_{sp}/c and c, as shown in Fig. 8–11 in the line b.

The effect of pH on the viscosity of amphoteric protein solution is obvious. Fig. 8–12 shows the relationship between the viscosity and pH of 0.2% protein solution. The electro-viscous effect is most obvious around pH=3 and pH=11, so there are two peaks. When the pH value reaches about 4.8, that is, close to its isoelectric point, the number of positive charges on the chain is equal to the number of negative charges. The molecular chain is highly crimped due to the reduction of repulsion, and the solution viscosity is minimized.

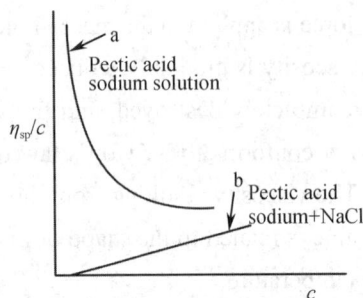

Fig. 8–11　The relationship between η_{sp}/c
and c of the macromolecular solution

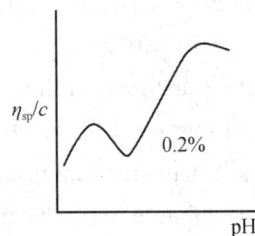

Fig. 8–12　The relationship between the
viscosity and pH of 0.2% protein solution

Section 5　Gel

5.1　Formation of gel

A **gel (凝胶)** is a semirigid colloidal system of at least two components in which both components extend continuously throughout the system. For example, when a warm sol of gelatin is cooled, it sets to a semisolid mass which is a gel.

There are two main methods to prepare gel. One method is the macromolecular solution gelation method, that is, take a certain amount of macromolecular material in the appropriate solvent and heating dissolved, standing, cooling, so that its automatic gelation. Another method is drying macromolecular compound to swell, which is used of macromolecular compound dissolved in the appropriate solvent, control the amount of solvent, so that it stays in the swelling phase to get the formation of gel.

5.2　Structure of gel

Gels may be classified into two types:

(1) Elastic gels are those which posses the property of elasticity. They change their shape on applying force and return to original shape when the force is removed. Gelatin, starch and soaps are examples of substances which form elastic gels. Elastic gels are obtained by cooling fairly concentrated lyophilic sols. The linkages between the molecules (particles) are due to electrical attraction and are not rigid.

(2) Non-elastic gels are those which are rigid e.g., silica gel. These are prepared by appropriate chemical action. Thus silica gel is produced by adding concentrated hydrochloric acid to sodium silicate solution of the correct concentration. The resulting molecules of silicic acid polymerise to form silica gel. It has a network linked by covalent bonds which give a strong and rigid structure.

5.3   Gelation and influencing factors

The process of a gel formation is known as **gelation (胶凝)**. Gelation may be thought of as partial coagulation of a sol. The coagulating sol particles first unite to form long thread-like chains. These chains are then interlocked to form a solid framework. The liquid dispersion medium gets trapped in the cavities of this framework. The resulting semisolid porous mass has a gel structure. A sponge soaked in water is an illustration of gel structure. The formation of the gel is facilitated by asymmetrical particle shapes, lowering temperatures, the addition of gelling agents (such as electrolytes), increasing concentrations of dispersed substances, and the prolonged storage time.

The worse the symmetry of the macromolecules, the better the gelation. Linear macromolecules such as gelatin, starch, rubber, pectin, and gum are easy to glue into a gel. Otherwise, symmetric spherical macromolecules do not gel in low concentrations. Protein molecules in the blood are spherical and do not gel easily, so they can flow smoothly in the blood vessels. The larger the concentration of macromolecular solution, the smaller the distance between macromolecules, the easier it is to bond with each other to form a network structure and cause gelation. The temperature has a significant effect on gelation. When the temperature rises, the macromolecules are not easy to cross link into the network structure due to the intensified thermal movement, and cannot undergo gelation. Therefore, low temperature is favorable for gelation.

5.4   Swelling and influencing factors of dry glue

Partially dehydrate elastic gels imbibe water when immersed in the solvent. This causes increase in the volume of the gel and process is called **swelling (溶胀)**. Swelling is the first stage of the dissolution of macromolecular compounds. For some substances in a certain solvent, such as raw rubber in benzene, with the development of swelling, it dissolves completely finally, which is called infinite swelling. But for other macromolecular compounds, such as vulcanized rubber, with the development of swelling the amount of fluid absorbed reaches the maximum, which is no longer continue to expand, this swelling is called finite swelling.

During the swelling process, in addition to the swelling of the volume of swelling substance, which is also accompanied by a thermal effect, this thermal effect is called swelling heat. Except for a few cases, swelling is usually exothermic. When a substance is swelling, it exerts a certain amount of pressure on the outside, this is called swelling pressure. This pressure can be very high in some cases. In the ancient swelling pressure was used to split rocks. Wooden blocks were inserted in the middle of cracks in the rocks and a large amount of water was injected. Therefore, swelling of wood fibers produced huge swelling pressure, which cracked the rocks. The pressure of swelling is used to mine the pyramid-building stones, known as wet-wood splints.

5.5   Syneresis and thixotropy

Many inorganic gels on standing undergo shrinkage which is accompanied by exudation of solvent. This process is termed **syneresis (离浆)**. The syneresis is very common phenomenon which can be found in paste, blood and jam. The aging cells losing water and the skin getting wrinkle also belong to syneresis.

Some gels are semisolid when at rest but revert to liquid sol on agitation. This reversible sol-gel transformation is referred to as **thixotropy (触变).** Iron oxide and silver oxide gels exhibit this property. The modern thixotropic paints are also an example. The characteristic of thixotropy is that the disassembly and recovery of gel structure are reversible. The thixotropy of gels is widely used in drug production. The thixotropy gels can be changed from gels to liquids as long as they are shaken a few times. It is very convenient to take them. Such as some eye drops, antibiotic oil injection is used in this form.

重 点 小 结

本章主要介绍了大分子化合物的基本概念、结构特点以及平均分子量的表示与测定方法，大分子溶液和大分子电解质的基本性质、渗透压、唐南膜平衡、黏度的概念以及它们的应用，凝胶的结构与性质。可以通过与普通小分子溶液的对照来理解大分子溶液及大分子电解质溶液的特性。

Object detection

Ⅰ. Select the correct option for the following problems (one option for each problem).

1. Consider a macromolecular mixture composed of 5 molecules of molecular weight $1kg \cdot mol^{-1}$, 2 molecules of molecular weight $3kg \cdot mol^{-1}$, and 1 molecules of molecular weight $4kg \cdot mol^{-1}$, which numbers are the number-average molecular weight and the mass-average molecular weight in $kg \cdot mol^{-1}$ respectively.

  A. 1.875, 3.153   B. 2.600, 3.153   C. 1.875, 2.600

  D. 2.600, 1.875   E. 1.000, 1.875

2. The intrinsic viscosity of a solution of polyisobutylene in cyclohexane is $0.0248m^3 \cdot kg^{-1}$. If $K = 3.3 \times 10^{-3} m^3 \cdot kg^{-1}$ and $\alpha = 0.70$, the viscosity-average molecular weight of the macromolecule is

  A. $2.74kg \cdot mol^{-1}$ B. $4.10kg \cdot mol^{-1}$ C. $7.52kg \cdot mol^{-1}$

  D. $17.84kg \cdot mol^{-1}$ E. $56.48kg \cdot mol^{-1}$

3. At 298.15K, plot Π/c of a solution of polystyrene in toluene as a function of polystyrene concentration c and obtain a straight line with the slope and intercept are 4.33 and 9.7, then the number-average molecular weight is

  A.$256kg \cdot mol^{-1}$ B. $572kg \cdot mol^{-1}$ C. $433kg \cdot mol^{-1}$

  D. $391kg \cdot mol^{-1}$ E. $175kg \cdot mol^{-1}$

4. At 298.15K, place the semi-permeable membrane filled with the $0.1mol \cdot L^{-1}$ macromolecular electrolyte solution R^+Cl^- in a $0.1mol \cdot L^{-1}$ NaCl solution, then in equilibrium the concentration of NaCl outside the membrane changes to

  A. $0.36mol \cdot L^{-1}$ B. $0.14mol \cdot L^{-1}$ C. $0.05mol \cdot L^{-1}$

  D. $0.24mol \cdot L^{-1}$ E. $0.45mol \cdot L^{-1}$

5. The fundamental difference in the properties of macromolecular solutions and colloids is

A. different viscosities

B. one is thermodynamically stable and the other is not

C. one is homogeneous ant the other is in a multi-phase

D. different sensitivities to the electrolytes

E. different osmotic pressures

Ⅱ. Try to answer the following problem.

How to sort the osmotic pressure of macromolecular solution, sol and micromolecule solution? Why?

Reference answers

Ⅰ. 1. C; 2. D; 3. A; 4. B; 5. C.

Ⅱ. Omitted.

Appendix
附　　录

表附-1　某些物质的标准摩尔生成焓、标准摩尔生成吉布斯自由能、标准摩尔熵及热容
（$p^{\ominus}$=100kPa，298.15K）

化学式	$\Delta_f H_m^{\ominus}$ / (kJ·mol⁻¹)	$\Delta_f G_m^{\ominus}$ / (kJ·mol⁻¹)	$S_m^{\ominus}$ / (J·mol⁻¹·K⁻¹)	$C_{p,m}^{\ominus}$/ (J·mol⁻¹·K⁻¹)
Ag(s)	0	–	42.6	25.4
AgCl(s)	−127.0	−109.8	96.3	50.8
Ag₂O(s)	−31.1	−11.2	121.3	65.9
Al(s)	0	–	28.3	24.2
Al₂O₃(α ,刚玉)	−1675.7	−1582.3	50.9	79.0
Br₂(l)	0	–	152.2	75.7
Br₂(g)	30.9	3.1	245.5	36.0
HBr(g)	−36.4	−53.4	198.7	29.1
Ca(s)	0	0	41.6	25.9
CaO(s)	−634.9	−603. 3	38.1	42. 0
Ca(OH)₂(s)	−986.09	−898.49	83.39	87.49
CO(g)	−110.5	−137.2	197.7	29.1
CO₂(g)	−393.5	−394.4	213.6	41.5
CCl₄(l)	−128.2	–	–	130.7
Cl₂(g)	0	0	223.1	33.9
HCl(g)	−92.3	−95.3	186.9	29.1
Cu(s)	0	0	33.2	24.4
CuO(s)	−157.3	−129.7	42.6	42.3
F₂(g)	0	0	202.8	31.3
HF(g)	−273.3	−275.4	173.8	–
Fe(g)	416.3	370.7	180.5	25.7
FeCl₂(s)	−341.8	−302.3	118.0	76.7

Continued

化学式	$\Delta_f H_m^\ominus /(kJ \cdot mol^{-1})$	$\Delta_f G_m^\ominus /(kJ \cdot mol^{-1})$	$S_m^\ominus /(J \cdot mol^{-1} \cdot K^{-1})$	$C_{p,m}^\ominus /(J \cdot mol^{-1} \cdot K^{-1})$
$FeCl_3(g)$	-399.5	-334.0	142.3	96.7
$FeO(s)$	-272.0	–	–	–
Fe_2O_3(赤铁矿)	-824.2	-742.2	87.4	103.9
Fe_3O_4(磁铁矿)	-1118.4	-1015.4	146.4	143.4
$FeSO_4(s)$	-928.4	-820.8	107.5	100.6
$H_2(g)$	0	0	130.7	28.8
$I_2(s)$	0	0	116.1	54.4
$I_2(g)$	62.4	19.3	260.7	36.9
$HI(g)$	26.5	1.7	206.6	29.2
$Mg(s)$	0	0	32.7	24.9
$MgO(s)$	-601.6	-569.3	27.0	37.2
$MgCl_2(s)$	-641.3	-591.8	89.6	71.4
$Mg(OH)_2(s)$	-924.5	-833.5	63.2	77.0
$Na(s)$	0	0	51.3	28.2
$Na_2CO_3(s)$	-1130.7	-1044.0	135.0	112.3
$NaCl(s)$	-411.2	-384.1	72.1	50.5
$NaNO_3(s)$	-467.9	-367.0	116.5	92.9
$NaOH(s)$	-425.6	-379.5	64.5	59.5
$H_2O(l)$	-285.8	-237.1	70.0	75.3
$H_2O(g)$	-241.8	-228.6	188.8	33.6
$Na_2SO_4(s)$	-1387.1	-1270.2	149.6	128.2
$N_2(g)$	0	0	191.6	29.1
$NH_3(g)$	-45.9	-16.4	192.8	35.1
$NO_2(g)$	33.2	51.3	240.1	37.2
$N_2O(g)$	81.6	103.7	220.0	38.6
$N_2O_3(g)$	86.6	142.4	314.7	72.7
$N_2O_4(g)$	11.6	99.8	304.4	79.2
$N_2O_5(g)$	11.3	115.1	355.7	95.3
$HNO_3(g)$	-133.9	-73.5	266.9	54.1
$HNO_3(l)$	-174.1	-80.7	155.6	109.97
$O_2(g)$	0	0	205.2	29.4
$O_3(g)$	142.7	163.2	238.9	39.2
$PCl_3(g)$	-287.0	-267.8	311.8	71.8
$PCl_5(g)$	-374.9	-305.0	364.6	112.8

Continued

化学式	$\Delta_f H_m^\ominus / (\text{kJ} \cdot \text{mol}^{-1})$	$\Delta_f G_m^\ominus / (\text{kJ} \cdot \text{mol}^{-1})$	$S_m^\ominus / (\text{J} \cdot \text{mol}^{-1} \cdot \text{K}^{-1})$	$C_{p,m}^\ominus / (\text{J} \cdot \text{mol}^{-1} \cdot \text{K}^{-1})$
$H_3PO_4(s)$	−1284.4	−1124.3	110.5	106.1
$H_2S(g)$	−20.6	−33.4	205.8	34.2
$SO_2(g)$	−296.8	−300.1	248.2	39.9
$SO_3(g)$	−395.7	−371.1	256.8	50.7
$H_2SO_4(l)$	−814.0	−690.0	156.9	138.9
$Zn(s)$	0	0	41.6	25.4
$ZnCO_3(s)$	−812.78	−731.52	82.4	79.71
$CH_4(g)$	−74.6	−50.5	186.3	35.5
$C_2H_6(g)$	−84.0	−34.0	229.2	52.5
$C_3H_8(g)$	−103.8	−23.4	270.3	73.6
$C_4H_{10}(g)$	−125.6	−15.7	310.2	97.5
$C_2H_4(g)$（乙烯）	52.4	68.4	219.3	42.9
$C_3H_6(g)$（丙烯）	20.0	62.72	266.9	−
$C_6H_6(l)$	49.1	124.5	173.4	136.0
$C_6H_6(g)$	82.9	129.7	269.2	82.4
$CH_3OH(l)$	−239.2	−166.6	126.8	81.1
$CH_3OH(g)$	−201.0	−162.3	239.9	44.1
$C_2H_5OH(l)$	−277.7	−174.8	160.7	112.3
$C_2H_5OH(g)$	−234.8	−167.9	281.6	65.6
$HCHO(g)$	−108.6	−102.5	218.8	35.4
$CH_3CHO(l)$	−192.2	−127.6	160.2	89.0
$CH_3CHO(g)$	−166.19	−128.86	250.3	57.3
$CH_3COOH(l)$	−484.3	−389.9	159.8	123.3
$CO(NH_2)_2(s)$	−333.51	−197.33	104.60	93.14

附录二

表附 −2　某些有机化合物的标准摩尔燃烧焓（ $p^\ominus$=100kPa, 298.15K ）

化学式	名称	$\Delta_C H_m^\ominus / (\text{kJ} \cdot \text{mol}^{-1})$		
		晶体	液体	气体
C	碳（石墨）	393.5		1110.2
CO	一氧化碳			283.0

Continued

化学式	名称	$\Delta_c H_m^{\ominus}/(kJ \cdot mol^{-1})$		
		晶体	液体	气体
CH_2O	甲醛			570.7
CH_2O_2	甲酸		254.6	300.7
CH_4	甲烷			890.8
CH_4N_2O	尿素	632.7		719.4
CH_3OH	甲醇		726.1	763.7
CH_3NH_2	甲胺		1060.8	1085.6
C_2H_2	乙炔			1301.1
$C_2H_2O_4$	乙二酸	251.1		349.1
C_2H_4	乙烯			1411.2
C_2H_4O	乙醛		1166.9	1192.5
CH_3COOH	乙酸		874.2	925.9
$CHOOCH_3$	甲酸甲酯		972.6	1003.2
$C_2H_5NO_2$	硝基乙烷		1357.7	1399.3
C_2H_6	乙烷			1560.7
C_2H_5OH	乙醇		1366.8	1409.4
C_3H_6	丙烯		2039.7	2058.0
C_3H_6	环丙烷			2091.3
C_3H_6O	丙酮		1789.9	1820.7
$C_3H_6O_2$	丙酸		1592.2	1626.1
$C_3H_6O_2$	丙酸		1527.3	1584.5
C_4H_8O	四氢呋喃		1527.3	2533.2
$C_4H_8O_2$	乙酸乙酯		2238.1	2273.3
$C_4H_8O_2$	丁酸		2183.6	2241.6
C_4H_{10}	丁烷		2856.6	2877.6
$C_4H_{10}O$	乙醚		2723.9	2751.1
C_6H_6	苯		3267.6	3301.2
C_6H_6O	苯酚	3053.5		3122.2
$H_2(g)*$	氢气			285.8
$C_6H_{12}O_6$	α–D葡萄糖	2802		
$C_6H_{12}O_6$	β–D葡萄糖	2808		
$C_{12}H_{22}O_{11}$	蔗糖	5645		

*氢气虽非有机物，但因常用于计算，故列入此表。

注：数据摘自CRC hand book of Chemistry and Physics, 100th Edition, 2019.

参 考 文 献

[1] 傅献彩，沈文霞，姚天扬，等.物理化学[M]. 5版.北京：高等教育出版社，2018.

[2] 天津大学物理化学教研室.物理化学[M]. 6版.北京：高等教育出版社，2017.

[3] 刘幸平，刘雄.物理化学[M]. 10版.北京：中国中医药出版社，2016.

[4] 何美，周华锋.物理化学简明双语教程[M].北京：中国石化出版社有限公司，2009.

[5] 周华锋，侯纯明，姚淑华.物理化学双语解题指导[M].北京：中国石化出版社有限公司，2017.

[6] Atkins P, Paula J D. 阿特金斯物理化学[M]. 10版（影印版）.北京：高等教育出版社，2019.

[7] Ira N. Levine. Physical Chemistry[M]. 6th Edition. The McGraw-Hill Companies, 2009.

[8] Hu Ying. Physical Chemistry[M].北京：高等教育出版社，2013.